COST AND COMPETITION IN AMERICAN MEDICINE

Theory, Policy and Institutions

Les Seplaki, Ph.D.

UNIVERSITY
PRESS OF
AMERICA

Lanham • New York • London

Copyright © 1994 by
University Press of America® Inc.
4720 Boston Way
Lanham, Maryland 20706

3 Henrietta Street
London WC2E 8LU England

Library of Congress Cataloging-in-Publication Data

Seplaki, Les.
Cost and competition in American medicine : theory, policy, and
institutions / Les Seplaki.
p.   cm.
1. Medical care, Cost of—United States.   2. Medical economics—
United States.   3. Competition—United States.   I. Title.
RA410.7.S47   1994
338.4'33621'0973—dc20   94–22105 CIP

ISBN 0–8191–9639–8 (cloth : alk. paper)
ISBN 0–8191–9640–1 (pbk. : alk. paper)

Table of Contents

PART ONE:
AN OVERVIEW OF ECONOMIC PREREQUISITES

PART TWO:
ANTITRUST MARKETS:
AN OVERVIEW OF THE PRINCIPLES

Chapter 8

Chapter 9

Chapter 10

PART THREE:
HEALTHCARE MARKETS

Chapter 15
The Physician Market Place

Chapter 16
Economic Coordination of Hospital-Physician Functions

Chapter 17
Competition and Cost Control in the US Pharmaceutical Industry

PART FOUR:
COMPETITION AND ITS ENFORCEMENT IN HEALTHCARE

Chapter 21
Competition Enforcement and Healthcare
Intermediation

Chapter 22
Competition in the Physician Sector

Chapter 23
Competition Enforcement in the Hospital Sector

Chapter 24
Structural and Regulatory Constraints on
Hospital Competition

PART FIVE:
HEALTHCARE COSTS, POLICY AND PROGNOSES

Introduction

This volume is about competition in healthcare markets, the enforcement of competition on the healthcare scene, and the apparent impact of competition enforcement on costs. While healthcare is generic and can be very technical in a noneconomic sense, competition is an economic concept and has been well defined, in terms of both its theoretical and its institutional dimensions.

The enforcement of competition in any market, while fundamentally statute based, has been imbedded in common law applications. That is, the standards and technical particulars of the enforcement have evolved in a long series of cases and opinions that emerged largely at the federal judicial level. However, while the enforcement process and procedure are fundamentally legal, the elements of the causes of action include essential economic considerations that have long been studied both theoretically and empirically.

This volume will attempt to generate a synthesis between the principles of competition enforcement in healthcare, those of the underlying economics, and healthcare costs. These are diverse, yet functionally related subjects. Competition enforcement policy cannot be understood without some knowledge of underlying economic theory. Competition enforcement in healthcare cannot be examined without reviewing the basic generic issues akin to competition enforcement in any market. Thus, in spite of its modal appearance, the volume should be viewed as one integral treatise, rather than a modal one. It attempts to bring together the essentials of industrial organization, neoclassical microeconomics, antitrust institutions anbd policy, and healthcare institutions and regulation, to shed some light, at least theoretically, and to some extent empirically, on the relationship between the fundamentals of economics, healthcare institutions and healthcare costs.

The underlying principles of the economics of industrial organization will be dealt with in a nut-shell in Part One. Inherently, it is an overview of the subject. The volume assumes some knowledge of basic microeconomics on the part of the reader. Hence, Part One presents the micro and industrial organization issues concisely, yet with a considerable degree of comprehensiveness, and the standard tools of micro analyses, such as graphs and equations, are omitted, for they may be found in any of the many dozens, perhaps hundreds, of pertinent microeconomics volumes in any college library. A reference section for each chapter provides ample direct guidance to pursue further readings on the micro and industrial organization, and indeed all other, issues involved. An examination of the notions of industry, market, and competition, is followed by a brief review of market structure determinants, such economies of scale, entry related issues, contestable markets and mergers. Chapter 3 reviews some basic product and factor market structures, followed by a birds-eye view of various measures of market and economic powers in Chapter 4, mergers in Chapter 5, and some major entry issues within the context of competition in Chapter 6.

Part Two explores the fundamental issues of "generic antitrust", once again with considerable brevity, in preparation for Part Four, the segment on antitrust enforcement in healthcare. After a review of basic antitrust principles and procedures in Chapter 7, the notion of the market, within the antitrust context is examined in Chapter 8, followed by two chapters on the issues of various market conduct and market structure (mergers) restraints.

In Part Three, Chapter 11 takes a close look at healthcare industry, and specific markets, as well as the nature of competition in those markets; after an overview of the healthcare industry, review of some current and historical cost data is presented. In particular, Chapter 12 examines the hospital market environment, followed by a specific look at hospital pricing techniques. Chapter 14 looks at the generic concept of "healthcare intermediation", that is, institutions and markets where healthcare services are mediated between providers and users. The physician market place, and physician-hospital interactions are looked at in Chapters 15 and 16. Finally, in Part Three, Chapters 17 and 18 examine the structure of competition and costs in the pharmaceutical and dental markets respectively.

Part Four examines in detail the principles, processes and institutions involved in the enforcement of competition in US healthcare markets; specifically, it analyzes recent antitrust enforcement experience in those markets, and attempts to draw some inference for a relationship between those enforcement efforts and healthcare costs. In the discussion of healthcare-specific policy issues, attempts were made to strike a balance between various points of view. Thus, Chapter 19 reviews antitrust principles but within the healthcare context, followed by a closer look at antitrust market definition issues in healthcare in Chapter 20. The following four chapters examine the history of antitrust implementation in various healthcare markets such as in relation to healthcare intermediaries (Chapter 21), physicians (Chapter 22), and hospitals (Chapters 23 and 24).

Finally, Part Five examines contemporary competition, cost and policy issues in the US and abroad with some emphases on the pending healthcare reforms, and their implications for various market, costs and competition. In this context, the cost and policy of AIDS are looked at in Chapter 25, regulatory issues and their impact on costs and competition are examined in Chapter 26, some essential healthcare cost and policy variables are compared on the international scene in Chapter 27, and finally, Chapter 28 focuses on the pending healthcare reforms.

The volume can readily be digested by anyone with a basic course in, or a fundamental understanding of, microeconomics principles, some industrial organization and a rudimentary familiarity with the institutional structure of the healthcare industry.

In the preparation of this volume, the author benefited from a variety of experiences and professional contacts. In particular, a Corporation Fellowship in Law and Economics at the Harvard Law School and the antitrust research conducted as well as graduate courses taken at Harvard by the author was particularly helpful in developing an understanding of antitrust theories and policies, as well as the interpretation of the cases. The author's recent two-year appointment as a Visiting Scholar in Economics and Public Health at Columbia University rendered the resources of Columbia's libraries, particularly the impressively endowed Armand Hammer Health Sciences Library, available for research. Many institutional and theoretical items dealt with in the medical sections of the volume benefited from discussions with Professor R. Callabio, MD., of Columbia. The discussion on the dental healthcare sector benefited from interactions with Professor Z. Marin, DDS, of NYU, and from a discussion with, as well as materials made available to the author from Professor H.B. Waldman, DDS. of the SUNY Stony Brook School of Dentistry. J. O'Donnell, D.Ph., of the Rush-Presbyterian Medical School in Chicago, and S. Ushiyama, D.Ph, a research executive in the pharmaceutical industry, were helpful with materials and suggestions in connection with the preparation of the chapter on the pharmaceutical industry. Stating that any errors or omissions remaining in the volume are the responsibility of the author is virtually needless.

PART ONE

AN OVERVIEW OF ECONOMICS PREREQUISITES

Chapter 1
INDUSTRIES, MARKETS AND THE MEANING OF COMPETITION

Conceptual Confusion and Relationships

The concepts of "industry" and "market" are fundamental for the study of competition in any economic arena. Yet historically, these terms have been used interchangeably and rather loosely, with often less than adequate attention paid to the differences in their meaning and application. In fact, "industry" has at times been used as a synonym for "market"[1]. Other terms, such as "line of business"[2], have also been substituted.

A concise, yet relatively functional, definition of "industry" included all firms concerned with the affairs of any one firm in the group, and concentrated on the similarities in trade practices and production technologies: "the chief characteristics of an industry are largely a matter of technique and processes; an individual business must be conceived as operating within an 'industry' which consists of all businesses which operate processes of sufficiently similar kind (...possession of substantially similar technical resources) and possessing sufficiently similar backgrounds of experience and knowledge so that each of them could produce the particular commodity under consideration.."[3]. A logical extension of this definition in a more modern context could include all firms into an industry group whose conducts have a substantial economic impact upon each other within the same planning horizon, regardless the degree of technological similarities. At any rate, within the context of competitive policy enforcement, "industry" definitions may enjoy considerably more latitude and freedom of choice than "market" does.

A "market" may also be viewed in a conceptual sense, with no specific analytical functions or purpose. For instance, we may consider a market to be any system of communications or arrangements whereby potential buyers and sellers interact with a view to transact. The actual consummation of transactions themselves is not required. Only the presence of a viable intent to transact is needed. Viable intent, on the other hand, assumes the presence of willingness as well as the economic ability to act on the part of both, the buyers and sellers. No specifically confined space, place, or physical delineations are needed for this definition. Hence, global and domestic markets for international currency transactions, professional services, securities and precious metals are readily embraced by this definition, as are domestic markets for specific commodities in a more traditional sense.

Definitional and conceptual confusions are enhanced by the multiple application of the term "market" in the economic literature. In one context, economists think of the market as the product-line and geographical delineation of a set of commercial activities involving a specific set of buyers, sellers and products. This approach is used, for instance, within the context of antitrust enforcement - as we will examine those issues later. In another context, the literature viewed markets as a set of specific conditions ("market structures") under which the market participants transact to attain certain rational goals such as profit maximization; conditions labeled as "perfect competition", "monopoly" and other specific sets of well defined circumstances fall into this alternative context. Standard microeconomic texts routinely examine these and related issues.

While to a certain extent conceptually independent, these two usages are not unrelated. Thus, we do not need to delineate the geographic boundaries of perfect competition to derive a profit maximizing level of output for a firm or for all of the firms. Nor do we normally apply a theoretical market model to measure, define, or delineate a product and geographic market for a medical service. However, if the need to make predictions regarding the behavior or performance of specifically delineated product markets arises, market structure theories may need to be utilized. Similarly, "the theory of the firm" by way of the examination of specific market structures and their behavior is often resorted to in the course of enforcing public policies aimed at controlling the competitive conduct of "real life" firms. Finally, the number of sellers, or buyers, in a specific market is an important structure determining variable and the latter, in turn, can be directly influenced by expanding the geographic parameters of the market. Hence, the interdependency in this regard at least is obvious.

Supply and Demand Dimensions

The supply and demand dimensions of the market are two major variables by which the market's size and identity are analyzed. An important area of examination is the sources of supply available to a specific group of buyers. Thus, we need to examine the significant alternative sources of supply to a defined group of customers of cars within a specific price range. Or, we may want to look at significant alternative sources of cardiac surgery (i.e. facilities with qualified professionals) available to, and used by, people within a specific county or other geographic area. Competition, in this context, is viewed by antitrust enforcers as the existence of a sufficient number of independent and significant competing suppliers.

Competition as a Generic Concept

Competition has had different meaning to different people, and at different times. It is widely used by lawyers and economists. Antitrust, as a tool of public policy, use terms such as "lessening of competition", or, "restraint of trade", or, "monopolize". Competition is the technical standard upon which the wrong is separated from the right, the acceptable is distinguished from the anti-social, and the legal is recorded versus the illegal. The courts have consistently viewed competition as the US economy's foundation. For instance, "the heart of our national economic policy has long been faith in the value of competition"[4], or, "the Sherman Act was designed to be a comprehensive charter of economic liberty aimed at preserving free and unfettered competition as the rule of trade"[5]. Competition has become a legal standard for evaluating economic activity. In fact, in most antitrust enforcement proceedings no meaningful conclusions can be arrived at unless "...one faces up to the problem of how to define competition"[6]. Nevertheless, the ambiguity in the general competitive concept serves some useful purposes in that it allows flexibility in the application of the law, and in the adaptability of the courts, to ever changing economic conditions and business practices.

While such classification is somewhat arbitrary, and subject to value judgment, professional and academic views of competition may be viewed in philosophical, legal, and economic contexts. *Philosophically*, competition may be viewed as a contest among certain parties. Although, as we will see in this volume, key related questions are who the "parties" are and what is the field of contest. In a specific goal oriented approach, competition has also been viewed as an effort to inflict injury to others[7]. Traditionally, and in more general terms, competition was seen simply a process of adjustment aimed at managing economic activity, and channeling resources to their most effective and efficient utilization if such opportunities exist. Where competition as a manager is not present, as in the traditional totalitarian socialist systems, its functions is simply replaced by the discretionary powers of administrative managers. At any rate, the ultimate function and target of competition within the context of public policy is attaining social, instead of private - whether individual or corporate, goals.

The realm of *judicial applications* concerns itself with regulating economic conduct either directly, or indirectly via regulating structure in order to attain certain economic goals. We will later examine systematically the statutes involved, at this point, however, we will note that competition in this context is construed as the right of an entity to enter into an endeavor, to engage in a production, business or professional process not proscribed by law. Competition may become a by-product of this right when more than one entities enter into the same type of endeavor and attempt to prevail under legitimate constraints. Through the legitimate exercise of competition, that is, by legally offering better or cheaper, or both, output, the entities have the right to inflict economic injury upon each other. These principles have been enunciated in a number of pertinent cases. For instance, the purpose of antitrust as a tool of public policy is "to protect competitive freedom, i.e. the freedom of individual business units to compete unhindered by the group action of others"[8]. Or, "... equality of opportunity is [reduced] if group power is utilized to eliminate a competitor who is equipped to compete"[9].

While it is assumed at this point that the reader has a fundamental familiarity with them, later in the volume we will provide a brief systematic overview of the various standard competitive models offered by the *economic literature,* namely perfect competition, monopolistic competition, monopoly, oligopoly, and workable or effective competition. We will note that all of these models have a common purpose which they attain with varying degrees of success, namely to predict rational behavior. Specifically, efforts are made to predict what will be produced, in what quantity, and at what cost and price, hence with what profit. These predictions, in turn, describe market conditions, productive efficiencies, varying firm conduct under correspondingly varying circumstances, qualitative and quantitative output combinations in relation to needs, and the level of research and development as well as technical progress. Perfect competition, a logical exposition of economic relations that had its highest level of acceptance during the 1920s and 1930s, is predicated upon highly abstract assumptions without which the desired logical consequences and ultimate conclusions could not be drawn. However, in order for the model to remain logically workable, some essential components had to be left out. Thus, time and inherent changes in technology, consumer tastes and methods of production, are excluded from the predictive model. Everything is certain and static within the context of a single commodity production and its associated production costs, with its transportation, sales, marketing, advertising and other related costs being assumed away. Mainly because no such marketing efforts are called for in a world of homogeneous products, and also because if they were taken into account, the model could not be used for precise predictions. One eminent economist indicated that perfect competition helps in understanding economic reality[10]. Many others disagreed by formulating and propagating alternative models of behavior and prediction.

Because of the abstractions in pure monopoly models, a number of oligopoly models, some more theoretical than others, were generated over the years, along with those of imperfect competition by way of attempts to emulate real firm behavior. Oligopoly models in general are based on the notion of interdependence and mutual indeterminacy among a few large rivals, in the absence of stabilizing assumptions regarding rival behavior. Once those assumptions are made, and, depending on the assumptions, some type of oligopolistic equilibrium solution is reached within the models. Imperfect competition, on the other hand, do resemble some attributes of perfect competition with modification for product differentiation, and consequent control of some degree over price and the firms' minimum markets share. However, in order to increase the model's predictive power and internal logical consistency, some quite unrealistic assumptions had to be made even in monopolistic competition, including perfect diffusion of competitive impact and identical production costs functions for the firms, which substantially reduced the model's applicability to reality. The model of "workable (or effective) competition" was offered as a policy-specific alternative, although it heavily bears the marks of perfect competition, and there is no convincing evidence that the courts have consistently accepted it as a policy target norm[11].

References

1   Robinson, J. "The Industry and the Market", *Economic Journal*, June 1956, pp. 360-61.
2   Cox, S.R. and Penn, D.W. "Industrial Organization Research and the Academic Economist", *Industrial Organization Review*, Vol. 2, 1976.
3   Wilson, T. and Andrews, P.W.S. *Oxford Studies in the Price Mechanism*, Clarendon Press, Oxford 1951, p.168.
4   *Standard Oil of Indiana* v. FTC 340 US 231, 248 (1951)
5   *Northern Pacific Railroad Company* V US 356 US 1, 4 (1958)]
6   Bok, D. C. "The Tampa Electric Case and the Problem of Exclusive Arrangement under the Clayton Act" *The Supreme Court Review*, University of Chicago Press, 1961, p.286.
7   Papandreou A. G. and Wheeler, John T. *Competition and its Regulation*, Prentice Hall, N.Y. 1954.
8   *Silver v NYSE* 373 US 341, 359-60 (1963)
9   *Wm. Goldman Theaters v. Loews* 150 F 2d 738,743 (1945)]
10 Stigler, G. *Essays in the History of Economics*, University of Chicago Press, 1965, pp.259-61]
11 Clark, J. M. "Competition, Static Models and Economic Aspects" *American Economic Review, Papers and Proceeding*, May 1955. Clark, John M. *Competition, Static Models, and Dynamic Aspects*, Brookings Institution, Washington DC 1961. Sosnick, Steve H, "A Critique of Concepts of workable competition" *Quarterly Journal of Economics*, September 1958.

Chapter 2
DETERMINANTS OF
MARKET STRUCTURE

Market, and often industry, structure points to the size distribution of firms. It gives us a barometer of economic power, where that power is utilized, and, when examined in conjunction with conduct, we also learn how it is utilized. Market structure is also a major concern for public policy. Regulatory and antitrust agencies typically concern themselves less with markets that have a large number of small firms than with markets containing a few large firms. This concern reflects the view that if markets are to perform in a socially desirable manner, if they are to contribute substantially to social welfare maximization, then market structure must follow a pattern of economic power diffusion. The extent of economic power diffusion depends on the largest firms' ability to raise price above the marginal cost of production without losing most or all of its business to its rivals. That is most likely to occur in markets with a few large firms, in highly concentrated markets. Such markets also give rise to collusive activities aimed at attaining the same high level of profits that a single monopolist alone could generate (joint monopoly profit maximization). The higher the level of market concentration the less likely an attempt at collusion will fail. Indeed, an inverse relationship was found between the number of firms in a collusive market and the likelihood of success for the collusion.[1]. This, however, does not necessarily exclude competitive behavior, possibly to the extent of perfect competition, even on the part two firms if they make appropriate assumption regarding rival behavior[2].

As general determinants of market structure, demand and cost conditions play a crucial role. Given a certain level of demand, a specific market size, the number and size of member firms will vary directly with the size of the minimum efficient firm. That is, under optimum conditions, the number of member firms will decline as minimum efficient firm size approaches the size of the market. Holding minimum efficient firm size (costs) constant, the number of member firms will vary directly with the size of the market.

Economies of Scale and Scope

The above indicates that as the average cost of production falls with increases in output, the number of firms will likely decline and market structure will become more concentrated. "Economies of scale" measures the relationship between the size of the production unit (firm, or single plant in the case of multi-plant operations) and the prevailing or emerging cost of production. This relationship is depicted by the production unit's long-run average cost curve. Some long-run average cost curves show no relationship between cost and output. No cost savings are gained by increasing the scale of production, therefore, market structure as a function of cost is undefined in this case. This would be an unusual case, since such situation would not justify the existence of a firm as a production unit. If any entity, no matter how small, could produce at the same cost as larger firms can, then consumers would simply meet their own needs for goods and would not have to purchase them from larger specialized firms who, otherwise, can produce them at a lower cost. Economies of scale by way of lower production (and transaction) costs through increased output are a prerequisite for the existence of business organization as production unit.[3]. On the other hand, if substantial economies of scale over an initial large output range can be had, so called "natural monopolies", where 100% market share (often protected by regulation) is needed to generate the lowest production costs. If, on the other hand, low output levels generate maximum economies, then, depending on the market size, a larger number of relatively small market participants are called for. Finally, in production processes where diseconomies of scale are delayed over a large output range, cost conditions normally do not indicate the desirability of specific firm size, beyond the initial small level where all economies are reaped.

Scale economies are grouped into two major categories, based upon their source: (a) technological, (b) non technological. Technological economies are generated largely by specialization of labor force and capital, and the presence of indivisibilities within production capacity mandating high optimum utilization rates for machines. Nontechnological economies include favorable terms of trade from suppliers of raw material, credit sources, transportation facilities, and advertising media[4].

Economies of scope constitute cost savings from producing several products in one plant rather than in correspondingly several plants. The scope of production is expanded, hence its cost is spread over a larger number and types of products, managerial skills, and marketing networks. In addition, any good will (reputation) that accrues to the firm's name benefits all products[5].

Over-expansion of production can yield "diseconomies of scale" and increasing average production costs. These emanate from the increasing layers of bureaucracy that accompanies firm expansion, increased burden of paper-work, and reduced managerial efficiency and concentration on expanded responsibilities over a much larger number of managerial functions. Planning becomes cumbersome, the number of transaction much larger, making coordination of a multitude of processes and goals much more difficult and costly[6].

A product of output-cost relationship measurement is the "minimum optimal scale" [MOS - also referred to as "minimum efficient scale", MES]. Minimum optimal scale is attained at the lowest possible output level needed to utilize all available economies in a specific market or industry[7]. Empirical studies appear to indicate that plant capacity, or the percentage of industry output, required to attain MOS has been relatively small in most industries[8]. In the alternative, efficient firm size was also viewed in terms of the ability to survive. This more generic view of efficiency-scale relationship suggested that a firm, or class of firms, can be considered most efficient not in terms of the level of their output or cost, but basically if they were able to maintain their statusquo in the industry, that is if they were to prosper.[9]

Barriers to Entry

Barriers to entry constitute competitive obstacles faced by actual or potential entrants into a market not faced by incumbent firms. More formally, it is defined as "the extent to which, in the long-run, established firms can elevate their selling prices above the minimal average costs of production and distribution.... without inducing potential entrants into the industry".[10] A net cost approach to this definition was taken by another prominent economist who defined barriers to entry "as a cost of producing any level of output which must be borne by a firm which seeks to enter the industry but is not borne by firms already in the industry"[11].

A major category of entry barriers is *product differentiation*. Product differentiation efforts are aimed at image and perception creation. They succeed when consumers perceive a product or service as favorably different from its competitors in terms of any characteristics. Furthermore, if successful, product differentiation can be a tool for established firms to protect, maintain and exercise market power, hence it has a direct and substantial impact on market structure.

Product differentiation may be generated by three major factors. First, objective variations in a product, or physical product attributes, such as size, taste, durability, packaging and so forth. Secondly, buyer ignorance of true quality differences among products and services make them vulnerable to differentiation efforts. In medicine, for instance, patient ignorance of the nature of product or service needed, particularly in local hospital markets, make them vulnerable to emotionally appealing, yet possibly insubstantial, advertisement campaigns. Thirdly, a possibly overlapping source category involves the emotional vulnerability of potential customers. Economists have tended to center their attention on the first two, delegating the third source to social researchers such as marketing people, or psychologists[12,13].

We have already discussed economies of scale. If present, these economies, also constitute major barriers of entry. In order reap the benefits of economies, that is, in order attain the minimum optimal scale of production, often large scale of production needs to be undertaken. That, in turn, requires major initial absolute amounts of capital outlays, which in itself deters entry [8]. High initial capital requirements may also act as entry barriers due to the cost or scarcity of initial capital. Since for a new entrant the project itself is untested, there is lack of experience, hence the risk is perceived to be higher. Higher perceived risk generates higher capital finance charges, higher cost of production, and given an established price level usually set by the incumbents, lower profit incentive to enter[14].

Control over essential factors of production may also constitute an entry barrier. A classic example of this situation was presented by the Aluminum Company of America which, through a network of patenting and later by long-term contracts, controlled the supply of bauxite, an essential raw material for aluminum production; there ALCOA was able maintain and perpetuate its dominant position in aluminum production markets. However, in addition to just controlling supply, entrenched incumbents may cause further problems to potential entrants by raising the cost of inputs, thereby reducing the potential profitability of entry, or the profit margin of firms already existing in the market. While the general theme is the same, the economics literature presents a number of versions of this entry barrier technique[15].

In some types of production, certain costs are incurred regardless whether production continues or ceases. These are called "*sunk costs*". These involve specialized investments geared specifically to the instant needs of commerce, and would include projects like pipelines, and strategically located distribution centers. Some economists argue that sunk costs also constitute an entry barrier[16]. These costs are given and assumed for the incumbents. They are already part of their cost structure. They already incurred them. However, for a new entrant it is a new cost that needs to be coped with, and its size may deter entry if, even barring predatory pricing on the part of the incumbent, the post entry market price is not expected to cover the new entrant's cost.

Incumbent firms may also practice so called "strategic entry deterrence". These involve actions on the part of incumbents designed to make entry unattractive to outsiders. One such type of action involves the incumbent setting price not at the normal profit maximizing level, but at a low enough level to dissuade new entry - "limit pricing". A "limit price" may thus be defined as the maximum price level, normally under the profit maximizing level, that an incumbent may charge without attracting entry. Another strategy that incumbents may apply is over investment in plant capacity implying a threat of drastic price cutting if entry occurs, particularly in the face an expanding market. [15]. A third strategy, a variation on the second, "brand proliferation". Over investment in production capacity allows the saturation of the market with a large number of brands and products of similar characteristics, leaving little or no prospects for successful marketing by a potential entrant.

The economic literature accounts for a number of additional types of entry barriers. These include government imposed regulatory constraints such as patenting, licensing, and exclusive franchising, and are imbedded in the governments intention to enforce the incumbent's property rights. [10, p.49]

Contestable Markets

During the early 1980s, the theory of contestable markets was introduced as a revolutionary development in the study of industrial organization, an "uprising in the theory of industry"[17]. It was claimed that this theory could also be readily utilized by government policy makers, particularly in the field of antitrust enforcement[18]. The scenario involves a situation where the status or number of incumbent firms is not important. Nor is the existence or absence of economies of scale. New entrants face the same cost conditions as incumbents do. Furthermore, upon exit, all expenses and costs can be recouped, and all assets can be salvaged at a price equal to their purchase price minus depreciation. There are no sunk costs. Incumbents must price their products at the competitive level, that is, at marginal cost. If not, new firms can enter uninhibited, collect existing profits, force price back down to marginal cost level, and then execute their costless exit. The industry equilibrium will remain at the competitive level regardless of the apparent market structure.

This notion of free entry and exit has already been presented in the literature back in the mid 19th century[19] and further discussed in the mid-1970s.[20]. Additionally, there are several problems with the theory for it to have any policy utility. The underlying assumptions have been found untenable. For instance, there is no realistic support for the zero sunk cost assumption. Since it is beyond our scope at this stage to examine these issues references are made to some of the extensive literature dealing with this subject[21]. The topic will be briefly revisited in the next chapter.

Mergers

Traditionally, we think of a merger as the complete acquisition of one firm by another. For purposes of public policy and antitrust, a merger takes place when one previously independent firm acquires at least a controlling block of ownership in another, resulting in the strong possibility that the acquired ownership will allow the acquirer to impose, or substantially influence, major management decisions at the acquired firm.

Mergers have been classified into three major, if somewhat overlapping, categories. A "horizontal" merger involves firms from the same competitive arena (market), where they were in direct competition with each other prior to the merger. The firms come from the same stage of a production process. The resulting amount of competition eliminated by a horizontal merger clearly depends on the market shares of the involved firms prior to the merger. "Vertical" mergers involve firms that have operated on different stages of a production process, hence were in direct or indirect supplier-customer type of relationship prior to the merger. In fact, since the parties to the vertical merger come from effectively different competitive markets, they may also be viewed as a type of "conglomerate" merger, since the latter is defined as one involving firms from different, often unrelated, markets. Conglomeration has been subcategorized into (a) pure - with the merging parties coming from totally unrelated markets with different production processes; (b) product extension - with the parties producing goods of a complementary nature, and (c) market extension - with the parties producing similar or even competitive goods, however, separated by geographical distance; thus, market extension merger involves conglomeration mostly in a geographical sense.

There are several reasons for mergers to take place. In the case of small sellers, failing business in terms of declining revenues and frequent losses may be a reason. A less important seller's motive to be bought out may relate to son Johnny being more interested in fast cars and related items, hence not to be trusted with the family business, causing the father to cash-in for a lifetime of efforts. Firms acquire other businesses for more earthly reason. Merger brings about growth, and size may have its fringe-benefits: replacement of old, possibly inefficient, management with a new one; ability to buy inputs at reduced cost with volume discounts; technical economies of scale discussed earlier, and, "self-aggrandizement" due to size. In addition, sellers may benefits from the "bloating frog effect": if one becomes larger, it costs more to buy one - a defense against being acquired[22]. By acquiring other businesses, firms spread their risk through diversification[23].

References

1   Stigler, G.J. "A Theory of Oligopoly", *Journal of Political Economy*, Vol 72, February 1964.

2   Cournot, A. *Researches into the Mathematical Principles of the Theory of Wealth*, Nathaniel T Bacon (1897 - originally published in 1838). McMillan, New York, 1927. Also see Stackelberg, H.v. *Marktform und Gleichgenwicht* (Vienna: Julius Springer, 1934), and Bertrand, J. "Theorie Mathematique de la Richesse sociale" *Journal des Savants* (September 1883).

3   Coase, R.H., "The Nature of the Firm", *Econometrica*, Vol. 4, November 1937.

4   Alchian, A.A. "Costs and Outputs", in Moses Abramowitz (ed) *The Allocation of Economic Resources: Essays in Honor of Bernard F. Haley*, Stanford University Press, Palo Alto 1959. Discussed various other sources of scale economies.

5   Nichols, L.M. "On the Sources of Scope Economies in US Manufacturing Firms", *Review of Industrial Organization*, Spring 1989.

6   Chandler, A.D. *The Visible Hand: The Managerial Revolution in American Business*, Harvard University Press, Cambridge MA 1977.

7   Bain J.S. *Barriers to to New Competition*, Harvard University Press, Cambridge MA, 1956.

8   Bain, J.S. "Economies of Scale, Concentration and the Condition of Entry in Twenty Manufacturing Industries" *American Economic Review* Vol. 44, March 1954.

9   Scherer, F.M. Beckenstein, A. Kaufer, E. and Murphy, R.D. *The Economics of Multi-Plant Operations: An International Comparison Study*. Harvard University Press, Cambridge, MA. 1975. Also see, Stigler, G.J, "The Economies of Scale" *Journal of Law and Economics*, Vol. 1, October 1958.

10 Demsetz, H. "Barriers to Entry" *American Economic Review* Vol 72, March 1982, p.47.

11 Stigler, G.J. "Barriers to Entry, Economies of Scale, and Firm Size" in George J Stigler *The Organization of Industry*, Richard D. Irwin, Homewood IL 1968, p.67.12 Caves, R.E. and Williamson, O.J. "What is Product Differentiation, Really?" *Journal of Industrial Economics*, December 1985. See also Waterson, M. "Models of Product Differentiation", *Bulletin of Economic Research*, January 1989, and Ireland, N. *Product Differentiation and Nonprice Competition*, Basil Blackwell, Oxford, 1987.

13 Britt, S.H. *Psychological Principles of Marketing and Consumer Behavior*, Lexington Books, Lexington MA. 1978.

14 Williamson, O. "Review of Bowman" *Yale Law Journal* Vol. 83, January 1974.

15 Salop, S.C. and Scheffman, D.T. "Raising Rival's Costs" *American Economic Review Papers and Proceedings*, Vol. 73, May 1983. Krattenmaker, T.G. and Salop, S.C. "Competition and Cooperation in the

Market for Exclusionary Rights" *American Economic Review Papers and Proceedings*, Vol. 76, May 1986. Also see Krattenmaker, Thomas G. and Salop, S.C. "Anticompetitive Exclusion: Raising Rivals' Cost to Achieve Power Over Price" *Yale Law Journal*, Vol 96, December 1986, and Campbell, T.J. "Predation and Competition in Antitrust: The Case of Nonfungible Goods" *Columbia Law Review*, Vol. 87, December 1987.

16   Baumol, W.J. and Willig, R.D. "Fixed Costs, Sunk Costs, and the Sustainability of Monopoly" *Quarterly Journal of Economics*, Vol. 96, August 1981.

17   Baumol, W.J. "Contestable Markets: An Uprising in the Theory of Industrial Structure", *American Economic Review*, March 1982, pp. 1-15. Also see Baumol, W.J., Panzar, J.C. and Willig, R.D. *Contestable Markets and the Theory of Industrial Structure*, Harcourt Brace Jovanovich, San Diego, CA. 1982.

18   Baily, E.E. "Contestability and the Design of Regulatory and Antitrust Policy" *American Economic Review*, May 1981, pp.178-83.

19   Chadwick, E. "Results of Different Principles of Legislation and Administration in Europe: of Competition for the Field, as Compared with Competition Within the Field of Service" *Royal Statistical Society,* 1859.

20   Crain, M.W. and Ekelund Jr. R.B. "Chadwick and Demsetz on Competition and Regulation" *Journal of Law and Economics*, Vol 19, April 1976, pp.149-62, pp.381-420.

21   Sheperd W.G. "Contestability v. Competition" in Jacquemin, A. *The New Industrial Organization*, Clarendon Press, Oxford, 1987. See also Vickers J. "Strategic Competition Among the Few" *Oxford Review of Economic Policy*, Autumn 1988, pp.39-62, Schwartz M. "The Nature and Scope of Contestablity Theory" in Morris, D.J. *Strategic Behavior in Industrial Competition*, pp.37-57, and Stiglitz, J.E. "Technological Change, Sunk Costs and Competition", *Brooking Papers on Economic Activity*, pp.883-937. Also see, Salop, S.C. "Strategic Entry Deterrence" *American Economic Review Papers and Proceedings*, Vol. 69 May 1979.

22   Greer, D.F. "Acquiring in Order to Avoid Acquisition" *Antitrust Bulletin*, Spring 1986, pp.155-56.

23   Sherman, R. *The Economics of Industry*, Little Brown, Boston 1974. Also see Bierman, H. Jr. and Thomas J.L. " Note on Mergers and Risk" *Antitrust Bulletin*, Fall 1975, p. 105.

Chapter 3
COMPETITIVE STRUCTURES IN PRODUCT AND FACTOR MARKETS

Economists have traditionally viewed firms as operating in some type of "market structure". Market structure in this context refers to the competitive environment within which firms rationally interact in order to minimize costs and maximize profits. Market structures can be viewed and compared in terms of some standard dimensions that are analytically applicable to each of them. These dimensions include (a) number of firms, (b) size of the firms, (c) pricing policy, (d) product composition, and (e) entry/exit conditions.

Based upon these dimensions, the structure of competition and the profit maximizing conduct of firms have been classified into the following fundamental categories: perfect competition, imperfect competition. Imperfect competition, in turn, includes monopoly, monopolistic competition, and oligopoly. In addition, largely for policy considerations, a modified version of imperfect competition, namely workable competition, has been introduced.

The time frames for much of the fundamental analyses in these markets center on the "short-run" and "long-run". The short-run in this context is viewed as any time period during which the firm alters output by changing the quantity of some of the factors of production while holding the quantity of other factors constant. Thus, in the short-run we deal with "variable" factors (e.g. labor), and "fixed" factors (e.g. capital, scale of operation, or capacity). In the long-run, we find only variable factors because the firm is assumed to be able change output only by varying all factors of production, that is, by changing the scale of operation and capacity. There are no specific time periods attached to these designations. They are defined and measured in terms of the behavioral patterns of the firm.

Another common text-book denominator for much of the market structure analyses is the assumption of "rationality" on the part of the firms. Rationality indicates that the firm is a profit maximizer, that is, will always seek out that level output at which it generates the highest attainable profit. The attainment of the highest level of profit has two conditions: (a) total revenue (TR) is greater than total cost (TC), and (b) marginal revenue (MR) is equal to marginal cost (MC). While the former is self-explanatory, the latter needs a little more attention. Marginal revenue is the increment in total revenue generated by a change (e.g. an additional unit) in output. Mathematically, it is the slope of the total revenue curve. Marginal cost, on the hand, is the increment in total cost for the same reason; measured by the slope of the total cost curve. At any output level where MR>MC, there is an incentive to expand as additional units of output generate a positive change in profits. On the other hand, where MR<MC there is no further incentive to expand as only negative changes in profits occur; however, there is an incentive to reduce output so long as MR<MC because the consequent reduction in cost is greater than that in revenues, improving the profit picture. Thus, with normal cost and revenue functions a rational firm will not only maximize profit where the two conditions are met, but will have also attained a stable equilibrium from which it has no incentive to depart. While the revenue functions differ between perfect and imperfect competition, the cost functions are typically assumed to be the same. Rational firm behavior for all market structure assumes the meeting of these two conditions, although with oligopoly, because of its peculiar characteristics, we will note various alternative scenarios, models, for equilibrium solutions. Because of the nature of this volume, designated to concentrate on the healthcare industry, with the coverage of neoclassical price theory at the fundamental level being presented only to place the study of health market competition in the proper economic environment, we will not elaborate further on the intricacies of these analyses. Standard microeconomic texts may provide   particularly interested readers with much further material and detail[1].

Perfect Competition

The perfectly competitive market is characterized by a number of restrictive assumptions. In fact, the assumptions are so restrictive that it is difficult to discern any significant rivalry among the firms. Furthermore, it has been difficult to find realistic examples that would fit the slate of perfect competition. It is a high level of abstraction in economic theory that provides a pure model for studying firm profit maximizing behavior. It is a normative standard for comparison and evaluation of the structure and performance of other, more realistic or less restrictive, market structures, for it is under perfectly competitive market conditions in all markets that society may have a chance for achieving optimum level of welfare.

The perfectly competitive (product and factor) market dimensions include a large number of firms, with each firm so small that not one of them can have any control over market price by altering production output or factor procurement quantities. Hence, the firms must accept the price dictated by the market, and at that price they can sell, or buy, any quantity they have the capacity to produce, or purchase. The firms produce and sell products that are identical ("homogeneous") in every respect. Thus, there is no reason, and there is nothing, to advertise. Entry into and exit out of the market will encounter no barriers. In other words, there is no difference between the costs faced by an incumbent and a new or potential entrant. The transaction cost associated with factor movements from one alternative use to another is zero, and factors of production remain equally productive in all of their alternative uses. Finally, information about prices, costs, product supply and demand is freely and instantaneously available to all buyers and sellers in all markets ("perfect knowledge"). Under these circumstances, it has been concluded that perfect competition is in fact characterized by an absence of effective competition[2].

In the short run, perfectly competitive firms can generate a profit, excess or "abnormal" or "accounting" profit, to the extent that price exceeds average cost at the equilibrium output level. In the long-run, the complete absence of entry barriers changes the picture drastically. Firms are attracted into the market. The result is the disappearance of excess profit due largely to the two effect that free entry generates: (a) price effect - the entry of new firms increases the supply of the product (the market supply curve shifts to the right), and with a given demand function, the price drops; in the same time (b) the cost effect shifts the average cost curve up due to the increased demand in the relevant factor markets. The outcome is that perfectly competitive firm profits are simply competed away in the long-run, and, if we can assume a neatly organized market where the dynamic process of factor movements in and out stops when the moment of long-run equilibrium has arrived, firms find themselves with their price just equal to the minimum point of their long-run average cost, with zero excess profit - left with only "normal profit". Normal profits are just enough incentives to stay in the market for those firms that are already in, but not enough for new ones to enter. Thus, in the long-run perfectly competitive firms earn no more and no less than their opportunity cost of being in that market. This state of affairs throughout all markets will stop inter-market factor movements even in the face of zero transaction costs. Intermarket factor incentives to migrate simply disappear, and society's productive resources are optimally allocated. Market price is equal to marginal cost, that is, to the opportunity unit cost of production - foregone earnings by not being in another opportunity are not higher than those actually earned. More comprehensively, the amount that consumers are willing to pay for a unit of the product is equal to the opportunity factor costs utilized.

When at least one of the perfectly competitive assumptions is relaxed, we are left with a type of imperfect competition. As we indicated earlier, this category includes monopoly, monopolistic competition, and oligopoly.

Imperfect Competition

Monopoly

A monopoly is a single firm market with a product without close substitutes, protected by barriers to entry. Hence, the monopolist has a virtually complete control over its price, constrained only by the possibility of potential entry if attracted by large profits, and by regulatory provisions, if present. [While the literature distinguishes between "pure" and "differentiated" monopoly, depending upon the availability or absence of relatively close substitutes, the purpose of our volume does not warrant getting into those details].

Since it constitutes the market, the monopolist's demand curve is its market demand curve - negatively slopped: if it wants to sell more, the firm must reduce price. Uninterfered from the outside, it seeks out the profit maximizing price and corresponding output levels, which, as explained above, will occur where the firm's marginal revenue equals it marginal cost. The price level will be higher, the output level lower, than in perfect competition. Specifically, the price level will be on the upper, elastic, portion of the demand curve, and the price charged will exceed marginal cost by an amount the size of which varies inversely with the price elasticity of demand itself.

In the absence of entry, the long-run monopolist can earn the same level of excess profit as the short run, however, less efficiently from its and society's point of view than perfect competition can. For instance, there are no specific safeguards, as in perfect competition, that the monopolist's long-run equilibrium output level will occur at the minimum level of the long-run average cost curve, or that the utilized plant will be of a socially optimal size operated at full capacity. Hence, in the long-run, the monopolist is not likely to achieve the allocative and production efficiency associated with perfect competition, since market price exceeds long-run marginal cost: the value placed on the last unit of output is greater than the perceived value of the factor input that produced it. A reallocation of resources to monopoly is called for, resulting in larger output at the level where marginal cost becomes equal to price.

The output restrictive higher price policy of the monopolist reduces consumer welfare (consumer surplus) substantially, using conventional micro text book analyses and standard minus forty-five degree demand curve, by about two thirds. Approximately one-third is lost completely: it exits from society, it is a "dead-weight loss". Roughly another third gets transferred over to the monopolist by way of the higher profit that it earns; so, while that is a loss to consumers, it is a gain by the monopolist, and not a net loss to society. Approximately (depending on the slope of the demand curve) the last third, will remain in the form of consumer surplus. Thus, society's welfare suffers a net reduction by about one-third, due to the monopolist's underutilization of resources. The result has been an increased attention to monopoly from policy makers, particularly within the context on antitrust policy, not so much for the size *per se*, but for the potentiality of competitive abuses both during the firm's growth period and after its maturation.

Monopolistic Competition

Located in mid-spectrum between monopoly and perfect competition, this competitive model assumes the presence of a large number of firms, each with minimum, but greater than zero, market power. The firm's market power emanates from its ability to slightly differentiate it product, or service, from others. The differentiation may be in terms of technical and performance characteristics, perceived or actual quality, location, and the like. While differentiated, the products remain close substitutes, allowing some pricing discretion on the part of firms the extent of which varies directly with the degree of successful differentiation. The retention of close substitutability limits the range within which a firm can alter price without drastic changes in its sales. In fact, even a small change in price will cause large quantity changes, due to the very flat, but not horizontal, shape of the firm's demand curve. However, while a firm is profoundly affected by its own price and output actions, its competitors, individually, will hardly notice the impact because the impact on the market as a whole is widely diffused.

Entry into the market is relatively easy, hence short-run profits are competed away in the long-run through increases in product supply and factor costs[3]. With a negatively slopped demand curve, the long-run average cost curve at the equilibrium output level will be tangent to the demand curve at a point to the left of the minimum. However, not as far left as it is in monopoly. Nevertheless, a monopolistically competitive firm will operate with somewhat sub-optimal size plant, and with less than full-capacity utilization. If product differentiation was eliminated, hence, the demand curve would become horizontal, as in perfect competition, optimal plant size with full-capacity utilization would be achieved. Consequently, while long-run equilibrium price is equal to average cost in equilibrium, and the firm is earning no more than "normal" profit (i.e. zero excess profit) as in perfect competition, price is higher than long-run marginal cost and, in contrast to perfect competition, output fall short of one corresponding to the minimum long-run average cost.

Oligopoly

Another market structure in mid-spectrum between perfect competition and monopoly is oligopoly. The classic, traditional, case of oligopoly assumes the presence of only two, or, at most, few firms. Each of these firms possess substantial market power. Competitive gestures (pricing, advertising, output changes) on the part of one have profound effects on others and are likely to solicit reactions. In fact, the oligopolistic firm cannot predict the outcome and final results of its actions, even upon itself, without assuming some, or none, rival reaction. Without making such assumptions, there is no unique oligopolistic profit maximizing equilibrium, such as we found in the other market structures.

Thus, "oligopolistic interdependence" requires a set of assumptions regarding rival behavior and reactions if any equilibrium solution is to be found. Indeed, much of the literature dealing with "oligopolistic solutions" attempt to provide just that, various models based upon various sets assumptions regarding rival reactions[4].

While traditional models typically assume a two-firm oligopolistic market, actual scenarios of oligopoly can deal with many firms, provided that only a few control the market (see for instance US food processing), with the rest of the firms considered merely as "fringe" operators none of which can have any significant impact on the market as a whole, or on the major players in the market.

Workable Competition

The various market structures briefly discussed above do not provide ideal policy targets. While perfect competition, in contrast to the various imperfectly competitive markets, can produce production and allocative efficiency, equity in markets and optimum social welfare, it is far too remote from reality. What may be most desirable for public policy is a combination of selected features from the various market structures tempered for the needs of society. Enters "workable competition". As a policy target, workable competition should have at least the following attributes: (a) the number of firms is consistent with scale economies and industry life cycle; (b) no artificial barriers to entry; (c) prices reflect product quality, and buyers should be fully aware of all pertinent information in that context; (d) rival reactions cannot be predicted with 100% certainty; (e) lack of collusion and other overtly anti-competitive or commercially deceptive conduct; (f) only the economically fittest should survive; (g) production should be efficient and profit levels adequate to reward investment and efficiency; (h) production should reflect consumer preferences[5].

Factor Markets

So far, we have placed our nut-shell discussion of the firm within the context of the out-going shipping or show room, its functioning in the final (output) product market. Let us now take a brief look at how the firm conducts itself through its receiving room, in the factor or input markets. Similar to output market conditions, the firm may find itself in various competitive conditions and related assumptions in factor markets.

The issues in this context involve the determination of factor prices, such as the wage of labor, and the return to other factors such as land, capital and entrepreneurial talent, and the optimum amount of factor utilization consistent with profit maximization in the final analysis. Thus, this aspect of neoclassical microtheory (the theory of the firm) deals with how the fruits of production are distributed among the various contributors to the production process.

The fundamental analyses assume that labor is rewarded according to its contribution to the production process. More specifically, it receives the market value of its marginal product; "value of marginal product" equals marginal physical product of labor times final product price in perfectly competitive factor markets, and "marginal revenue product" = marginal physical product of labor times marginal revenue in imperfectly competitive factor markets. The firm will consider it well advised to hire labor in these markets up the input level where labor price (wage) is just equal to the dollar value of labor's contribution as described above: "the marginal productivity theory of wages"[1].

Contestable Markets

During the early 1980s this theory was advanced regarding the functioning of markets and the implied application of antitrust policy to anticompetitive structure and conduct in those markets[6]. According to the theory, a market's performance is controlled by external factors, such as completely uninhibited entry predicated upon no difference between the potential entrants' and incumbent's cost functions and production as well as marketing capabilities. Once having entered into the market, a new firm can maneuver into a gainful position without having to concern itself with existing rivals. And, if things do not work out, the cost of exit from the market is zero, as all moneys expended upon entry can be recovered and sunk costs are nonexistent. Thus, a contestable market is one where hit-and-run entrants can prosper, and before the existing firms wake up to the fact and attempt to put on pressure, the winner is gone with the loot. The implications for antitrust policy and competition enforcement are clear. In this type of market, the most important controlling factor is potential competition; that alone can secure a nearly perfectly competitive performance for society because both excess profits and inefficient production are eliminated by hit-and-run entry. So, long-run equilibrium will be the same as in perfect competition.

The theory's tenure of acceptability turned out to be short. It has been criticized on various grounds, especially by its assumptions of zero sunk costs, and non-reactive incumbents. If these assumptions are relaxed even to a small degree, the theory cannot survive[7]. Additionally, empirical studies have found a high degree of association between the level of prices and profits on the one hand and high concentration and entry barriers on the other. In the airline industry, a point of example offered by the authors of contestable markets, rates have been found to be up to 50% lower than in markets where the number of competitors was five or more. These essentially defy the validity of market contestability[8].

References

1   Nicholson, W. *Intermediate Microeconomics and its Application*, 5th Edition, Dryden Press, Chicago, 1990. Varian, H. *Intermdediate Microeconomics: A Modern Approach*, 2nd Edition, W.W. Norton & Co. New York, 1990. Jehle, J.A. *Advanced Microeconomic Thoery*, Prentice Hall, Englewood Cliff, NJ 1991.

2   Hayek, F.A. "The Meaning of Competition", in *Individualism and Economic Order*, Henry Regnery, Chicago, 1948. See also, Schumpeter, J.A. *Capitalism, Socialism and Democracy*, 3rd Ed. Harper & Rown, New York 1950; and Knight, F.H. *Risk, Uncertainty and Profit*, University of Chicago Press, Chicago, 1971.

3   Chamberlin, E.H. *The Theory of Monopolistic competition*, 8th Ed. Harvard University Press, Cambridge MA. 1962. Also see, Robinson, J. *The Economics of Imperfect Competition*, MacMillan, London 1969. Sraffa, P. "The Laws of Return Under Competitive Conditions", *Economic Journal*, Vol. 36, December 1926, pp. 535-50. Moss, S. "The History of the Firm From Marshall to Robinson and Chamberlin: The Source of Positivism in Economics" *Economica*, Vol. 51, August 1984 pp.307-18.

4   Cournot, A. *Researches into the Mathematical Principles of the Theory of Wealth* (Nathaniel Bacon transl.) MacMillan, New York, 1927 (originally published in 1838). Stackelberg, H.von *Marktform und Gleichgewicht* Julius Springer, Vienna 1934. Bertrand, J. "Theorie Mathematique de la Richesse Sociale" *Journal des Savants* September 1883, pp.499-508. Sweezy, P. "Demand Under Conditions of Oligopoly" *Journal Of Political Economy*, Vol. 47 University of Chicago Press, Chicago 1939, pp.568-73. Hall, R. and Hitch C.J. "Price Theory and Business Behavior" *Oxford Economic Papers*, Vol. 2 May 1939 pp.12-45. See also, Stigler, G.J. "The Kinky Oligopoly Demand Curve and Rigid Prices" *Journal of Political Economy*, Vol. 55, October 1947, pp.434-49. von Neuman J. and Morgenstern, O. *Theory of Games and Economic Behavior*, Princeton University Press 1963. Friedman, J. W. *Oligopoly and the Theory of Games* North-Holland, Amsterdam 1977. Ordeshhok, P.C. *Game Theory and Political Theory: An Introduction* Cambridge University Press, Cambridge 1986. Shubik, M. *Game Theory in the Social Sciences* MIT Press, Cambridge MA. 1982, and *A Game Theoretic Approach to Political Economy* MIT Press, Cambridge MA 1987. Nash, J.F. "The Bargaining Problem" *Econometrica*, Vol. 18, April 1950, pp.155-62.

5   Scherer, F.M. and Ross, D. *Industrial Market Structure and Economic Performance,* 3rd Edition, Houghton Mifflin Boston 1990 pp. 52-55. Clark, J.M. "Toward a Concept of workable competition" *American Economic Review* Vol. 30, June 1940 pp. 241-56. Sosnick, S. "A Critique of Concepts of workable competition" *Quarterly Journal of Economics*, Vol. 72 August 1958, pp. 380-423.

6   Baumol, W.J. "Contestable Markets: An Uprising in the Theory of Industrial Structure" *American Economic Review*, March 1982, pp.1-15. Baumol, W.J., Panzar, J.C. and Willig, R.D. *Contestable Markets and the Theory of Industrial Structure* Harcourt Brace Jovanovich, SanDiego CA 1982. Baily, E. "Contestability and the Design of Regulatory and Antitrust Policy" *American Economic Review*, May 1981, pp. 178-83. Shepherd, W.G. "Contestability v. Competition" *American Economic Review*, September 1984, pp.572-87.

7   Vickers, J. "Strategic Competition Among the Few" *Oxford Review of Economic Policy* Autumn 1988, pp.39-62. Schwartz M. "The Nature and Scope of Contestability Theory" in *Strategic Behavior and Industrial Competition* by Morris J.D. et al (eds), Clarendon Press Oxford 1986, pp. 37-57. Stiglitz, J.E. "Technological Change, Sunk Costs and Competition" *Brookings Papers on Economic Activity*, No. 3 1987, pp.883-937.

8   Gilbert, R.J. "The Role of Potential Competition in Industrial Organization" *Journal of Economic Perspectives*, Summer 1989, pp. 107-27. Moore, T.G. "US Airline Regulation" *Journal of Law and Economics*, April 1986, pp.1-28. Baker, S. H. and Pratt J.B. "Experience as a Barrier to Contestablity in Airline Markets" *Review of Economics and Statistics* May 1989, pp.352-56. Call G.D.and Keelre, T.E. "Airline Dergulation Fares and Market Behavior: Some Empirical Evidence" in *Analytical Studies in Transport Economics* Daughety A (ed), Cambridge University Press, New York 1985. Breshnahan, T.F. Reiss P.C. "Do Entry Conditions Vary Across Markets?" *Brookings Papers on Economic Activity* No. 3 1987 pp. 833-869.

Chapter 4
MEASUREMENT OF ECONOMIC AND MARKET POWERS

An entity possesses *economic* power when it is able to produce a designed effect upon others. The existence of economic power is always a matter degree, and is constrained by a variety of available options such as innovations, advertising, lobbying, and many other factors. *Market* power rests in the ability of setting or influencing prices within a specifically delineated market, or in the ability of controlling rivals' actions, or both. Market power can be generated by product differentiation that induces brand switching, even in the face of stable prices; by the market share of one or of a group of firms; and, by barriers to entry which tend protect the statusquo of the incumbent firms. In addition, firm growth, and vertical as well as conglomerate integrations may also affect market power[1].

Excess Price Index

Some, relatively more realistic, measurements of market power were developed during the early 1930s and 1940s. One, the Lerner Index, depicts market power by way of the difference between price and marginal cost expressed as proportion of price itself. Since in perfect competition the difference is zero, market power is also zero. In a profit maximizing monopoly, on the other hand, price far exceeds marginal cost, yielding a substantial index[2]. While the simplicity of this index as a method of market power measurement is appealing, its application may be inhibited by measurement problems relating to marginal cost. Furthermore, the index might be viewed as a measurement of the *impact* exercised by market power, rather than that of the market power itself. Thus, if a monopolist chooses not no maximize profit and keeps price artificially low for, say, trying to pre-empt entry, its Lerner Index would be quite low, indicating not a lack of monopoly power, but rather a lack of the exercise of monopoly power. It could, however, be argued that threat of entry prompting a monopolist to keep prices substantially below the profit maximizing level is in itself an offset to monopoly power, hence the index, though indirectly, reflects upon that offset in the latter scenario.

Excess Profit Index

Another attempt to measure market power focused on excess profits[3]. The amount of excess profits here is thought to reflect directly upon the existence of market power. Excess profits were defined as total revenue reduced by costs, depreciation, and prevailing opportunity costs.

q Ratio

Originally developed for macro applications in investment analyses, it defines a firm's market power as the ratio of market value to replacement cost for assets[4]. As the degree of market competition increases, the value of q approaches 1. As the value of q remains above 1, and related directly to the extent it does, net return on investments in assets remains positive (market value > replacement cost), hence the incentive for new firms to enter increases, or for existing firms to expand, and, in the absence of barriers, entry will continue until q will be equal to 1. Entry barriers, on the other hand, will secure and protect monopoly rent for existing firms with market power, subsequently capitalized into the market value of the firm, leaving q values well above 1.

Concentration Ratio

An essential yardstick for public policy implementation has for some time been the state of industrial or market concentration, that is, an examination of the market power possessed by a number of the largest firms, expressed as a percentage of the total volume of business in some specifically delineated market. Part Two will review some of the principles involved in market definitions, delineations, and measurements in antitrust. At this juncture, we note that a delineated market will, in a predefined geographic area, likely contain directly competing firms, producing relatively or absolutely high substitutes, priced within the same range, using similar production processes. A properly delineated geographic and product market will include all economic forces and factors that substantially impact upon the economic decisions of the participants, and exclude those that do not.

The *concentration ratio* has been used by academics and public policy enforcers for decades as a measure of firm size distribution in a market. It was normally expressed in terms of sales, likely because of the relatively ready availability of data in that category. However, other financial or operating dimensions could have also been useful though less than perfect: employment may not reflect size due to optional factor substitutability with capital; asset data may be biased by prevailing accounting methods; but, even sales data may be unduly biased by some prevailing price differences.

Concentration ratio ranks a certain number of the distinctly largest firms and expresses their share in terms of percentage of the total market. The number of the largest firms thus focused upon has normally been between four ("four-firm concentration ratio") and sixteen, with four and eight having been the most frequently used. In fact, for US Justice Department merger policies during the 1960s and 1970s, the four-firm concentration ratio was relied upon. The value of the ratio ranges from a theoretical zero, for perfect competition, to 1.0 in markets where the designated number of firms control the entire market. The value of the concentration ratio varies directly with the market share controlled by the designated number of firms.

While the utilization of the concentration ratio yields relatively simple and quick measurements, it obscures the size distribution among the chosen firms. A four-firm concentration ratio in market "A" may be 95%, the same as in market "B". However, in market "A" the largest firm may have a 93% market share, with the three others dividing the rest of the 2% equally among themselves. In "B", each of the four firms have a 23.75% market share, indicating a much more even distribution of market power, hence a likely greater degree of competition, among the dominant firms than in "A".

The Hirschman Index

During the mid-1940s an, at that time, obscure index was developed by way of a study of international trade issues that involved summing the square of all individual elements in a series[5]. A few years later, an unpublished dissertation at Columbia utilized it within the context of studying concentration in the US steel industry[6]. In economics, the index simply sums the square of all member firms' market shares in a delineated market, thus taking account of the share of all market participants; not just the largest firms, as does the concentration ratio. Additionally, taking the square of all single firm market shares actually highlights the share of the larger firms. The value of the index varies directly and proportionately with the extent that the market departs from a situation of perfect equality among the participants' market shares. If the industry contains only one firm, with a market share of 100%, the index attains a value of 10,000 (i.e. 100 squared). If all of the firms have identical market shares, then the index is equal to 10,000/n, where n is the number of firms.

The index allows us to uncover and reflect upon data regarding individual member firms whose market-shares are hidden by the concentration ratio. For instance, in a four-firm market of equal shares the index is equal to 2,500 (i.e. 10,000/4, and the sum of the squares of the four 25% market shares). In another market of four-firms, with one firm having 95%, and the other three having approximately 1.67%, the index yields approximately 9,033 (approaching the 10,000 level), indicating the much greater inequality of market share distribution.

By the mid-1980s, the US Department of Justice accepted this index as a measure of concentration[7], and designated markets with an index of 1,000 or less as "unconcentrated", needing a 200 point or more rise in the index to merit a Departmental challenge of a merger, and markets with an index of 1,800 or more as "concentrated", needing only a 100 point merger generated rise in the index to attract close attention from the Department[8].

While the H-index is presently the most widely accepted one, other yardsticks of market concentration have also been advanced that are worth a brief mention. The *entropy* index, derived from physics, is somewhat more complex than the H-index, although it relies on the same information. It is the antilog of the negative of the weighted sum of the logged reciprocals of individual market shares, with latter being the weights themselves. Another yardstick, the *Gini Coefficient,* based on the principles of economics course concept dealing with income distribution, namely the Lorenz Curve, measures the distribution of market shares. It relates the cumulative percentage of firms to their cumulative market shares, and compares it with a norm of perfect distribution.

References

1   Rothschild, R.W. "The Degree of Monopoly", *Economica,* February 1942, pp.24-40. Presents a theoretical discussion of a market power measurement method. See also Papandreou, George, A. "Market Structure and Monopoly Power", *American Economic Review*, September 1949 pp.883-97. Triffin, Robert *Monopolistic competition and General Equilibrium Theory*, Harvard University Press, Cambridge MA 1940.

2   Lerner, A.P. "The Concept of Monopoly and the Measurement of Monopoly Power" *Review of Economic Studies*, June 1934, pp. 157-175.

3   Bain, J.S. "The Profit Rate as a Measure of Monopoly Power" *Quarterly Journal of Economics*, February 1941,pp.271-93.

4   Tobin, J. "A General Equilibrium Approach to Monetary Theory" *Journal of Money, Credit and Banking,* Vol.1, February 1969, pp. 15-29, and "Monetary Policies and the Economy: The Transition Mechanism", *Southern Economic Journal*, Vol. 44 Janury 1978, pp. 421-31. Tobin, J. and Brainard Williams C. "Pitfalls in Financial Model Building" *American Economic Review Papers and Proceedings*, Vol. 58, May 1968, pp. 99-122. Tobin, James and Brainard, W.C. "Asset Markets and the Cost of Capital" in Balassa, B. and Nelson, R. (eds) *Economic Progress: Private Values and Public Polcies* (Essays in Honor of William Fellner) North-Holland, Amsterdam 1977.

5   Hirschman, A.O. *National Power and Structure of Foreign Trade*, University of California Press, Berkeley, CA 1945]

6   Herfindhal, O.C. *Concentration in the Steel Industry*, PhD dissertation, Columbia University, New York NY. 1945.

7   US Department of Justice, *Merger Guidelines*, June 14, 1982.

8   Adelman, M.A. "Comment on the 'H' Concentration Measure as a Numbers Equivalent", *Review of Economics and Statistics*, Vol. 51, February 1969, pp.99-101. Also see Stigler, George J. "The Measurement of Concentration" in George J. Stigler, *The Organization of Industry*, Richard D. Irwin, Homewood IL 1968.

Chapter 5
STRUCTURAL MARKET TRANSFORMATION:
A Birds-Eye View of Mergers

The structure of an industry may be viewed in a static and in a dynamic context[1]. Statics view the currently prevailing degree of integration either among firms that directly compete with each other or those that operate at different stages of the production process, or among firms or markets that produce goods that are non-competing either by virtue of the product's nature, or of the geographical dimensions. The dynamic interpretation of these issues concerns itself with changes in these production dimensions, and views the integrated dimensions of the production process over a period of time. Integration by way of structural transformation may be classified into three major, somewhat overlapping, categories: horizontal, vertical and conglomerate.

Horizontal, Vertical and Conglomerate Integration

Horizontal transactions involve two or more firms from the same directly competitive environment. The degree of competition eliminated by such mergers depends on the respective firms' market shares. Since firms party to these transactions were functioning at the same production stage, these mergers may also be labeled as *uni-stage*.

Multi-stage mergers, involving firms from different stages of the same production process, are considered vertical integration. A "downstream" version of this merger takes place in the direction of the final product (manufacturer acquiring a wholesaler, or the latter a retailer and so forth). The opposite for "upstream", in the direction of raw material sources. Only firms that operate at the same production stage compete with each other horizontally as each production stage constitutes a separate market. Hence, a vertical merger is a multi-market merger, unless the merging firms operate at both of the involved production stages, in which case the merger takes on both vertical and horizontal characteristics[2].

Since they involve different markets, vertical mergers also have diversification qualities, hence could be included with the third category of mergers, conglomeration. Conglomerate mergers involve firms from different geographical or product markets, or both. A somewhat arbitrary and overlapping classification groups conglomerate mergers into three categories - product extension, market extension, and "pure". Firms party to the product extension merger produce essentially complementary goods that extend rather than compete with each other. In market extension mergers, the participating firms may produce competing products, however, competition prior to the merger was barred by geographical separation and related costs; conglomeration takes place by way of geographics rather than products. Conglomeration of the "pure" type entails firms from completely different product and geographical markets, and is likely to involve firms with different production processes.

Historical Backdrop

Pior to 1950, horizontal mergers were frequent, and not horizontal mergers were simply beyond reach. The judicial remedy, Section 7 of the Clayton Act in its original form, could not adequately cope with them. The subsequent 1949 Celler-Kefauver Amendment extended the scope of the Act and rendered it relatively potent. Hence, until the 1980s, very little of significance occurred by way of horizontal mergers, and, as we shall see later in the volume, industrial and judicial pre-occupation seemed to shift to other types of mergers. During the 1980s, and in a somewhat diminishing pattern to date, much of the thinking was dominated by the "Chicago School", leaving caretaking in the market to the firms themselves: mergers, even among major competitors in the same market, are thought to be a possible source of economic efficiency ultimately benefiting the consumer, hence government is well advised to stay out of it. Major acquisitions in this spirit included cash-loaded oil companies, the 1988 acquisition of Kraft Foods by Philip Morris for a meager $13 billion, and Kodak's purchase of Sterling Drug for $5 billion.

The Motives for Mergers

The reasons for the parties to merge, to acquire, or to be willingly acquired, tend to differ among the transactions. The desire to *grow* will motivate an acquisition. Stockholder-owners want to maximize their dividend income, while non-owner management wants to pursue growth for maximizing its personal utilities emanating from size. Over some, initial and mid-range, production stages growth may bring with it increases in income (the shape of standard cost functions from micro principles texts will indicate the reasons for this). In addition, while in some cases size dimensions (such as assets, sales, and employment) and mergers may positively correlate, sales of the newly merged company may not exceed the sum of the sales of the pre-merged companies. While mergers can take place on the expense of sales by the new firm, compared with the combined sales of the pre-merged firms, there seems to have been a correlation between the motive to grow and conglomeration, particularly where the target market for diversification displayed a much higher growth rate than the merging firms' original source markets[3].

Accounting and tax considerations may also motivate mergers. Earnings-per-share may be viewed as a corporate performance barometer. It can be elevated by accounting either statically, or dynamically to show substantial growth patterns for shareholder consumption, so long as "generally accepted accounting practices" are observed. One way to portray favorable earnings is through consolidation, burying losers into winners. Another is to redistribute outstanding shares so as to increase E/S, because a reduced number of outstanding shares (S) will increase the value of the ratio even in the face of constant or even declining earnings (E); e.g. payment for merger transactions can be made by way of non-common stock instruments, such as convertible bonds, warrants, rights, and other issues[4]. Thirdly, a mid-year merger can look good if subsequent earnings pictures are elevated, by including the acquired company's profits (especially if the acquiring company was a loser that year) for the entire year, or by altering the acquired company's depreciation accounting to generate additional profits. Finally, the cost of acquisition can be recorded lower if the cost of non-tangible assets (e.g. good will) is excluded from the purchase price.

Tax savings can facilitate a merger decision. A "loss-carry-over", or unused depletion allowance, of the acquiring company can be utilized against the positive earnings of the acquired company. Or, by way of a debt-equity switch, the payment for the new company will be made with debentures instead of equity, increasing the E/S ratio, deferring debt payments until the debt matures, and paying for the acquired firm with interest (before-tax income) instead of dividends that can be paid out only after taxes. Additionally, any accumulated cash reserves on the part of the acquired firm can be distributed through the merger constituting a return on capital thus taxed at a possibly lower capital gains rate, rather than a possibly higher prevailing rate.

Since investors may value a firm's stocks in terms of its growth potential, a merger can project such a *growth potential*. Assume company B earns $200, with 200 common stocks outstanding, with an E/S=1. They target company S for acquisition, also with E/S=1, and issue 40 shares to pay for the merger. Assume B's share price at $100, and S's at $20, and the two P/Es (price-earnings ratios) at 100 and 20 respectively. After the merger, B's earnings will $400 with only 40 more shares outstanding and a total of 240. The new E/S=1.67. If investors attribute the same growth potential to the new firm as they did to B, they will bid up the new firm's share price to about $160-$170, so as to maintain the same P/E. Its reputation increased, B can now make another acquisition with even fewer of its shares, enhancing further its E/S ratio, and also its P/E ratio through the likely favorable reaction by the market. So long as the market subscribes to B's anticipated growth, it can enter into further merger agreements generating higher P/E and E/S ratios for itself.

Conglomerate mergers are often motivated by *risk reduction*. Risk may simply be viewed as significant variations in earnings measured by standard deviations[5]. Conglomerate mergers may reduce risk by spreading it over several markets, hoping that low performance in some will be offset by better performance in others. However, empirical studies have not been able to conclusively confirm this outcome. In fact, there does not appear to be empirical confirmation of a potentially increased profitability attributed to mergers either. Mergers may not even be more profitable than other types of investment[3]. Some studies found at best neutral, and even a negative, relationship, between profitability and mergers[6]. Merger's appeal emanates from the fact that, compared to internal expansion, it is a less expensive way to grow, faster, and largely precludes the risks of entering a new market *de novo*. Merger simply takes over existing facilities, personnel, technology instead of creating new ones. Thus, the extent of cost disadvantages, if any, is substantially reduced. In addition, the acquired firm may be paid for by installments, financing the acquisition from income earned along the way, rather than by lump-sum outlays. Risk is once again minimized.

The motive of increasing m*arket power* may be behind mergers, especially horizontal ones. In fact, the turn-of the century merger wave produced some of the presently existing industrial giants in oil and sugar refining, tobacco, cement, alcoholic beverage distilling, and others. The new firm that emerges is likely to be larger than either one of the older firms. However, whether the new firm's market power will be significantly and effectively be larger than the sum of the pre-merged firms' depends on the degree of complementarity between merged resources[7]. In general vertical mergers in either direction tend to increase market power by foreclosing competitors in the markets involved. Finally, conglomerate mergers may increase market power through the financial "deep-pocket" policy of the acquiring firm utilized for the benefit of the acquired firm.

Deterrents to Merger

There are a number of factors which tend to cause second thoughts before or during merger consummation. If politically subscribed to by the prevailing administration, philosophically accepted, and enforced, the *antitrust laws* have shown themselves to be potent deterrents to horizontal mergers in particular. Since the 1960s, with some exceptions during the 1980s, the Government has been fairly consistent in successfully invoking the power of Section 7 of the Clayton Act. The US Department of Justice has issued a number of Merger Guidelines, in 1968, 1982, 1984, and most recently in April 1992. The latter, the first one issued jointly with the Federal Trade Commission, will be briefly reviewed at the end of this chapter.

Transaction costs constitute another major deterrent to mergers. Basic minimum brokerage costs are likely to be doubled by tender solicitation and acceptance of securities. There are administrative and legal costs. Substantial professional, legal and accounting, time may be devoted to the transaction yielding implicit costs if in-house talent is used, and explicit costs if consultants are utilized. These costs may amount to about 5% of the acquired firm's value[8]. If the merger is contested, efforts are duplicated, and transaction costs multiply.

Finally, a group of *regulatory* deterrents should be mentioned. Rule 10b-5 of the Securities and Exchange Act places stringent rules on the manner and method of application for mergers, and, if not abided by properly, could result in a reversal of the transaction, with the accompanying costs. The 1968 Williams Act, amended in 1970, mandates information disclosure conditions for the parties to a merger, once again carrying the risk that if not abided by, reversal and even prosecution may follow.

The US Department of Justice and The Federal Trade Commission 1992 Horizontal Merger Guidelines

This new set of guidelines articulate five elements of analysis to determine whether to challenge a merger: (a) market definition, measurement and concentration - has always been essential if not fundamental for the determination of the anticompetitive impact of the merger; (b) potential adverse competitive effects of the merger; (c) entry; (d) efficiencies; and, (e) failure of existing assets. For the first time, the guidelines also concentrate on the circumstances under which a merger might lead to the unilateral (in addition to coordinated) exercise of market power. The term "coordinated interaction", rather than "collusion", is utilized allowing for the possibility of a merger causing even a tacit collusion. Entry is given added emphases. The guidelines provide a framework for analyzing whether entry is timely, likely, and sufficient to prevent or offset an anticompetitive merger.

The Guidelines do not discuss to any significant extent the horizontal effects of non-horizontal mergers. Furthermore, the enforcement foundations and policies for non-horizontal mergers have not been changed since published in 1984. The main thrust of the 1992 Guidelines is to elaborate more clearly on how horizontal mergers may adversely affect competition, and the way particular market factors interact with those effects. Furthermore, the new horizontal guidelines sharpen the distinction among the various types of supply responses to mergers. Finally, as mentioned above, the competitive impact of potential entrants, into the market where the merger was consummated, is given careful attention. This aspect of the Guidelines will be reviewed in the following chapter on entry.

References

1   Seplaki, L., *Antitrust and the Economics of the Market,* Harcourt, Brace, Jovanovich, San Diego, CA. 1982, Part Six, Chapter 1, pp. 385-401.
2   *Brown Shoe Co. v. US* 370 U.S. 307 (1962) gives a classic example of this situation.
3   Hogarty, Thomas, F. "Profit from Mergers: The Evidence of 50 Years", *St.John's Law Review*, Vol. 44, July 1970, pp.378-91. Hogarty, Thomas, F. "The Profitability of Corporate Mergers", *Journal of Business*, Vol. 43, October 1970, pp.317-27. Gort, M. "New Evidence on Mergers", *Journal of Law and Economics*, Vol. 13, July 1970, pp.167-84].
4   *Accounting Principles Board*, May 1969. The APB of the American Institute of Certified Public Accountants issued a policy whereby E/S must be displayed on the face of the income statement for ready scrutiny. Furthermore, corporations with securities that could be considered dilutive are required to post two E/S ratios: the "primary earnings per share" showing E/S with all common stocks considered, and "fully diluted earnings-per-share" without such restrictions.
5   Alberts, William W. "The Profitability of Growth by Merger" in Alberts, William W. and Segall, John E. *The Corporate Merger*, The University of Chicago Press, Chicago IL. 1966, pp. 262-72.
6   Reid, Robert S. *Mergers, Managers and The Economy*, New York, 1968, Chapter 8, and Kelly, Edward *The Profitability of Growth Through Mergers*, Unpublished PhD Dissertation, Columbia University, 1965.
7   Weston, John F. "The Nature and Significance of Conglomerate Firms" *St. John's Law Review*, Vol. 44, July 1970, p.70, and Stigler, George J. "Mergers and Preventative Antitrust Policy", *University of Pennsylvania Law Review*, Vol 104, April 1955, pp.178-84].
8   Steiner, Peter O. *Mergers*, University of Michigan, Ann Arbor, MI 1975

Chapter 6
FACTOR MOBILITY AND MARKET COMPETITION

The purpose of public policy regarding market competition, particularly in merger and monopolization cases, is to determine if a firm, or group of firms by way of overt or covert cooperation, has or is likely to attain market power. We already equated market power in terms of ability to maintain price above competitive level by output restriction. We also noted that in perfect competition a firm's market power is zero because in the long-run it must price its product at marginal cost that includes a return on capital necessary to retain the firm in the market. Thus, the greater is the extent, and the longer, a dominant firm, or group of dominant firms, can keep price above marginal cost, without losing a significant amount of its sales, the greater is its, their, market power.

A constraint upon the pricing and output actions of existing dominant firm(s) in a market is the presence and entry intentions of firms not yet in the market, or of firms already in the market but operating on the "fringe" with no significant market power. Thus, the extent of market power on the part of existing dominant firms is determined by the ability of existing fringe competitors to expand capacity promptly, or by the ability of outside firms to quickly enter into the market without significant cost disadvantage. In fact, even with a market share smaller than that normally considered to be a source of monopoly power, a firm or firms can act as dominant entities by keeping price substantially above competitive level if fringe competitors or potential entrants must mount significant obstacles in their efforts to expand or enter.

Thus, entry is of considerable importance for assessing existing market powers. In a broad sense, because it is not only the intentions and cost advantages or disadvantages of potential *new* entrants into the market that is important. The ability of already existing small firms with no present market power, but with the potential of expansion within the market under the proper conditions, is also important. Consequently, when we speak of "entry" within the context of competition enforcement by public policy, we speak of the flow of resources *into the dominant firms' sphere of operation* in a market regardless whether that flow is originated *de novo* by firms from outside the market, or from previously existing non-dominant firms already within the market.

Definitions

The courts and economists have been dealing with the concept of "entry" and, therefore, what constitutes "barriers to entry" for over four decades. In its application to policy, entry had a minimal role for many years. Ease of entry, even in a horizontal merger case, was almost irrelevant. The Federal Trade Commission rejected ease of entry as a factor mitigating an otherwise anticompetitive horizontal merger transaction by saying "... the existence of potential competition does not justify or excuse elimination of actual competition"[1]. During the past fifteen years or so, entry has become a fundamental and often decisive issue in merger[2] and even monopolization and conspiracy cases[3]. Even in predatory pricing cases, the issue of entry can play an important role, that is, if ease of entry essentially precludes successful predation[4].

In economics, the concept of entry, and barriers to entry, first received prominent attention in the mid-1950s[5]. Bain started an as yet unresolved debate as to what are those market conditions that could validly be considered as barriers to entry, and, therefore, which markets are easy to enter and which are more difficult, or even impossible, to enter. Bain interpreted entry barriers by first identifying the effects of barriers and then pointing to market conditions that brings about those effects. He considered entry barriers to be present when incumbent firms could charge above cost prices without attracting entry..."..the extent to which, in the long-run, established firms can elevate their selling prices above the minimal average cost of production and distribution without inducing potential entrants to enter the industry"[6]. Thus, entry barriers exist in any market where economic profits are earned by existing firms, and they, in turn, according to Bain, emanate from advantages in production costs, economies of scale, and product differentiation.

The "Chicago School" theory argues for a subset of Bain's variables as entry barriers: only the long-run advantages in production costs enjoyed by existing firms (generated by unequal access to inputs, patents, tariffs, and regulatory constraints) should be viewed as barriers to entry. Such advantage will allow the existing firms to raise price above marginal costs without attracting new entrants. This view disregards advantages in product differentiation, economies of scale, and large capital requirements as valid entry barriers[7].

An examination of the relevant market's history might, or might not, shed light on prevailing barriers to entry. If data reveals considerable in/out traffic for a market in response price changes, relaxation of regulatory constraints, or cost changes, or, in the absence of *de novo* entry fringe firms demonstrated notable expansions, it may reasonably be concluded that entry barriers are not significant. However, even under these circumstances, significant entry barriers may be at play if the expansion of fringe firms or the entry of new ones take place only in the face of inefficient incumbency. The barriers are there, but the expanding fringes and the new ones succeed in spite of the higher cost of production they may face because of the existing firms' inefficiency.

What about markets that show minimum or no entry or fringe expansion? Are we to conclude that substantial barriers are at play? May be not, especially with low prices and minimum profits which only a high degree of competition can generate. Instead of entry barriers, there is competition that does not make entry appealing. If, on the other hand, profits, real prices and demand were high and rising, all scale economies were utilized by existing dominant firms, and technology was relatively stagnant, entry should have historically taken place. If it did not, there may be valid reasons to seek and identify entry barriers.

Recognized and Unrecognized Entry Barriers

If the a potential entrant would face no entry barriers, the monopolist, or group of existing firms with monopoly power, would have to charge competitive price, and the monopoly power would dissolve. The extent of any existing entry barrier, therefore, can be measured by the difference between monopoly price and the long-run competitive equilibrium price, which, in turn, depends upon the price elasticity of demand[8].

As indicated earlier in the volume, a source of entry barrier is *economies of scale*. If the relationship between the market demand curve and the long-run average cost curve is such that only a small specific number of firms, say two, can share in the market and each produce at a price at or above average cost, then new entrants will be precluded by potential cost conditions[9]. When, under these circumstances, only one firm can efficiently produce for the entire market, we have a "natural monopoly" situation. However, economies of scale may not be viewed as entry barriers, if we accept Professor Stigler's argument to the effect that existing firm(s) face the same cost conditions as potential entrants - scale economies are equally available to all members of the market, therefore, they should not be viewed as entry barriers. Barriers to entry, according to Stigler, must be viewed in terms of some net costs disadvantage that accrues only to the potential entrant, and need not be born by incumbents[7]

Another source of entry barriers is *capital requirements*. It is predicated upon the assumption that potential entrants may not be able to raise large amount of capital to enter, hence the incumbent's monopoly profits are protected. However, it is also predicated on the assumption that potential entrants need, in fact, to raise capital in lump-sum, or even at all. These obstacles may be overcome by leasing, acquiring used equipment, or simply dispensing capital by installment.

Exclusive possession of indispensable resources can some time act as an entry barrier. Raw materials, specialized managerial talent. *Licenses and patents* can act as entry barriers into markets for some commodities, the marketing and delivery of energy and other regulated sectors, and into certain endeavors and professions. *Advertising* may be subject to economies of scale, can be viewed as a capital cost with long-term returns, hence may be considered as an entry barrier[10]. However, it has been argued that advertising may be an entry inducing rather barring factor: new firms can use advertising to inform customers of their product's availability; without advertising, distribution networks would have to be expanded yielding an increase in long-run average costs; scale economies of production could be reached much slower because quantity would not expand as fast to attain the needed level. Thus, a lack of advertising would increase long-run average cost for every one, not just potential entrants[11].

Product differentiation has been viewed as a plausible entry barrier. A brand name, for instance, might prevent market penetration. The new firm's compensating marketing costs, as well as its average total costs may be too high, causing it difficulties in the competitive arena. It all may add to needed start-up capital. On the other hand, product differentiation may be viewed as a "....means of competition that serves the public, providing minimum assurances of quality, and catering to a real consumer desire for product improvement and variation"[12]. Thus, a market may be rendered more competitive, easier to enter, with product differentiation due to its affect on buyer attitudes. Dissatisfaction with prevailing suppliers will find ready outlet in alternative sources of a product or service. In other words, the more standardized are the products, the less incentive is there for buyers to seek alternatives, assuming legal entry barriers away.

Two other entry barriers may be worth mentioning in this brief prelude treatise to the main body of the book. *Excess capacity* has sometimes been viewed as a source of entry barrier, due to the large amount of specialized equipment already at the existing firms' disposal, representing considerable sunk costs. Discretionary lower prices may effectively discourage new competition. Another, related barrier entails *limit pricing* on the part of the incumbents. "Limit price" in this context may be defined as the maximum possible price that does not encourage or initiate entry, but still generates some monopoly profits. The potential entrant must consider the further price impact of its entry in the face of incumbents keeping output constant, and if the new firm attempts to offset the price depressing affects of increased output by reducing its offering, then it will need to cope with higher costs, due to the likely U-shape of its long-run average cost curve. The amount by which limit price can exceed minimum long-run average cost is determined by the cost disadvantage experienced by new firms, and by the extent that new entry depresses price[13].

A variant consideration involves the so called *Sylos Postulate* which attributes an expectation to potential entrants that incumbents will maintain output in the face of the entry threat. In that case, entry will nevertheless occur if the difference between the set limit price and the incumbent's long-run average total cost is greater than the cost advantage that existing firms enjoy over potential entrants[14].

Entry in the Light of the 1992 Merger Guidelines

In April 1992, the US Department of Justice and the Federal Trade Commission released their first joint Merger Guidelines, focusing on horizontal mergers. The document is meant to update the 1984 US Justice Department Merger Guidelines, and a statement issued by the Federal

Trade Commission in 1982 concerning horizontal mergers. At this juncture, we will take a quick look at the current guidelines in so far as they directly involve entry related issues[15].

A merger is not expected to have any significant impact on, or upon the exercise of, market power if the *threat* of committed entry into the relevant market is *real* enough to prevent profitable sustained price increases above pre-merger levels; in fact, such threat of entry may even prevent a merger from taking place. The threat of committed entry is real if it can be expected to be (a) timely, (b) likely, and (c) sufficient in magnitude, character and scope to deter or offset any significant anticompetitive impact of the merger. The threat of entry is real when it is easy, that is, where there are no significant barriers. The absence of barriers is indicated by passing the tests of timeliness, likelihood and sufficiency. When these tests are passed, no antitrust concern or even further analyses are called for. "Committed entry" in this context is defined as new competition requiring substantial sunk costs upon entry and exit.

In order to pass the test of *timeliness*, entry must significantly impact upon relevant market price within two years from the initial planning. Firms having had serious entry plans prior to the merger, will be included among the incumbents. Thus, entry, or adjustments to pre-existing entry plans, induced by the merger may be examined as possibly deterring and offsetting the merger's anticompetitive impact. In a durable goods market, if buyers anticipate entry, they can be expected to postpone purchases by expanding the life of goods already possessed, shifting the demand curve to the left in the face of possible negative supply shifts, thus countervailing, at least temporarily, any possible anticompetitive results from the merger. Under such conditions, even if entry is expected to occur beyond two years, the Government will consider entry "timely" provided its pro-competitive impact can be felt within the two year period, and beyond.

An entry is viewed *likely* if it generates reasonable profits for the entrant at pre-merger prices, and if such prices can be sustained by the entrant. Furthermore, entry is likely if the potential entrant can expect to procure upon entry a share of the market which is at least equal to the minimum viable scale (MVS), without depressing price below the pre-merger level. MVS is the minimum average annual sales level that the entrant needs to sustain for profitability at premerger price levels; thus, at MVS, long-run average cost equals to premerger price levels - not to be confused with minimum efficient scale, MES, that is, the output level generating the minimum long-run average cost, discussed earlier in the volume. MVS depends upon expected revenues at premerger prices (or at reliably projectible prices that would have prevailed if the merger did not materialize), and upon the various costs of entry, including some fair rate of return on invested capital should the venture and sunk costs cannot be recovered. MVS is expected to vary directly with the size of entry level fixed costs, with the proportion of entry level fixed costs represented by sunk costs, with marginal costs at low initial output levels, and with the length of time involved in the delay before market acceptance allows full plant utilization.

A new firm may succeed upon entry if it can benefit from the incumbent's monopolistic output reduction which may exceed five percent, if the price increase due to monopoly power is at least five percent. It will also benefit from sharing in any market expansion, especially if the existing firms are subject to capacity constraints and the new firm's products have relatively strong appeal. Vertical integration and forward contracting are additional opportunities through which potential entrants may ultimately benefit. These can work in reverse as well. Potential entrants may negatively be benefited from market declines, prior supplier commitments to incumbents, and preemptive sales increases by existing firms.

These factors also impact on the *sufficiency* of entry, which is important if the new firms are to have the desired competitive effects upon a more concentrated market that is likely to be caused by a merger.

References

1 *Ekco Products Co*. 65 FTC 1163, 1208, affirmed 347 F.2d 745 (7th Cir. 1965)]

2 *US v. Waste Management Inc*., 743 F2d 976 (2d Cir.1984). *US v. Calmar Inc*. 612 F.Supp. 1298 (D.N.J. 1985). *Echlin Manufacturing Co*. 105 FTC 410 (1985).

3 *Ball Memorial Hospital Inc. v. Mutual Hospital Ins* 785 F.2d 1325 (7th Cir 1986). *International Distribution Centers Inc. v. Walsh Trucking Co*. 812 F.2d 786 (2d Cir). cert denied 107 S.Ct. 3188 (1987)].

4 Joskow, P. and Klevorick, J. "A Framework for Analyzing Predatory Pricing Policy" *Yale Law Journal*, p.213-15, July 1979.

5 Bain J.S. *Barriers to New Competition*, Harvard University Press, Cambridge MA. 1956]

6 Bain, J.S. *Industrial Organization*, 2d ed. John Wiley & Sons, New York, NY 1968, p. 252]

7 Stigler, G.J. "Barriers to Entry, Economies of Scale and Firms Size" in Stigler, George J. *Organization of Industry*, Richard D. Irwin, Homewood IL. 1968, p.67]. Demsetz, H. "Barriers to Entry" *American Economic Review*, Vol. 72, March 1982, p.47. Also see Gilbert, R.J. "Mobility Barriers and the Value of Incumbency" in Schmalense R. and Willig, R. *Handbook of Industrial Organization*, Vol 1., pp.475-535, Schmalensee, R. "Ease of Entry: Has the Concept Been Applied too Readily" *Antitrust Law Journal*, Vol. 56, 1987 p.41. Salop, J. "Measuring Ease of Entry" *Antitrust Bulletin*, Vol 31, 1986, p.551. Salop and Simons "A Practical Guide to Merger Analysis", *Antitrust Bulletin*, Vol. 29, 1984, p.663. Ferguson, J.M. *Advertising and Competition: Theory, Measurement, Fact* Ballinger, Cambridge MA 1974, pp.10-12.

8 Mueller, D.C. "The Persistence of Profits Above the Norm", *Economica*, Vol. 44, November 1977, pp.369-80] .

9 Dewey, D. "Industrial Concentration and the Rate of Profit: Some Neglected Theory" *Journal of Law and Economics*, Vol. 19, April 1976, pp.67-78.

10 Comanor W.S. and Wilson T.A. "Advertising, Market Structure and Performance" in *Advertising and Market Power*, Harvard University Press, Cambridge MA 1974, Ch 4. See also, Palda, K.S. *The Measurement of Cumulative Advertising Effects*, Prentice Hall, Englewood Cliffs NJ 1964.

11 Telser, L. "Some Aspects of the Economics of Advertising", *Journal of Business*, April 1988, and Telser, L. "Advertising and Competition", *Journal of Political Economy*, December 1964.

12 Kahn A.E. "Standards for Antitrust Policy" *Harvard Law Review*, September 1953, p.36

13 Bain, J.S. "Pricing in Monopoly and Oligopoly" *American Economic Review*, Vol. 39, March 1949, pp.448-464. Gaskins, D.W. "Dynamic Limit Pricing: Optimal Pricing Under Threat of Entry" *Journal of Economic Theory*, Vol. 3, September 1971, pp.302-22, and Spence, M.A. "Entry, Capacity, Investment and Oligopoliy Pricing" *Bell Journal of Economics*, Vol. 8, Autumn 1977, pp.534-44.

14 Sylos-Labini, P. *Oligopoly and Technical Progress*, Harvard University Press, Cambridge MA 1969.

15 US Department of Justice, News Release, Thursday, April 2, 1992, *Justice Department and Federal Trade Commission Issue Horizontal Merger Guidlines*, pp. 47-54.

PART TWO

ANTITRUST MARKETS IN GENERAL:

AN OVERVIEW OF THE PRINCIPLES

Chapter 7
ANTITRUST PRINCIPLES AND PROCEDURES

The perfectly competitive market model provided economists with an ideal frame of theoretical analysis as to how markets should function with the utopian outcome of optimum social welfare by way of some perfect allocation of resources among all of their alternatives so that no further adjustments in the markets were possible without a net reduction in social welfare. In reality, a number of critical perfectly competitive assumptions cannot be satisfied so as to allow real-life markets to meet consumer needs. Furthermore, even if the assumptions were met, there is no assurance that all essential economic and social values would be secured. Thus, the dispute as to the extent to which market forces should be replaced by government policy, even if the latter is assumed to be flawless, will almost certainly be perennial.

Some Gaps in the Competitive Framework

Even if the crucial assumptions of a competitive market are met, some gaps and their social consequences remain. For instance, while perfect competition meets consumer tastes, those tastes are weighted by the *financial resources* of the consumers themselves, the latter depending upon the ownership of the amount and nature of resources. Final outputs are unequally distributed according to financial means, that is according to initial output distribution. The statusquo tends to perpetuate itself. Thus, a perfectly competitive model would have to be stratified for each level of initial resource distribution.

Consumers act according to their income, and, according to their *preferences*. Those preferences may not be perfect, or even rational. Perfectly competitive outcomes may thus be biased by prevailing consumer preferences. In that case, government polices may be called upon to "keep in line" those preferences according some sets of social value judgment. The consumption of some types of goods and services is simply discouraged by taxation and other legal rules, others are encouraged by subsidization, and by non-direct financial means such as education and information dissemination.

Some economic entities impose costs or benefits upon others. The recipients of such benefits do not have to pay for them, and nor do the generators of costs upon others. These costs and benefits are known as *externalities,* as the beneficiaries, or victims, perceive these from external sources. Thus, some producers discharge toxic materials or air into the environment, causing costs, expenses and negative utilities to others, without having directly to pay for them. The market simply ignores these factors, hence they do not directly enter into the rational calculations of the producers or of the consumers. Other goods and services can be obtained at an absolutely zero price by the additional user. These are called *public goods* and include items such as national defense, police services, general knowledge disseminated by science, or specific knowledge produced for tuition paying students by private colleges also made available to the public, and so forth. When an additional person acquires a unit or more of these, no other individual need be deprived of it. There are no explicit or implicit costs involved. Since no private firm could or would rationally produce these public goods at zero marginal costs that would secure a zero efficient price, governments normally assume the role of the supplier for public goods.

Another competition impeding problem, *economies of scale*, has already been discussed. The presence of economies of scale mandates that a product be supplied to the market by production units, or by a single production unit, in large enough quantity that will allow the producer to travel down low enough on its long-run average cost curve to benefit from the cost saving associated with large output. The presence of a large enough number of firms to allow effective, or perfect, competition will likely prevent each producer from attaining the necessary output level needed to generate these cost savings. Hence, government regulation may be called upon to secure entry only to a number of producers which is the minimum required to supply the market. Finally, the perfectly competitive set of assumptions run into problems in real life because of the *number of firms* is often small enough for effective collusion to take place, and, there is *imperfect knowledge* on the part of both the buyers and the sellers as to the nature of available goods and factor proportions, respectively. In addition, we already noted that *entry barriers* protect incumbents, and prevent desirable factor mobility, and, it as well as other factors, can cause producers to deviate from profit maximization as their primary goal, even in the unlikely event of consumers always making the most rational decision.

Competition May Not Always Be The Best Solution

Inventions need to be rewarded with exclusivity. *Patents* provide that protection for a period of time, usually for seventeen years. Thus, patents impose a legally sanctioned monopoly. In the case of *natural monopoly,* discussed earlier, competition is replaced by monopoly or oligopoly, depending upon the size of the market to be served, and that imperfectly competitive structure is protected by regulation presumably in the interest of the consumer. For social and financial reasons, some *states* control the distribution of liquor, insurance, and other socially sensitive operations. In some sectors of the economy, in the production of nuclear substances and devices, for instance, the *federal government* has exclusive rights of production and procurement.

Labor unions, *"organized labor"*, may be viewed as a direct aberration of the competitive process - that among the suppliers of labor, the members of various segments of the labor force. Yet, at least by designation, these organizations are viewed as protectors of their individual members' rights, and they deal with management, rather than their members individually.

Legislative Background

Antitrust statutes, and the subsequently emerged antitrust case (common) law embody two fundamental principles[1]. One, proscription of private competitive restraints is in very general and sweeping terms, without enumerating specific acts or situations of concern. Two, this very general language of the few statutes that constitute the foundation of the body of antitrust rules need to have been interpreted by the enforcing agencies and by the courts by way of thousands of prior cases over the years in order to generate those rules that appear to prevail in subsequent cases.

The language of the statutes was designed to be vague and general in order to avoid placing industry in a straight jacket of specificities, and to avoid encountering violations by firms that may not have been specifically listed hence could not be dealt with. The need to interpret the statutes also allowed considerable discretion to the enforcing agencies and the courts. The courts, in particular, were in the position to definitively interpret the rules in the statutes and essentially formulate mandates for further conducts. In fact, the courts appear to enjoy more independent discretionary power in the field of antitrust than in any other area of their endeavor.

The Statutes in a Nutshell

The *Sherman Act* of 1890 is the first congressional commandment embodying the competitive objective of the antitrust laws. In broadly phased terms, the Act prohibits unreasonable restraints upon and monopolization of trade. It delegates broad powers to the courts to interpret and apply proscriptions on a case-by-case basis, in civil and criminal actions brought by the enforcement agencies or private litigants.

More specifically, *Section 1* of the Sherman provides that ".. every contract, combination in the form of trust or otherwise, or conspiracy, in restraint of trade or commerce among the several states, or with foreign nations, is declared to be illegal.."[2]. On its face, the section seems to condemn contract, combination or conspiracy. In order for it to apply, some type of cooperative relationship between two or more persons must be present, and substantial enough to restraint interstate or international trade or commerce. *Section 2* focuses on "... every person who shall monopolize, or attempt to monopolize, or combine or conspire with any other person or persons to monopolize any part of the trade or commerce among the several States, or with foreign nations....."[3]. In essence, the section proscribes the intentional acquisition, or attempted acquisition, of market dictatorial powers in actual or potential restraint of competition by individual entities, or by a group of entities pursuant to conspiracy.

Both of these sections embody the fundamental principles of antitrust enforcement, namely, dealing with the issues in a comprehensive manner through rather vague language, and delegating the final interpretation and decision to the courts. This was summed up in a 1940 case as follows: "The prohibitions of the Sherman Act were not stated in terms of precision or of crystal clarity and the act itself does not define them. In consequence of the vagueness of its language... the courts have been left to give content to the statute"[4].

Two other major statutes, the Clayton (1914) and the Robinson-Patman (1936) Acts, along with the Federal Trade Commission Act (1914) constitute much of the antitrust statutory foundation beyond the Sherman Act. While the Sherman Act proscribes *de facto* restraints, ones that have already materialized, the others tend to focus on anticompetitive conduct that will likely result in substantial restraints, although also termed in very general language. In addition, some sections have been, for all intents and purposes, replaced by major amendments. Thus, *Section 2 of the Clayton Act* has been substantially amended by the *Robinson-Patman Act* to effectively proscribe price discrimination in restraint of trade. The practice of concern involves unjustifiably charging different prices to different competing customers for the same product, thus placing one or more customers in a market competitive advantage, or disadvantage, in relation to the others "....where the effect of such discrimination may be substantially to lessen competition or tend to create a monopoly in any line of commerce, or to injure, destroy, or prevent competition with any person who either grants or knowingly receives the benefit of such discrimination, or with customers of either of them.."[5]. Defense to the alleged conduct of discrimination, however, may be shown by the discriminator by way of correspondingly different applicable costs, downward competitive pressures on prices in the relevant markets, and in terms of other variables. Discriminatory conduct may take the form of outright price differences, or any other direct or indirectly impacting conduct (rebates, advertising allowance, and so forth) that yields substantially unequal financial results for the participants.

Section 3 of the Clayton Act essentially covers two major areas of contracting between seller and buyer: (a) exclusive dealings and total requirements, involving exhaustive supply arrangements thus precluding the seller's competitors from selling to the same buyer, and (b) tying arrangements whereby a seller with monopoly power in product A attempts to transfer that power to its market for product B, where it otherwise would not have a significant market power, by way of using product A as the "tying product", and product B as the "tied product" -

potential buyers of A are induced to also buy B, "... on the condition, agreement or understanding that the lessee or purchaser thereof shall not use or deal in the goods.... or other commodities of a competitor or competitors of the lessor or seller where the effect of such lease, sale, or contract for sale or such condition, agreement or understanding may be to substantially lessen competition or tend to create a monopoly in any line of commerce"[6].

Mergers are at the center of attention in *Section 7 of the Clayton Act*. Amended in 1950 by the Celler-Kefauver Act, the section proscribes the acquisition by a corporation of "the whole or any part of the stock or .. assets of another corporation engaged also in commerce where in any line of commerce in any section of the country the effect of such acquisition may be substantially to lessen competition, or tend to create a monopoly" [Clayton Act section 7]. While the original law of 1914 was restrictive to essentially horizontal mergers with local competitive impact only, hence left vertical and conglomerate merges uncovered, the post-1950 amended statute covers all types of merger activity among corporations with substantial and potential anticompetitive impacts in any business and in any region of country. A classic opinion that traces the evolution of merger statutes, as well as some of the fundamental issues and reasoning, rather thoroughly involves firms in the shoe manufacturing and retailing markets[7].

The Federal Trade Commission Act of 1914, substantially amended in 1938, 1973, and 1975, supplements the Sherman and Clayton Acts. In particular, Section 5 of the Act provides that "unfair methods of competition in or affecting commerce, and unfair or deceptive acts or practices in or affecting commerce, are declared unlawful"[8]. While by appearance, and substance, the Act overlaps with the Sherman and Clayton Acts, and gives the Commission power to proceed against conducts involved in those laws, it gives the Commission power to proceed beyond the realm of the fundamental antitrust statutes due to the inclusion of terms such as "unfair or deceptive acts or practices" whether or not they directly involve competitive acts "In a broad delegation of power it empowers the Commission, in the first instance, to determine whether a method of competition or the act or practice complained of is unfair. The Congress intentionally left the development of the term "unfair" to the Commission rather than attempting to define the many and variable unfair practices which prevail in commerce"[9].

The Rationale For Antitrust Enforcement

The Greek philosopher, Aristotle, enunciated the virtues of private property and the private incentives that emanate from it for the benefit of society as whole. Some two hundred years ago, Adam Smith expounded the virtues of the "invisible hand" of competition in the market place as the ultimate managerial force for corporations, instead of the discretionary powers of a single authority. Thus, the *economic rationale* for antitrust enforcement is the preservation of as much competitive power as possible within the constraints of the market place. "The Sherman Law and the judicial decisions interpreting it are based upon the assumption that the public interest is best protected from the evils of monopoly and price controls by the maintenance of competition"[10]. Those who venture their resources in creating an enterprise should be rewarded for their toils and be protected from competitive abuses in the market.

The preservation of a Jeffersonian society of many independent entities was evidently Congress' *political motive* for enacting the antitrust laws. In denouncing the concentration of economic wealth, Senator Sherman reminded Congress that if we in this country will not endure a king or an emperor, "we should not submit to an autocrat of trade"[11]. The Acts passed after 1890 were designed to check the power of large buying and selling organizations, to slow down increasing industrial concentration, and to arrest as early as possible practices that may result in anticompetitive restraints and monopoly. "Throughout the history of these statutes, it has been constantly assumed that one of their purposes was to perpetuate and preserve, for its own sake and in spite of possible costs, an organization of industry in small units which can effectively compete with each other"[12]. While size *per se* has not been viewed as contrary to society's interests, the abuse of size for competitive advantage has always been frowned upon.

Finally, the Federal Trade Commission Act was enacted in 1914 to ensure that *ethical* business entities were not abused by devious commercial practices. In 1938, the Act was amended to extent protection to consumers as well as competitors, by including deceptive and unfair commercial practices.

Enforcement Procedures

The antitrust statutes delegate considerable discretion to the enforcement authorities. It appears that Congress sought to provide various cumulative enforcement remedies to a number of enforcement options. The US Department of Justice was initially empowered to bring civil and criminal actions. Subsequently, the Federal Trade Commission became active in Clayton Act and FTC Act cases involving probable and unfair restraints. Thirdly, section 4 of the Clayton empowers private litigants to seek remedies under most of antitrust statutes, enhanced by the prospects of a treble damage recovery. The Justice Department may simultaneously, but not typically, bring civil and criminal actions. The FTC may pursue involuntary and voluntary proceedings. And, private litigants may seeks injunctive or compensatory relief, or both. The courts have recognized the wide discretion given to government agencies to initiate enforcement proceedings: "Just as the Sherman Act itself permits the attorney general to bring simultaneous civil and criminal suits against a defendant based on the same misconduct, so the Sherman Act and Federal Trade Commission Act provide the government with cumulative remedies against activity detrimental competition"[13].

The *Justice Department*'s Antitrust Division enforces the laws within its jurisdiction primarily as public prosecutor seeking to compel compliance in adversary proceedings. It basically functions as a litigating arm of the executive branch of the government by enforcing policies that reflect the current views of the administration in power. It acts upon an external information source or upon the results of an internal study. Its information discovery efforts may include fundamental industry research, FBI investigation, civil investigative demands, and, in criminal actions, formal grand jury proceedings. If subsequent action is taken, a criminal actions are designed to be penal, while civil actions aim at preventing future violations. Criminal proceedings may culminate in fines upon corporate and individual defendants for each violation, and may also result in incarceration for persons involved. Civil actions are basically proceedings in equity, are terminated in settlement by way of a consent decree that outline the defendant's mode of conduct for the future.

Proceedings by the *Federal Trade Commission* tend to be less formal and more administrative in nature. It typically acts upon complaint and by its own initiative pursuant to research. The results of its investigation are reported to the Commission itself which, in turn, may informally request compliance from the entities involved, or, may attempt to compel compliance by way of a quasi-judicial complaint, heard by an administrative judge. The judge's decision may be appealed to the Commission, whose decision in turn may be reviewed by the courts.

Private actions may be directed at treble damages, or at injunctive reliefs. Their potential financial impact upon a defendant may be more profound than those of the government, due to the automatic punitive damages included in the treble damage recovery. While private persons do not have explicit standing to sue under the antitrust laws, competitors, customers, licensees, suppliers and even minority shareholders have been procedurally accommodated. These actions tend to be particularly potent when they come in the wake of a ultimately successful US Department of Justice action previously contested by the defendant.

References

1   Seplaki, L., *Antitrust and the Economics of the Market*, Harcourt Brace Jovanovich, San Diego CA. 1982, pp. 2-13.

2   *Sherman Antitrust Act*, Section 1, 26 Stat. 209 (1890), as amended, 15 U.S.C.A. sec. 1 (Supp.1, 1975)

3   *Sherman Antitrust Act*, Sec.2, 26 Stat. 209 (1890), as amended, 15 U.S.C.A. sec. 2 (Supp.1, 1975)

4   *Apex Hosiery Company* v. Leader. 310 US 469, 489 (1940)

5   *Robinson-Patman Price Discrimination Act*, sec 1, 49 Stat 1526 (1936), 15 U.S.C.A. sec 13 (1970)].

6   *Clayton Act*, Sec. 3, 38 Stat 731 (1914), 15 U.S.C.A. sec 14 (1970)]

7   *Brown Shoe Co.* v US, 370 US 307 (1962)

8   *Federal Trade Commission Act*, Sec. 5, 38 Stat. 719 (1914), 15 U.S.C.A. sec 45 (Supp 1 1975)

9   *Atlantic Refining Co.* v. Federal Trade Commission, 381 US 357, 367 1965)]

10 *US v Trenton Potteries Co.* 273 US 392, 397 (1927)

11 *Congressional Record*, 21st Congress, 1st Session, 1890, p. 2,457

12 *US v Aluminum Co. of America*, 148 F.2d 416, 429 (2d cir.1945)

13 *FTC v. Cement Institute*, 333 US 683, 694 (1948)

Chapter 8
BASIC ISSUES OF THE MARKET IN ANTITRUST

W e noted earlier that our economic system is based largely upon economic management by competition in the market. To facilitate the efficacy of this general system of economic management, Congress passed a body of broadly worded rules, the antitrust statutes. The statutes themselves were reviewed earlier. In this chapter we will take a brief look at some important economic dimensions of most of the antitrust statutes, specifically the role of the market, its definitions, meaning, function, and consequent interpretations. While we will refer to some of the pertinent concepts again, the reader is reminded to relate back to Chapter Four where we briefly focused upon some market and monopoly power measurement tools.

Congress passed procompetitive antitrust laws on the assumption that a competition based economic system is most likely to enhance social welfare: consumers will have a choice from a wide range of goods and services at low prices, while producers can take advantage of a fair distribution of all business options. The spirit of antitrust legislation views the anticompetitive exercise of horizontal and vertical market power as obstacles to attaining these desired social goals. Some conduct, such as horizontal price fixing and market division, are considered evil enough that they are *per se* assumed to be an unreasonable impeachment of competition, and require no proof of relevant market, or market power. In other instances, market power and competitive restraints by way of abusing that market power must be proven, hence the market must be delineated. Thus, while very important, market definition in antitrust litigation is merely a means to the end, rather than the end in itself. To prove legal responsibility, the firm's market power over price, output, and the conduct of potential entrants needs to be shown. At least in theory, the *firm's conduct* itself could indicate the presence of market power by way of its predatory conduct, price discrimination, excessive profits or profit margins, or its supply and demand elasticities. However, the acquisition of adequate evidence for, and proof of, these conduct variables under actual market conditions, is very difficult[1], compelling the courts to proceed towards the identification and measurement of market power by way of first defining the relevant product and geographical markets.

Notably, none of the antitrust statutes in their language refer to the term "market". The term has evolved as the product of judicial and economic thinking in the course of the analyses, trial, and appeal of thousands of antitrust cases during the past century, in particular, during the past five decades. The need to clarify the notion of the market stems from at least three sources. First, even if we determine with certainty what "competition" means (see the brief treatise in Chapter one), only those products can be in competition with each other that are demanded or sold in the market. In other words, we cannot ascertain the presence of competition, unless we also ascertain the product or service arena of the competitive activity. The second need for the identity of the market emanates from a fundamental prerequisite under the antitrust laws: determination of the presence or absence of the market or monopoly power on the part of a firm or of a group of firms - the presence of that power predisposes the firm or firms for further scrutiny, while its absence essentially clears them of any illegal activity, in spite of some wrong doings. The third, and somewhat related, need for knowing the identity of the market emanates from the necessity to identify under the law injury to competition in the market by the conduct of firm(s). In general, a definition of the market may follow that of the *US Department of Justice, 1984 Merger Guidelines* which essentially depicts an economic market or industry as being a product or set of products, or a service or set of services, within some geographical area, where the price charged, quantity sold, or quality selected by any seller substantially influences the prices, quantities, or qualities of the products sold by other firms. The closeness of the market relationship between two or more firms directly varies with the impact of a firm's decisions upon the decisions of other firms if thought to be in the same market.

Market and Standard Industrial Classification

As discussed in Chapter One, occasional synonymity and confusion is read into the concepts of the "market" and "industry". If the members of a group of firms produce commodities or services that possess the required degree of substitutability, and they produce no other goods, then it is probably accurate to equate the concept of the market with that of industry, provided that the goods or services are interchangeable from the perspective of a given set of consumers, and the goods fall in the same price range. That these qualifications are necessary is clearly illustrated by the US Census Bureau's Standard Industrial Classification, or S.I.C., system and its application to market delineation efforts.

The SIC system has been generated by the US Department of Commerce, Bureau of Census to categorize firms and their plants according to the product they produce or the manufacturing methods they employ. In total, the SIC code may have seven digits, although usually the first four are used for purposes of industrial organization studies. Between the first and fourth digits, the degree of similarity between the firms' products of concern increases with each added digit. SIC codes have been used for antitrust empirical market delineation in the past[2], although they do not allow for the geographical dimensions of the market. Thus, SIC codes do not classify by region, only by product lines. Consequently, the only geographical boundary that the SIC system recognizes is the national one. For many antitrust issues, that would not suffice.

In addition to the Bureau of Census SIC system, the Federal Trade Commission, the Internal Revenue Service, and the International Trade Commission have their own product or business classification systems utilized for their own specific purposes. They closely resemble the SIC from which they were largely developed in the first place. The IRS systems produces business/firm classification based on tax related financial data. The ITC's product classification is utilized for its Tariff Schedules of the United States, designed for custom officers, rather than industrial studies by economists. The FTC database, the "line-of-business" classification (LOB), divides industrial production into 260 categories, at about the 4-digit detail level in the Commerce Department's SIC system, and has been considered useful by some prominent industrial organization economists[3], although the confidential designation of the data, and the limited time period of four years (1974-77) covered, precludes it from general utilization by the economics profession outside the FTC.

A typically utilized SIC code contains four digits, where the first digit indicates the crudest classification basis, with every digit added constituting a refinement. The foundation for the SIC system appears to contain two main elements: similar utilization patterns at the consumer level, and similar production technology at the producer level. Furthermore, while it was initially designed to classify products at the plant level, it has also been applied to firms, based on the firm's product that represents the largest proportion of its total output, even if the firm is a diversified one. The system is revised periodically to reflect changes in the economy. For most lines of business as well as for governmental and non-profit enterprises it provides a standard terminology and code number normally up to four digits. The first two digits indicate the major industry grouping. These major groupings are divided into nine categories: 01-09 for agriculture; 10-14 mining; 15-17 contract construction; 19-39 manufacturing; 40-49 transportation, communication, electric, gas, and sanitary services; 50-59 wholesale and retail trades; 60-67 finance, insurance, and real estate; 70-89 services; and 91-94 government. The application of the SIC code system may be illustrated by the example of sewing machine manufacturers. SIC code 36 designates electric machinery, equipment, and supplies. Code number 363 designates household electric appliances, and, extended by one more digit will take us to sewing machines with the code number 3635. Since some product lines cross several SIC code categories, individual designations may be somewhat arbitrary. For instance, some of the packaging industry falls into five SIC two digit categories: 26 - paper and allied products, 28 for chemical and allied products, 32 - stone, clay and glass, 33 - primary metal industries, and 34 - fabricated metal products.

The Market in Antitrust Statutes

The identity and size of the relevant market is more significant under some antitrust statutes than under others. Thus, the definition of the relevant market, and some firms' market share in that market to determine the extent of individual or joint monopoly power, in *Sherman 2* cases is normally viewed important, although the language of the statute refers only to "any part of the trade or commerce" without mentioning anything like the "relevant market". Hence, some debate among legal scholars as to the timing and extent of market definition in Sherman 2 cases may be noted. For instance, one view is that "... market definition becomes crucial only when there are no other discoverable facts establishing the existence and degree of market power more directly and with tolerable accuracy"[4].

Importance is attached to market delineation and the market share of the firms involved in, and of the newly emerged firm pursuant to, a merger in *Clayton 7* cases. The method of market definition in merger cases is normally viewed to be the same as in monopolization cases, although, once again, questions have been raised whether or not the rigor of analysis need to be at the higher level often applied for Sherman 2 cases. *Sherman 1* proscribes horizontal collusive conducts. In cases proving *per se* offenses (where no other remedial or mitigating circumstances are considered), no market definition is normally required. In cases which invoke the *rule of reason,* calling for further analysis of pertinent facts and circumstances in order to determine the reasonableness of the restraint, market power of the conspirators may play some role.

Under the *Robinson-Patman Act* 1(a), price discrimination by a firm with monopoly power may lessen competition in a market of its customers. In addition to the need to determine whether or not the discriminator has monopoly power in its own market, the extent of the competitive restraint needs to be estimated by delineating the market where the competitive impact may have occurred, or to determine if there was adequate competition in the first place.

Market delineation and market power measurements may not be as important in other situations. Thus, if under Clayton 3, an exclusive dealings contract involves a substantial amount of business, expressed as percentage of the total business in the area, the conduct may be found anti-social even if the seller has no competitors. On the other hand, if under the same Statute a tying contract is being tested, and particularly when the tying item is a service, instead of a "commodity" specified by the Clayton Act, the Government may use the Sherman Act to determine if the firm of concern has a monopoly power in the market for the unpatented tying item, and if so whether or not it abused, by transfer to the tied item's market, that power to the detriment of competition in that market where it presumably had no prior monopoly power. In those situations, market delineation, and market share measurements are essential. Patent protection in the tying product's market automatically assumes the existence of monopoly power. In cases involving price fixing by a group of firms, the conduct is illegal *per se* regardless of the market share held by the group, and whether or not they were in direct competition with each other prior to having entered into the conspiracy. The fact of conspiracy presupposes a violation of Sherman 1, with no further consideration of any other factors or circumstances by the court called for.

Delineating Criteria For Antitrust Product Markets

The statutes utilize a considerable number of terms pertaining to market delineations thus allowing substantial flexibility to dealing with various industries, product types, production processes, cost conditions, pricing methods, distribution systems, consumer and producer attitudes, potential competition, and other dimensions of market activity. Some of the standard criteria considered in pertinent market delineation efforts include product contents and performance, the amount and nature of consumer utilities derived from the product or service, absolute prices, price ratios, changes in the latter two, vertical integration, entry conditions, interindustry conduct, average cost comparisons, product derivation and technology, interchangeability measured by the cross-elasticity of demand, and geographical consideration.

In terms of *product contents and performance*, similar physical content of the product may be of relevance for market definition, although its application has not been consistent. In a well-known case, the court sought to define the market for cellophane by including all flexible wrapping materials with physical attributes somewhat different from those of cellophane. The market was defined in broad terms favoring the defendant[5]. Just a year later, another case appeared to ignore the product contents and performance of various types of paint in spite of obvious similarities among them, and exclusively included in the market only paint for automobiles, excluding all others, this time favoring the plaintiffs[6]. Thus, the relevance of the product content and performance criterion appears to have been reduced by some type of ultimate utility criterion. Nevertheless, in a major case involving the aluminum industry just after World War II, the question was whether the market should include secondary and scrap aluminum, in addition to virgin aluminum, ingots. The court's answer excluded the former two, leaving ALCOA with a power of over 90% to monopolize the aluminum reduction market, leading to divestitures and ALCOA's exclusion from government contracts for a period of time[7]. At about the same time linen rugs were excluded from other kinds of rugs[8], and precious metal watches from nonjeweled one[9].

The *ultimate utility criterion,* similar to product contents and performance in that it concerns itself with the way consumers use the product, received considerable application in industries such as advertising, news dissemination, and transportation. In one case, the questions addressed the inclusion of morning newspapers with evening ones into the same market[10], while another scrutinized the difference between industrial steel wool and household steel wool[11], and yet another looked at different fuel types based on their utilization by industry[12].

Either absolute or relative *price differences* may make a difference in a decision whether to include two goods into the same market. Thus, in one case the court found a small absolute, but at that time substantial relative, price difference of 5 cents between two brands of cigarettes large enough to place them in separate markets[13].

The extent and uniformity of *vertical integration* achieved by firms may be pertinent to the decision of placing them in the same market. In a relatively early case, the court had at least two alternatives available to it in which cans were produced or sold to canners. One pertinent variable could have been the volume of cans sold by can producers, the other would have included the latter plus the cans produced and sold by the canners who produced part of their own supply, thus reducing the markets share of the can producing defendant[14]. Another merger was considered harmless on the basis of vertical integration related issues[15]. A substantial part of the defense in another case, involving GTE's acquisition of Western Utilities where the concern was the foreclosure of GTE's competitors from selling to the acquired firm, rested on the vertically integrated relationship between Bell Systems and Western Electric[16].

We have explored the significance of entry barriers. Market delineation deliberations may include the consideration of *potential entrants*, in addition to incumbents. Factors to be considered in this context would need to include the nature and extent of the barriers, such as cost differences, and the presence of legal barriers. In fact, with relatively insignificant transportation costs, significant potential competition may emerge from a totally different geographical area.

Potential competition received relatively little attention, and was declined as a decisive factor, in two cases from the mid-1950s involving the FTC in one, and the US Department of Justice in the other[17]. A few years later, the amount of analysis devoted to this factor appears to have increased, but its consideration still has not been decisive[18]. Nevertheless, the perceived significance of potential entry within the context of relevant market delineations increased, and, still a few years later, this consideration has found its way into a market definition itself; the market is "...an area in which the parties to the merger or acquisition compete, and around which there exist economic barriers that significantly impede the entry of new competitors"[19]. The issue continued to gain respect. In fact, some attempts were made to differentiate between ease of entry on the one hand, and entry barriers on the other, in terms of their relevance to market definition. The market power of incumbents may already constitute an implicit entry barrier. If this is compounded by explicit barriers, then potential entry can be restricted to the extent of an undertaken merger substantially restraining competition. In[20] P & G's size and advertising capabilities were considered substantial enough entry barriers to disallow the merger.

Markets may be delineated in certain cases based upon significant differences in the *average cost* of production. If cost differences are large enough to potentially allow the low cost firms to drastically underprice their products to the extent that they will not be in the same price range with the rest, the large price differences will more than offset whatever degree of substitutability may be present among the goods, hence may place them in a different market within consumer perception. Thus, close substitutes may not be in the same product market if there are drastic price differences. "... substitutes should be disregarded, even if indistinguishable in character, use or consumer preference, whenever their cost of production substantially exceeds that of the product allegedly monopolized"[21]. Cost differences may come about as a result of production destination. Thus, a tire manufacturer produces and sell tires to automobile manufacturers and, indirectly via wholesalers and jobbers, to the retail market. Depending on the relative volumes and specifications, these two groups of tires could be produced at substantially different costs, sold at substantially different prices, and designated to different markets. Based upon these factors, they could be viewed as being in different markets[22]. This approach was quite different from one that segregated markets on the basis of *product derivation*, or production technique, although the application of the latter appears to have lacked consistency. In one case, gasolines produced by different methods were held in the same market[23], while another one viewed corn starch to be in a separate market from other starches[24], and a later one considered parchment paper to be in a market separate from all other papers serving the function[25].

A frequently relied upon criterion for market delineation has been the *cross-elasticity of demand* and consumer perceived *substitutability* among the goods. The many opinions that relied upon this criterion also used terms of the same meaning like "reasonable interchangeability", or, "fungability". The notion of elasticity is a general one. When applied to economics, it normally denotes a relationship of responsiveness between changes in some independent variable and the resulting changes in a designated dependent variable. The simple concept of the (point or arc) elasticity of demand with respect to price pervades micro texts, and measures consumer responsiveness in terms of percentage changes in quantity demanded for a specific commodity to percentage changes in the price of that *same* commodity. The cross-elasticity of demand is a close cousin in that it also measures consumer responsiveness in terms of quantity to a change in price, but it does so by involving not only one but two commodities. Thus, it measures the relationship between a percentage change in the price of one commodity, and the resulting percentage change in consumer demand for the other commodity. The size and sign of the cross-elasticity coefficient (the ratio of a percentage change in the demand for one commodity to the percentage change in the price of another) indicate the magnitude and nature, respectively, of the relationship between the two commodities. The degree of substitutability between two commodities is thought to vary directly with the size of a *positive* coefficient (negative coefficients indicate a relationship of complementarity). In general, and theoretically, if this positive coefficient is high enough - historically without specific quantitative thresholds, between two commodities, they belong in the same product market. As implied, the problem is to set a specific level of coefficient, or even a range of coefficients, that may be considered as cutoff point for market delineation. Unfortunately, the cases have not been determinate in this regard. In fact, until the 1950s, no more than lip service was paid by the courts to substitutability or cross-elasticity. Subsequently, they became recognized as an essential ingredient in the process of antitrust market delineation. The court's interest was indicated by "...a relevant market cannot meaningfully encompass an infinite range. The circle must be drawn narrowly to exclude any other product to which, within a reasonable variation in price, only a limited number of buyers will turn; in technical terms, products whose cross-elasticities of demand are small..."[10]. Or, "... the market is composed of products that have reasonable interchangeability for the purpose for which they are produced ... it seems to us that DuPont should not be found to monopolize cellophane when that product has competition and interchangeability with other wrappings..."[5].

It appears from the cases that the courts have been fairly ready, at least since the 1950s, to accept substitutability from the consumer's perspective as a criterion for market definition. *Substitutability from the producers' perspective* ("supply substitutability") was a less noted criterion. Supply substitutability entails speedy and inexpensive changes within the output portfolio of a firm, thus being readily able to adjust to the needs of a specific market, particularly to those of a new market. An important prerequisite for its relevance to the assessment of antitrust markets is the absence of significant entry barriers. With a high degree supply substitution, a market must be viewed not only in terms of the existing firms, but also those with the capability of entering should price, demand, and cost conditions economically warrant it. Conditions can be accommodating by the very phenomenon which concerns public policy enforcers, namely the abuse of power by a firm already existing in the market. If that power is abused by a "traditional" way of increasing price and reducing output, consumers will turn to new supply alternatives (demand factor) which, if available (supply factor), could reduce the existing firm's ability to take advantage of its market power; in essence, the market can be viewed as having been expanded by the ability of outside firms to replace part or all of their existing output with goods that will accommodate the monopolist's migrating customers. Thus, this is basically a notion of entry, enhanced by the assumption that the potential entrant can move with facility because of inexpensive and rapid retooling or output substitution. The supply substitution criterion for market assessments views a firm not yet in the relevant market not in terms of its specific existing portfolio of goods (or services), but rather in terms of its readily and inexpensively (or at least profitably) attainable scope of output potentials, hence its ability to enter into new markets.

In some cases [e.g. DuPont, 1957; and Brown Shoe], in addition to the relevant market, the definition of which having been predicated upon reasonable product interchangeability measured by the cross-elasticity of demand [as in DuPont, 1956], a subset of products, with special characteristics and uses, have been identified and viewed as being capable of having their own competitive environment, and a subject of antitrust concern.

Geographical Dimension
of the Relevant Market

In addition to the product dimension criteria, the territorial issues of the relevant competitive process need also be ascertained: the *geographical dimension* of the relevant market. When delineating the geographical dimensions of a carefully defined *product* market, we attempt to identify a protected area which includes a sufficient number of sellers which in unison have enough monopoly power to substantially raise price and hold the new price level for a while without attracting resource entry from the outside, or expansion by existing firms from within, that would restore prices to their earlier level. Its significance has been noted in a large number of decisions. Thus, a geographical market separates one region from another in terms of competition among product providers. The relevant area may be a small community, county, or the entire country - and, for some products, such as crude oil production, the globe. There are a number of variables considered when delineating the geographical dimensions of an antitrust market. Transportation costs, in whatever ratio they are absorbed between the seller and the buyer, in the light of prevailing prices, production costs and market conditions, often play an important role. In general, given product prices and production costs, there tends to be a negative relationship between freight-cost and the geographical extent of the market. Product perishability, local regulations, and customer buying patterns may also play an important role.

In general, the main determinants of a geographic market are price relationships and empirical sales patterns, probably in that order. "When prices and price movements in two territories are closely correlated, a single market definition is strongly indicated.... with a high correlation of the amount and direction of price changes [being] ordinarily enough ... in most cases they will be quite sufficient, particularly where one has data for an extended period of time"[4]. While theoretically plausible, practical implementations of this type of analysis is fraught with potential problems. It may be difficult to identify the best single price in each region for the analysis; same applies to the transport cost item. Furthermore, regions may have different freight absorption policies, making objective price correlations dubious. Even if the "best" price and freight cost item in each region can be identified, firm competitive policies may make them difficult to procure in a reliable form, or at all.

In addition, price level and pattern comparisons assume that prices and transportation costs move only as a result of competitive forces. However, similar and highly correlated price levels and movements may also be due to price discrimination practiced by a monopolist in different geographic markets with similar demand elasticities; or, dissimilar prices and price movements could also be found in the same geographic market, but in different market segments with different demand elasticities, due to, once again, to monopolistic third-degree price discrimination. Last, but just as significantly, two completely different geographic markets could display similar price patterns by way of a high correlation due simply to a common reaction to changes in some external factors, regulatory forces - especially in health care markets, or to independent changes in demand and supply in otherwise completely different markets.

The courts' view of geographical market dimensions seems to have varied over the years from very broad to rather restricted markets. In some cases, the geographical dimensions of the market turned out to be decisive in the final outcome of the case. Thus, in a relatively recent case, the geographical market for banking services was seen as not extending beyond a four county area surrounding[26]. Another case allowed for various alternative market areas, the State of Wisconsin, the tri-state area of Wisconsin, Illinois and Michigan, and the entire country, only to find a violation of Clayton 7 in each of these areas[27].

References

1   Jorde, R. "The Seventh Amendment Right to Jury Trial of Antitrust Issues",
     California Law Review, Vol. 69, July 1981, p.36. See also Pitofsky, R.
     "The Political Content of Antitrust", *University of Pennsylvania Law
     Review*, Volume 127, Fall 1977, p.1076, and, Sullivan L.A. "Economics
     and More Humanistic Disciplines: What are the Sources of Wisdom for
     Antitrust" *University of Pennsylvania Law Review*, Vol. 125, Spring 1977,
     p. 1214. And, Landes, W. and Posner, R. "Market Power in Antitrust Cases",
     Harvard Law Review, Fall 1982, p. 937.
2   Weiss, L.W. "The Concentration-Profit Relationship and Antitrust" in
     Goldschmid, Harvey J. et. al. *Industrial Concentration: The New Learning*,
     Little Brown, Boston 1974.
3   Schmalensee, R. "Do Markets Differ Much?" *American Economic Review*,
     June 1985, pp. 341-51].
4   Areeda, P. and Donald F. Turner, *Antitrust Law*, Little Brown & Company,
     1978, pp.355-58
5   *US v E.I. DuPont* de Nemours & Co. 351 US 377 (1956), p.404
6   *US v E.I. DuPont* de Nemours & Co. 353 US 586 (1957)
7   *US v. Aluminum Company of America*, 148 F.2nd 416, 425, and 91
     F.Supp.333 (SDNY 1950)
8   *US v. Klearfax Linen Looms Inc* 63 F.Supp. 92 (D.C. Min. 1945)
9   *Hamilton Watch Co. v. Benrus* 114 F.Supp.307, 314 (D.C. Conn.1953),
     aff'd 206 F.2d 738 (1953)
10   *Times-Picayune Publishing Co. v. US* 345 US 584 (1953), p. 612.
11   *Brillo Manufacturing*, in the Matter of, Doc 6557 (1963)
12   *US v Reading Co.* 253 US 26 (1920)
13   *American Tobacco et al* v. US 328 US 781 (1946)
14   *US v. American Can Co.*, 234 F.1019 (1916)
15   *US v. Columbia Steel* et al. 334 US 495 (1948)
16   *US v GT&E* Civ. No. 64-1912 (SDNY 1964)
17   *Crown Zellerbach Corp*, In the Matter of doc 6189 (1957). And US v.
     Bethlehem Steel Corp, 1968 F. Supp. 576 (1958)
18   *Brown Shoe Co* v US 370 US 294 (1962)
19   *US v Pabst Brewing Co.* 384 US 546, 556 (1966)
20   *FTC v. Proctor and Gamble*, 386 US 568 (1967). Potential competition by
     way of entry issues were also prominent in US v. Continental Can 378 US
     441 (1964), and US v Penn-Olin Chemical Co. 378 US 158 (1964), aff'd
     389 US 308 (1967)
21   *US v Corn Product Refining Co.* 234 F. 964 (SDNY 1916)
22   *Champion Spark Plug Co*, In the Matter of, 50 FTC 30 (1953)
23   *Standard Oil of Indiana v. US* 283 US 163 (1931)
24   *US v. Corn Product Refining* 249 US 621 (1919)
25   *Story Parchment Co. v. Paterson Parchment Paper Co.* 228 US 555 (1931).

26   *US v. Philadelphia National Bank* 374 US 321 (1963)
27   *US v. Pabst Brewing Co.* 233 F.Supp. 475 (1964), 384 US 546 (1966), 296 F.Supp. 994 (1969)

Chapter 9
MARKET POWER
CONDUCT RESTRAINTS

The previous chapter has systematically, though briefly, outlined the basic issues related to the definition of markets in antitrust enforcement. This chapter will take a brief look at various measurement issues in horizontal and monopolistic conduct restraint cases. Once the relevant market has been delineated, market or monopoly power exists which may actually have been, or potentially could be, abused to the detriment of competition, hence, presumably, social welfare. Thus, the fundamental concept of "market power" is essential. As indicated earlier, market power may be defined simply as the possessing firm's ability to *profitably* reduce output and raise price above the competitive level, that is, "...without losing so many sales so rapidly that the price increase is unprofitable and must be rescinded"[1] The terms "market power", "monopoly power" and some times "economic power", are often used as alternatives in the economic literature.

Unless we are in the theoretical sphere of perfect competition, firms, all firms, have some market power. Thus, the antitrust issue centers not on the mere existence of market power, but on the extent, and actual as well as potential competitive impact of it. In antitrust cases, this power has been measured and utilized by first delineating the relevant market in its product and geographic dimensions. Then, the defendant's market share is computed. Finally, an opinion is generated, presumably based on past cases, as to whether or not the monopoly power, suggested by the calculated market share, is substantial enough that, if unconstrained, and abused, it did have, could have, or there is a dangerous probability that it will have, a significant anticompetitive impact. Chapter Four looked at some of the economic theories pertaining to the measurement of market.

Cartels

A classic formalized horizontal market conspiracy with respect to price, and demand and supply allocations, is a *cartel,* designed to eliminate competition in terms of its target variables. In order for a cartel to succeed, some structural and behavioral conditions need to be met. First, its likely success, and cost of administration, varies inversely with the number of members. Secondly, the existence price increase accommodating market conditions, such as low demand elasticties are also conducive to cartel success. Thirdly, member loyalty to the cartel by way of abstaining from cheating is fundamental, and can be monitored much easier with fewer cartel members. In this connection, additional cartel problems may arise if new firms enter the industry but do not join the cartel. Furthermore, while the cartel's main goal is to coordinate pricing, production, supply, and allocate demand and other market activities in order to reap monopoly-like profits, the administrative and transaction costs of running a cartel are likely to be much higher than operating a single firm monopoly, with consequently lower profit margins.

The structural and behavioral conditions for a cartel's success are often not met. An ideal cartel could function effectively for prolonged periods of time if its members (a) controlled 100% of the market, (b) were approximately the same size, (c) would possess similar cost conditions, hence efficiency, and, (d) their products were either identical or very similar. If the members controlled a 100% of the market, the cartel could raise price by reducing output as would a single firm monopolist. Uniformity in costs, efficiency and products would facilitate the setting of an acceptable price, and similarity in size would allow for easier market demand allocation. The most likely problem, cheating, would be reduced as the number of cartel members gets smaller, and theoretically eliminated if individual firm prices would be communicated by way of secret bidding, with only the final results announced[2]. Given real market circumstances, much of the above is economic utopia, and most cartels do not succeed.

Disloyalty by way of cheating in cartels can take various forms. One possibility is price discrimination. Thus, secret rebates have been one way to get around an otherwise agreed upon cartel price. Another way was to concentrate on the production of goods that for some reasons or another were left out of the cartel agreement; for instance, merchandise with some blemishes, labeled as "seconds", priced lower than regular items, but still sold at a profit, hence intentionally produced, and favored by customers because of a relatively lower price, in larger quantities than regular goods included in the cartel agreement[3].

Attempts at cartels have, nevertheless, been frequent and persistent. They were supported by certain arguments in favor of such arrangements. The more notable of these procartel arguments included the opponents of "ruinous" cut-throat competition in capital intensive industries with proportionately much higher fixed costs and corresponding production capacity. In such situations, the firms have a very strong incentive to compete for incremental business by price reductions which still generated income higher than variable costs that could be applied to already existing fixed costs. However, if prices are lowered to a level where no contributions to fixed costs can be made, a gradual erosion of production capacity will result. Cartelization has been seen as a primary way to prevent this predicament.

Price fixing may also be thought of as preserving market statusquo for all firms, inefficient or not, hence retaining employment opportunities for the pertinent segment of the labor force. A macroeconomic argument, amounting to the reduction of unemployment by formal or informal price fixing cartels. The validity of the argument obviously depends on the components of the trade-offs between these macro benefits, and the already belabored costs of competition avoidance. In addition, the macro argument for price fixing is sometime augmented by the consideration of the additional funds generated by price fixing that can be made available to research and development, that price fixing facilitates long-term planning and reduces some market uncertainties, and that the additional income secured by price fixing will possibly insure the production of a higher quality output. In all of these instances, once again, we are faced with substantial trade-offs between the social costs of the cartel and the economic benefits that may accrue to the direct participants.

Trade Associations

A form of horizontal constraints that have been under scrutiny by a number of cases in industry and medicine was by way of *trade association* and society practices. At this juncture, I will quickly review the issues pertaining to industry. A trade association, in general, is a member supported entity designated to collect, process, and disseminate economic, industry and firm specific information for the benefit of its members. Trade associations may promote cooperative research, joint market surveys and market research, advertising and publicity, and joint publication of trade journals. Conducts used as an instrument of competitive restraint included certain types of statistical dissemination, price reporting systems, standardization practices, and cost accounting manuals. Useful industry-wide statistical dissemination include production levels, capacity and excess capacity data, market conditions, and inventory levels so as to advise members whether to alter prices or change production levels in the face of stock accumulation or shortage. Past, current, and projected price information has at times also been disseminated, asserting that such information contributed to competition rather than restraining it. However, those as well as standardized cost-accounting methods could lead to uniform pricing, or, at the least, the elimination of unimpeded price competition.

Joint Ventures

There may be agreements among competitors not inherently anticompetitive, monopolistic, or harmful to customers. By way of some agreements, a group of firms can carry on an activity at a more efficient scale, reduce transaction costs and free rider problems. *Joint ventures* could achieve these benefits without necessary economic harm. A joint venture is an agreement among a number of firms to conduct certain activity which they may or may not undertake by themselves. Some joint ventures could be made up of competitors, while others of completely non-competing firms. Price fixing and output restriction are possible motives for competing firms to enter into this type of agreement. However, because of the *per se* antitrust rule application to such conduct and the severe penalty, the achievement of certain economies is a more likely reason. In fact, the most frequent justification for joint ventures appears to be its enabling participating firms to achieve a minimum optimal production scale, hence produce at a much lower long-run average cost than if they functioned on their own. Economies in marketing may be a reason for joint ventures; while individual firm output may not be large enough to warrant a full-time sales agent in a territory, the combined output of joint venture participants could.

Joint ventures in research and development endeavors have been generally condoned. While uneconomical, and financially even prohibitive to individual firms, some research projects can be undertaken jointly. In addition to the pulling of resources necessary to finance the research project, free rider problems also tend to be solved, since firms participating in the project not only benefit from it, but also share in their cost[4]. Similar point can be made regarding joint ventures in advertising, normally undertaken by producers' association, instead of individual producers of, say, potatoes or beef.

A competition restraining consequence of joint ventures may occur by way of the exchange of price information among firms who would otherwise be competitors. The fundamental economics of this phenomemon is easy to envisage. The nature and volume of price information available to suppliers and consumers differs in each market. Yet, in essence, the degree and nature of price competition itself is based upon the nature and extent of the availability of price information to all participants of trade. One extreme in this context may assume that the seller knows only his cost, the buyer knows only his reservation price (the maximum price that he would be willing to pay), but that neither the buyer nor the seller knows the prevailing market price - the market is the least efficient, and the transaction is resolved, the price found, by way of negotiation. The other extreme would have many buyers and sellers, all being fully aware of current prices, with price negotiations absent. The buyers and sellers are fully aware of their trading options, and those not willing to receive or pay the market price will simply stay out of the market. In real life, there does not appear to be a gradual transition from imperfection to perfection in the markets. Thus, the degree of efficiency and practiced competition in a market does not directly, and even less likely proportionately, vary with the amount of available price information. On the contrary, the availability, and exchange, of price information among competitors can facilitate collusion. This latter consideration may be of concern with some joint ventures.

Concerted Refusal to Deal

A horizontal conduct restraint that does indicate the need for some type of market delineation, and market share measurements, is *boycott, or concerted refusal to deal*. This conduct entails a group of participants at one level of the production process (manufacturing, wholesaling, or retailing) who attempt to foreclose their competition by coercing, usually spanning two levels of the process, their trading partners not to deal with the indicated competition. Thus, the conduct may involve a group of garment manufacturers, functioning under an association name, coercing retailers into not carrying garments manufactured by their competitors by a threat of supply termination. If the participants have a substantial share of the particular line of garments involved, hence are in the position to place a substantial weight behind their threat, they can successfully implement the boycott, and foreclose their competitors from selling to the retailers involved (a conduct, *per se* illegal under Sherman 1). The same conduct may be directed against potential competitors that may emerge from a different production process. Thus, for instance, manufacturers intending to enter a new (wholesale) market at another stage of the same production process and become competitors to their existing wholesale customers may be boycotted by a group of the existing wholesale customers into abandoning the idea of this vertical expansion, thus protecting themselves from the potential competition of their presently manufacturing, but potentially vertically integrating, suppliers[5].

The significance of market delineation and market power studies in cases of this type rests with showing that the coercing group, the boycotters, have sufficient market power in their line of business to successfully implement the boycott, and thereby force the objects of the boycott to yield to their wishes. Otherwise, it can be assumed that the objects of the boycott may act on their own volition, for if they did not wish to abide by the boycotters' wishes, they could simply turn to alternative supplies of the products involved. We will review at greater detail refusal to deal activities in healthcare later.

The Oligopoly Dilemma

In an overt horizontal conspiracy, the firms display their conduct explicitly, and the court draws its conclusion from that conduct. Explicit *per se* rule applied conspiracies have been concluded from business conduct involving overt price fixing agreements. Toilet bowl manufacturers argued that the prices resulting from the conspiracy were reasonable, only to face the court's response "The reasonable price fixed today may through economic and business changes become the unreasonable price of tomorrow"[6]. An agreement among a number of midwestern oil producers, with some 80% control of the market, to implement a marketing program designed to put a floor under already depressed prices for oil by way of mopping up surplus oil from the market yielded a classic and subsequently often applied definition of price fixing from the court: "Any combination which tampers with price structures is engaged in an unlawful activity. Even though the members of the price fixing group were in no position to control the market, to the extent that they raised, lowered, or stabilized prices they would be directly interfering with the free play of market forces ..... Under the Sherman Act a combination formed for the purpose and with the effect of raising, depressing, fixing pegging, or stabilizing the price of a commodity in interstate or foreign commerce is illegal *per se*"[7].

The issues relating to monopolization, that is, the abuse of excessive market power, allow the analyst to deal with determinate situations. One firm's market share, and its conduct in view of that market share, is examined. Solutions regarding the firm's profit maximization or other behavior are determinate, and other than inter-industry demand shifts, entry, and potential rival expansion activity, the analysis fairly readily, if not automatically, yields a determinate result.

The analysis of oligopolistic competitive behavior is fraught with complexities. The perennially difficult questions deal with possible market power jointly, but tacitly and subtly, exercised by firms without discernible conspiracy in US manufacturing industries pervaded by oligopolistic markets. Is monopoly shared? Thus, it is a major element of concern in connection with horizontal conduct restraints. As indicated in Chapter Three, an industry may be considered oligopolistic when any one of a few firms possess a large enough share of the market to have a material impact on the market price. While the classical oligopoly is viewed as containing a few (typically two) large firms only, modern oligopolies may be populated by a few (from three to eight, or even more) large firms, along with many smaller ones with discernible market impact. Since each of the large firms possess substantial market influence, they have a profound influence on each other. They are *interdependent*. The final outcome of action on the part any one firm cannot be predicted without making assumptions regarding the rival reaction. Furthermore, the firms are aware of this interdependence, and must take these rival reactions into the consideration of their own actions. The number of firms with market influence, and their combined market share, for oligopoly to exist have not been clearly demarked in the economic literature. The range may include the classic duopolistic situation with two firms possessing 100% market share, transiting through the more modern oligopoly of four firms controlling 100% of the market, and further moving through the scope with several large firms controlling a predominant (say, 95%-95%) market share, with a few noninfluencial ones around, to some theoretical limit number of firms (say, nine or ten), still sensitive to each other's actions and reactions, controlling the market among themselves, with a host (possibly hundreds) of smaller ones operating on the fringes. Thus, given these possible ranges, oligopolies can be classified, based on traditional structural factors, into a variety of concentration degrees. Oligopoly Type I, where the largest 8 firms control at least 50% of the market, and the largest 20 firms at least 75%, and Type II where the largest 8 control about 33% with the largest 20 some 75%.[8]. Other structural factors that substantially contribute to oligopolistic rival interdependence include demand elasticities, and similarity among the rivals' cost functions as direct determinants, and the degree of product differentiation as an inverse determinant.

Public policy is ultimately concerned with the performance of these markets in view of society's interests. Performance, in turn, has been causally related to the structure and conduct of the markets. The inherently consistent competitive model accommodates the analyst with a readily discernible relationship among structure, resulting conduct, and reasonably predictable performance. Monopoly is also relatively easy to deal with. While a monopolist may not always take full advantage of his structural uniqueness by maximizing profits, if he does not, for instance, due to potential entry pressures, his conduct and the resulting performance, can be reasonably predicted. In oligopoly, public policy is not accorded the same analytical comforts. In fact, as we indicated earlier in the volume, there is some disagreement among economists as to what determines oligopolistic structure in the first place. Some (in the "Chicago School") believe in the importance of production scale economies, and in the need to be large to benefits from them by way of attaining, or at least approximating as closely as possible, the minimum efficient scale. Under this hypothesis, firms existing in the market will strive to produce a large enough level of output to minimize cost along their long-run average cost curve, and price at high enough level maximize profits. All this goes on in the shadow of firms lurking around the outside perimeters of the market ready to enter at the first sign of potential profitability for them, imposing pricing, cost and profit constraints on the incumbents. This analysis is obscured by the fact that economies of large scale production normally refers to plant operations rather than to the entire firm, and, minimum efficient *plant* operation may occur at much lower levels of output than it would for the entire firm. Consequently, the measurement of firm output as an indicators of the presence or absence of scale economies would, given the market size, likely yield higher long-run average costs. Or, putting it differently, looking at firm, instead of plant, output, the notion of minimum efficient scale can be highly exaggerated. Studies have shown that while individual dominant *firm* market shares in automobile and cigarette manufacturing have been substantial, in the vicinity of 55% and 30%, respectively, the most efficient plants need not have exceeded 5% of the total market [9]. Thus, firms much larger than what the most efficient scale would dictate have survived over the years. In fact, hundreds of small firms, much smaller than what the most efficient scale of operation would dictate, have also survived. Economies of scale, therefore, cannot be the only answer. There must be other entry barriers to oligopolistic industries, which protect small, as well as the large, companies from additional competition. The upshot of this theoretical predicament for policy makers is that oligopolistic concentration may be reduced, or its increase may be arrested, without impinging upon production efficiencies. How that impacts upon oligopolistic performance is another question.

Performance is largely a function of conduct. Thus, we need to at least glance at the impact of structure on oligopolistic conduct, an issue of considerable complexity. An important conduct variable is the setting product prices. When acting in that capacity, the oligopolist must cast a weary eye on its rivals' reactions. Back to interdependence. The interaction becomes complex, and indeterminate, when we attempt to ascertain some sort of *individual* oligopolistic price conduct that will lead to the profit maximization of each firm. The profit maximizing price of any one of the oligopolists would compromise the profit maximizing efforts of its rivals, particularly if we assume that each oligopolist would match its rivals' prices. When we add the assumption that they are aware of this interdependence, the ultimate solution, by way of *individual* actions, on the part of the oligopolist becomes rather perplexing. Thus, the natural solution to think of is to maximize profits as a result of a joint effort. The object, at least theoretically, is to maximize profits for the group[10]. In fact, there are a number of classic theoretical studies convinced of this type of oligopolistic joint profit maximizing price behavior[11]. The rationale is simple. If entry barriers are protective enough, intra-market price competition is self-defeating, both in terms of profits and market shares. Mutually beneficial intra-market competition must take non-price forms, such as advertising and product differentiation. The price at which each firm of the group will sell needs to be set at the profit maximizing level. The concern for the enforcers of public policy is the manner of actions, and interactions, whereby the joint profit maximizing price is determined.

Price leadership, whereby firms voluntarily and without coercion, and in their self-professed and declared economic interests, follow the price actions of a traditionally recognized price leader, has been considered by the courts as socially acceptable[12]. Other, much more tacit, conduct was found to be objectionable under the label of "*conscious parallelism*". Thus, a group of motion picture distributors, with a substantial share of the Texas and New Mexico markets, were denied the opportunity, by joint action, to impose specific prices on their exhibitors[13], and a dominant group of tobacco product manufacturers were found essentially, although tacitly, to have functioned within a cartel in terms of their price actions when attempting to cope with low priced entrants[14]. In another case, the court stated, "Here all that was done was a request by each defendant from its competitor for information as to the most recent price charged or quoted, whenever it needed such information and whenever it was not available from another source. Each defendant on receiving that request usually furnished the data with the expectation that he would be furnished reciprocal information when he wanted it. That concerted action is of course sufficient to establish the combination or conspiracy, the initial ingredient of a violation of Section 1 of the Sherman Act"[15].

The assessment of oligopolistic performance is not an easy task. A problem rests with discrepancies between the economic notions of costs and profits, and those for the same performance dimensions recorded by the accountants. Yet, the only formal source of data available to the economist for assessing individual firm performance are the firms' accounting records. Attempts at "reconstructing" those records in order to generate data easier to reconcile with the basic concepts of economic theory are fraught with all sorts of interpretive and consistency problems[16]. Even if measurable in a manner consistent with economic theory, the causes of profit need to be ascertained. While some literature attributes higher profits to higher levels of concentration, the relationship is rarely perfect, and the number of caveats and qualifications overwhelm the desire to feel comfortable about these relationships[17]. Instead of a direct and simple relationship between the levels of concentration and profit, other factors, such as firm size, advertising, and research and development activity could have an equally strongly impact.

Notwithstanding data and fundamental relationship measurement issues, some oligopolistic performance problems have become more or less clear. The underlying problem appears to be related to oligopolistic price rigidities. In most models of oligopoly, the firms' reluctance to compete in terms of price yields an artificial rigidity in market price, rendering it nonresponsive, or responsive with considerable delays, to changes in market conditions and costs. Instead of price, competitive dimensions, such as advertising, style changes, customer relations, and so forth, that often generate economic waste assume greater importance[18].

Monopolistic Conduct and Monopoly Power

In a general sense, the Sherman Act concerns itself with two sets of broad issues, trade restraint and monopoly. Traditionally, monopoly indicated a firm having to cope with no product substitutes, the notion of "pure monopoly". Indeed, most of the cases concentrating on monopoly issues do concentrate on one firm as the culprit. These have been noted as *single firm monopolies*. As we noted in the previous section, monopolistic power and control over the market need not be attributed to a single firm. A group of oligopolists may tacitly act together and exercise their joint power over the market: the notion of *shared monopoly*. Monopoly issues lend themselves to three general categories of investigation. The market, once again, needs to be delineated, and market shares calculated. Secondly, given the market share of the firm, its size needs to be assessed in view of potential competitive abuses; the presence of monopoly power is scrutinized. Thirdly, having identified the firm with monopoly power, past and present conduct needs to be sorted out to ascertain whether they are consistent with social interests.

An issue central to Sherman 2 is that of *monopoly power*. Its presence or absence has been viewed in terms of the market share of the firm, with a threshold of around 66%, based on the 1945 ALCOA decision. Thus, monopoly power does not necessarily mean monopoly. It simply indicates the presence of a large enough market power which, if abused, has, or could have, or will, result in competitive restraints. The competition restraining abuse of monopoly power indicates *monopolization*. Thus, monopolization is the relationship between monopoly power and the conduct of the firm possessing that power. As indicated earlier, monopoly power can be assessed not only in terms of numerical market shares, but can also, at least, be indicated if not proven, in terms of the conduct of the firms involved, by way of pricing, profit levels, and importantly in terms the presence or absence potential entrants. We have already dealt with the role of entry as a competitive factor extensively.

An issue that is closely related to, although not necessarily inherent in, monopolization relates to *attempts to monopolize*. Its meaning and application has often been plagued with confusion. The cases normally associate attempts to monopolize with the presence of a "dangerous probability" for the existence or emergence of monopolization, or with an indication of the intent to monopolize. ".... the employment of methods, means and practices which would, if successful, accomplish monopolization, and which, though falling short, nevertheless approach so close as to create a dangerous probability of it..."[19]. Thus, the anticompetitive results of the attempt to monopolize are both intended, with intent inferred from conduct such as predatory pricing, and probable[20].

Predatory Pricing

A conduct of monopolization, *predatory pricing*, has attracted considerable attention among economists and legal scholars. Its interpretation, and policy application, have been controversial, and were plagued with confusion. Traditionally, this conduct has been viewed simply as an attempt by a firm with monopoly power to lower price below cost, finance the losses with its resources attributable to its monopoly power, and, after having successfully driven its competitors out of the market, raise price back to the monopolistic profit maximizing level. A source of confusion has been the difference between predatory pricing, on the one hand, and aggressive price competition, on the other. Issues that arose related to profit margins pertinent before, during, and after predation, and applicable cost measurements. The length of time during which the price level is to be artificially depressed for predation is also of essence[21]. It may be that predatory pricing may occur even if a firm does not drop its price below average cost, but only low enough to generate a profit margin nontraditional or unacceptable by industry standards. The same intent can be inferred from this type of conduct, particularly if, after the departure of competitors, price is raised back up to its previous level, as from the classic predatory gesture of pricing under costs. Incidentally, predation can also occur in terms of non-price related conduct, such as excessive advertising that cannot be matched by smaller rivals, accompanied by issues of confusion similar to those indicated by pricing predation.

Predation costs money. In fact, the predator may view his efforts as an investment that is expected to yield future returns. The predator sacrifices a certain amount of current revenues in exchange for an expected much larger amount after the competitors are driven out (assuming no additional costs incurred by successful, and even unsuccessful, legal challenges). Thus, in order for predation to be profitable, the predator must have a greater amount of financial ammunition than his competitors at whom the predation is aimed, and the predation must be followed by a recapture of losses, plus the necessary additional income that warranted the effort in the first place. Meeting the first condition is needed for the predator to avoid financial suicide. The second condition must be assessed in terms of expected return on the effort, and in the light of the possibility that the predator, even after having successfully driven out its competitors, the subsequently attained monopolistic price level will attract new ones into the market depriving the predator of much of the return on his efforts. Hence, in the long-run, predation may only increase the velocity of firm turnover in a market, instead of the monopoly power of the predator.

Cases in Monopoly

Market definition and market power measurements are essential, often decisive, in monopolization cases. If the firm under scrutiny does not have monopoly power, as generally as that may be defined, it cannot, by definition, monopolize the market. Some of the major cases, a few already mentioned, rather clearly illustrate how the courts have dealt with this issue in the past. In the ALCOA case[22], emphasizing market power over conduct, the court looked at three alternative levels of market power, and after discarding 33% as showing a lack of power, and regarding 66% as being on the borderline, accepted a 90% alternative as a clear indication of the presence of monopoly power. Another case *a priori* precluded the absence of market power on DuPont's part simply by delineating the pond so large that the biggest fish had to be, relatively, very small in it "... we conclude that cellophanes interchangeability with the other materials mentioned suffices to make it as part of this flexible packaging material market"[23], hence possess no monopoly power.

In a subsequent landmark case, an approximately 80% market share was viewed as evidence of sheer monopoly power, and, by way of paying careful attention to *conduct accompanying power*, market power abuse was seen by the court largely through an elaborate entry barring leasing system through which the defendant marketed it products[24].

Vertical Conduct

Vertical restraining conduct involves firms operating at different stages of the production process. We have already defined a production *process* as the sum of all production *stages* through which a product must proceed from the most initial raw material stage to the final retail stage at the consumer level. Each production stage constitutes a separate *market* for antitrust purposes. Thus, a part of the final consumer product may be traced back from the retail outlets to the wholesaler, jobbers, rolled steel ingot, unrolled steel ingot, and to the mining of the coke and iron. A *vertically integrated* firm operates at more than one production stage. Firms that are not vertically integrated transact with each other, incurring the possibility that those transactions may result in trade restraints.

An issue of significance within the context of these transactions centers on the extent that firms in the upper market stage of the production process can control the conduct of firms in connection with product distribution in the lower market stages. A manufacturer has the option of owning and operating its own distribution system, for a considerable amount explicit and opportunity cost. In order to avoid these costs, and to concentrate on functions at which he is probably much more efficient, namely production, the nonvertically integrated manufacturer delegates the distribution functions to other firms. The delegation of distribution functions can take a variety of forms in terms of the degree to which the manufacturer relinquishes title to his product after transferring them to the distributor. In most instances, the first stage distributor is given title thus eliminating the manufacturer's need to bill on broader spectrum or to incur the expenses of maintaining its own inventory. Giving up title is accompanied by giving up certain elements of control over the distribution process.

In generic terms, vertical competitive restraints may occur when the manufacturer or upper stage distributor dictates, and by coercion enforces, or attempts to enforce, some terms within the lower distribution process. These terms may include pricing, or nonprice constraints such as attempting to prescribe customer groups, or constraining the lower distributor's inventory portfolio of competing product. In addition, vertical restraints can include such nonprice constraints as tying agreements, exclusive dealings, and total requirements contracts.

Vertical Price Restraints

Vertical price control by manufacturers, or *resale price maintenance*, has been around in illegal, legal, and once again, since 1976 illegal, form for the past half century. It entails a higher stage operator, a manufacturer, setting the price of its product at lower stages of the production process, after passing title, and normally attempting to enforce those prices by various types of sanction. Normally, for retail price maintenance to be effective, the products involved need to be clearly distinguishable and highly advertised, and nonperishable, except for consumer durables whose price is often altered by trade-ins. The manufacturer's incentive for maintaining resale price is to minimize price depressing competition at the retail level, maintaining the image of the product, sustain dealer support by securing a minimum profit for the dealer, and avoiding the product being used as a loss-leader (closely related to product image preservation).

For dealer benefits, resale price maintenance eliminates dealer level price competition, maintains a price level for the product higher than it would be without retail price maintenance[25], and increases dealer profit margin. A negative by-product may emerge by way of increased entry and substitute availability, causing higher access capacity of production and correspondingly higher costs, thus ultimately reducing profits.

A brief review of the judicial history of resale price maintenance provides an interesting picture. Early cases condemned resale price maintenance as basically efforts to fix price[26]. Political lobbying, the emergence of the fair trade movement, and even the support of the judiciary[27] sparked considerable interest in legalizing resale price maintenance (or, as it was called, "fair trading"). California passed the first fair trade statute in 1931. The California example, and a 1936 Supreme Court decision[28] caused a proliferation of permissive atmosphere for retail price maintenance through the country. In 1937, Congress passed the *Miller-Tydings Amendment* to Sherman 1 by removing vertical price contracts from the realm of price-fixing, provided the States where the transactions occurred also sanctioned them, and, provided that the goods were in open competition with substitutes. In order to include into a vertical price contract all retailers of a product in a state, whether or not they signed a contract with the manufacturer, not just the retailer that did sign, in 1952 Congress passed the *McGuire Act* as an Amendment to Section 5 of the Federal Trade Commission Act. Finally, 1976 saw the repeal of both federal statutes, rendering resale price maintenance to be exactly what it is: illegal horizontal price fixing imposed from above[29].

Nonprice Vertical Restraints

This type of conduct is normally enforced by commodity based contractual agreements. Their most common form entails tying contract, and exclusive dealing contracts. A *tying contract* incorporates a tying product, normally one in which the seller already has substantial monopoly power, and a tied product. The sale of the former is conditioned upon the buyer also purchasing the latter in some quantity. The contract is the result of already existing monopoly power in the tying product, and is not designed to create it. What it does attempt to create is an increased market power for the seller in the tied product. In fact, the contract extends the market power from the tying product to the tied product. The price effect of tying contracts is that the price of the tying good is lowered while that of the tied good is raised. This may be the result of the monopolist's inability to increase his monopoly power by maintaining or raising the price of the tying good along with coercing the buyer into purchasing the tied product as well. This becomes particularly evident in monopolistic price discrimination by way of tying agreements[30]. While price discrimination may be practiced in terms of the tying product, the contract generates price differentials for the tied combination of both goods. Thus, the monopolist lowers the price of the tying product below the profit maximizing monopolist's level, and raises it for the tied product above the competitive level. In this manner, the revenue extracted from the buyer, the buyer's expense, will vary directly with the intensity of the buyer's need for the tied product.

While the pattern of tying contracts reflected by much of case history suggests that the contracts were undertaken to extend monopoly power from the tying good market to the market for the tied product, these agreements may be motivated by a number of other factors as well. For instance, a seller may argue technical reasons for tying two products together, particularly in the case of complex mechanical devices and their service, components and parts. Finally, in markets where the two products are complements, and if the production of both products require major capital investment, tying contracts may also act as entry barriers, since a potential entrant will need to possess the capital to produce both goods. In any case, the contracts may not only act as instruments of monopoly revenue maximizing price discrimination, but will inevitably result in the foreclosure of the seller's competitors in the tied product market. The delineation of the market for the tying product, the proof of monopoly power of the seller in the tying product in view of his lack of same power in the tied product is likely to indicate the motive for the transaction.

Contracts requiring the buyer to deal only with the seller in terms of the contracted product, *exclusive dealing contracts*, restrain competition by way of foreclosing the seller's competitors from selling to the seller's customer to the extent of the volume, or market proportion, of the trade involved in the contract. The transaction's anticompetitive impact focuses on the existence of the contract, and on the proportion of the total market involved, for voluntary actions of exclusive deals on the part of either the buyer or the seller are not viewed as antisocial. At any rate, exclusive dealing contracts also have trade advantages for the parties involved. The seller has a secure market, allowing him to budget accordingly, cushioning the impact of trade fluctuations, and possibly reducing marketing and shipping costs. The buyer gains from a secured and scheduled supply source at a contracted price, reduced inventory costs, and predictable input costs.

There is a large number of landmark cases involving tying contracts. Many of them have been decided under the *per se* rule of illegality under Sherman 1. A relatively recent case involved the issue of market delineation and market power measurement in medical markets[31] and will be dealt with later in the book. Some earlier classic cases, however, well documented the significance of market considerations. As early 1936, IBM was found to have extended its monopoly power in computer hardware to the market for punch cards (instruments of data input used extensively at that time) relying on safety and performance factors[32]. A few years later, an attempt to transfer monopoly power from patents on salt dispensing machines to the dispensed salt pellets themselves, by requiring lessees of the machines to also acquire the unpatented pellets from the machine's lessor, was considered illegal *per se* under the Sherman Act[33].

Cases on *exclusive dealing contracts* also considered the market and market shares involved. In a case involving a contract between an electricity generating utility and a coal supplying company, the court rejected the notion of illegality under the antitrust laws simply because while the absolute amount of business involved in the contract was relatively large, the percentage of the total market the contracted amount represented was small[34].

References

1   Landes, W. M. and Posner, R. A. "Market Power in Antitrust Cases", *Harvard Law Review*, Vol. 94, 1981, p.937.
2   Hay, J. R. and Kelley. W.B. "An Empirical Survey of Price Fixing Conspiracies", *Journal of Law and Economics*, Vol. 17, 1974, p.13
3   McGee J., "Ocean Freight Rate Conferences and the American Merchant Marine", *University of Chicago Law Review*, Vol. 27. 1960, p. 191. See also *Standard Oil Co. v. US* 221 US 1 (1911), pp.32-33, and *US v Trenton Potteries Co.* 273 US 392, (1927) p. 405.
4   Kitch, E. "The Law and Economics of Rights in Valuable Information" *Journal of Legal Studies*, Vol. 9, 1980, p.683. Also see Antitrust Guide Concerning Research Joint Ventures, No. 992, *Antitrust and Trade Regulation Reporter*. Vol. 1, December 4, 1980.
5   *Fashion Originators Guild of America v. FTC*, 312 US 457 (1941), was a classic case in point.
6   *Trenton Potteries v US* 273 US 392 (1927)
7   *US v. Socony-Vacuum Oil Co.,Inc* 310 US 150 (1940)
8   Keysen C. and Turner, D. *Antitrust Policy*, Harvard University Press, Cambridge MA. 1959, Ch. 2
9   Dorfman, R. *The Price System*, McGraw Hill, New York, 1964, p.97
10 Asch, P. *Industrial Organization and Antitrust Policy*, Revised Edition, John Wiley & Sons, 1983, pp. 60-66
11 Stigler, George "A Theory of Oligopoly", *Journal of Poltical Economy*, Vol. 72, 1964, p. 44. Stigler, George "The Kinky Oligopoly Demand Curve and Rigid Prices" *Journal of Political Economy*, Vol. 55, 1947, p. 432. Markham, Jesse "The Nature and Significance of Price Leadership" *American Economic Review*, Vol. 41, 1951, p. 891. Fellner, William *Competition Among Few*, Alfred A. Knopf, New York, 1949, chapters 1 and 7. Phillips, Almarin, *Market Strcuture, Organization and Performance*, Harvard University Press, Cambridge MA. 1962, chapters 2 and 3. Baumol, William *Business Behavior, Value and Growth*, MacMillan, New York, 1959
12 *US v. United States Steel Corp*, 251 US 471 (1920), and US v. International Harvester 274 US 693 (1927)
13 *Interstate Circuit Inc. v US* 306 US 208 (1939)
14 *American Tobacco Co. v US*. 328 US 781 (1946)15 *US v. Container Corporation of America* 393 US 333 (1969)
16 Bain, Joseph "The Profit Rate as a Measure of Monopoly Power", *Quarterly Journal of Economics*, Vol. 55, 1941, p.271
17 Brozen, Yale "Significance of Profit Data for Antitrust Policy", and Peltzman, Sam "Profit Data and Public Policy", both in Weston and Peltzman (eds), *Public Policy Toward Mergers*, Cambridge University Press, Boston, MA. 1968

18   Scherer, Frederick, M. and Ross, David, *Industrial Market Structure and Economic Performance*, Third Edition, Houghton Mifflin Company, Boston, 1990, Chapters 6 and 10
19   *American Tobacco v. US*, 66S.Ct. 1125, (1946), p. 1127
20   Turner, Donald, F. "Antitrust Policy and the Cellophane Case", *Harvard Law Review*, Volume 70, 1956, p. 281
21   McGee, John S. "Predatory Price Cutting: The Standard Oil of New Jersey Case", *Journal of Law and Economics*, Vol. 1, 1958, p.137. Telser, Lester C. "Cutthroat Competition and the Long Purse", *Journal of Law and Economics*, Vol. 9, 1966, p. 259. Areeda, Phillip and Turner, Donald F. "Predatory Pricing and Related Practices Under Section 2 of the Sherman Act" *Harvard Law Review*, Vol 88, 1975, p.697. Scherer, Frederick, M. "Predatory Pricing and the Sherman Act: A Comment", *Harvard Law Review*, Vol. 89, 1976, p. 868. Areeda, Phillip and Turner, Donald, F. "Schere on Predatory Pricing: A Reply", *Harvard Law Review*, Volume 89 1976, p. 868
22   *US v Aluminum Co. of America*, 148 F.2d 416 (1945)
23   *US v. E.I. DuPont De Nemours & Co.* 351 US 377, (1956) p.389
24   *US v. United Shoe Machinery*, 110 F.Supp. 295 (D.Mass 1953), aff'd 347 US 521 (1954)
25   *Council of Economic Advisers*, Annual Report, 1969, p.108
26   *Dr. Miles Medical Co. v. John D. Park & Sons*, 220 US 373 (1911) ,
27   Brandeis, Louis, Justice "Cutthroat Prices: The Competition that Kills", *Harpers Weekly*, November 25, 1913
28   *Old Dearborn Distributing Company v. Seagram Distillers Corp* 299 US 183 (1936)
29   Seplaki, L., *Antitrust and the Economics of the Market*, Harcourt Brace Jovanovich, San Diego, CA. 1983, Part IV, Chapter 1. Frankel, M. "The Effects of Fair Trade: Fact and Friction in the Statistical Findings", *Journal of Business*, July 1955, and, Telser, Lester "Why Should Manufacturers Want Free Trade?", *Journal of Law and Economics*, Vol. 3, 1966, p.86.
30   Ferguson, John M., "Tying Arrangements and Reciprocity: An Economic Analysis", *Law and Contemporary Problems*, Vol. 30 1965, p. 552. Burrus, B.R. "Tying Arrangements and Reciprocity: A Lawyers Comment on Professor Ferguson's Analysis" *Law and Contemporary Problems*, Vol. 30 1965, p. 581. Bowman, William S. "Tying Arrangements and the Leverage Problems", *Yale Law Journal*, Vol 67, 1957, p. 19. Turner, Donald F. "The Validity of Tying Agreements Under the Antitrust Laws", *Harvard Law Review*, Vol. 72, 1958, p.50. Singer, Eugene "Market Power and Tying Arrangements", *Antitrust Bulletin*, Vol. 8, 1963, p.653. Burstein, M.L. "The Economics of Tie-in Sales", *Review of Economics and Statistics*, Vol. 42, 1960, p.60. Adams, Walter J. and Yellen, J.L. "Commodity Bundling and the Burden of Monopoly", *Quarterly Journal of Economics*, Vol. 90, 1976, p.475. Porter, Michael, E. *Interbrand Choice, Strategy and Bilateral Market Power*, Cambridge, Ma. 1976, ch 6.

31 *Jefferson Parish Hospital District No. 2 v. Hyde* 466 US 1 (1984)

32 *IBM v. US* 298 US 131 (1936)

33 *International Salt v. US*, 332 US 392 (1947). See also *Northern Pacific Railway Co.* v. US, 356 US 1 (1958), and US v. *Jerrold Electronics* 187 F. Supp 545 (1960), and United States Steel Corp v. *Fortner Enterprises*, Inc 429 US 610 (1977).

34 *Tampa Electric v. Nashville Coal*, 365 US 320 (1961). See also Standard Oil Co. of California v US 337 US 293 (1949).

Chapter 10
MARKET POWER
IN MERGERS

In Chapter 5, we reviewed the principles of mergers and some of the more general motives that often lead to them. In this Chapter, we take another look at the issues from the point of view of market power. We are also going examine in some more detail the 1992 Merger Guidelines.

A merger involves control acquisition in one entity by another. The form of the merger was essential prior to the 1950 amendment to the Clayton Act. In its original enactment, Clayton 7 applied to stock purchases, but not to assets acquisitions. Hence, stock acquisitions were examined under Clayton 7, while asset acquisitions, particularly if the newly emerged firm came upon substantial monopoly power, were scrutinized under Sherman 1 and 2 [see e.g. US v. Columbia Steel Co, 334 US 495 (1948)]. A 1980 amendment extended the reach of Clayton 7 beyond corporations to all "persons" whether or not incorporated.

Horizontal Mergers

If the parties to the merger transaction come from the same product and geographic markets, we have a *horizontal merger*. This type of merger will have at least two necessary consequences: (a) the number of firms in the market will reduced by at least one, and (b) the new merger produced firm will have a larger market share than either one of the premerger parties to the transaction. The reduction of the number of firms in the relevant markets in turn may facilitate collusion, or other types of oligopolistic behavior. Thus, a concern for merger policy has been merger generated reductions in market output and increases in consumer prices. Thus, in the transition from lower to higher concentration by way of mergers in a market, the issue of oligopolistic behavior due to increasing collusion becomes of concern much earlier than that of monopolization related issues. Merger policy, particularly as promulgated by a series of merger guidelines, were designed to avert both the collusion and monopolization problems.

Mergers are not treated by the courts under the *per se* rule. Instead, the *rule of reason* normally applied. The reason is that, under some circumstances and assumptions, some mergers may be deemed to be beneficial to society. The most common reason for allowing a merger rests with the expectation of post-merger higher production and distribution efficiencies by way of allowing the merging firms together to reach the *minimum optimal scale* of their operation faster than they would by internal expansion. In addition, expansion by merger allows the firms to acquire additional productive assets with greater facility, and also mitigates the social costs that would be incurred if firms not acquired would file for bankruptcy [the reader is reminded of Chapters 2 and 6, where economies of scale are reviewed]. In addition to scale economies, merger generated larger size may also increase efficiency by facilitating vertical integration. Thus, large retailers may secure their own supplies, and large distributors or manufacturers can invade lower distribution channels with much greater facility. Nevertheless, the degree to which horizontal mergers can increase efficiency depends on the industry involved. In some cases, such as retail grocery chains, horizontal mergers may substantially increase consumer welfare. Other situations, such as small restaurants, may remain more efficient on their own[1] At any rate, it would probably be impossible to clearly classify all mergers into undisputed groups on the basis of whether they are socially desirable or not. There would likely be overlaps with many horizontal mergers generating both efficiencies and socially undesirable oligopoly and monopoly effects. So, the priorities are not always clear. Market power and collusion consequences of a merger may be weighed as considerations more important that those relating to efficiencies, or, vice versa. Or, ironically, mergers may be suspect because they may create efficiencies, thus jeopardizing the welfare of the post merger firm's competitors[2].

The cases have not followed a consistent path. In the early 1960s, a horizontal merger between competing retailers of shoes was considered unacceptable because of the danger that the post merger more efficient (and also much larger) firm would put smaller existing firms into competitive jeopardy[3]. A few years later, a merger involved the third and the sixth largest grocery chains in the Los Angeles area, with a combined market share of the merging firms in the vicinity of 7%. The largest firm in the market, not involved in the merger, had a share of 8%. Nevertheless, the court noted a *trend* toward concentration in the market with the chains acquiring individual entrepreneurs, and disallowed the merger[4]. Finally, a case where geographic and product market power turned out to be decisive factors involved the merger between two commercial banks in Philadelphia where a decline in the number of commercial banking units has been observed for many years prior to the merger in question, to the point where by the time of the merger (around 1960) the seven largest banks in the area controlled some 90% of the commercial banking business. Having defined the relevant product market as community consumer banking, the relevant geographic market as the Philadelphia area, and having noted that the merging firms were already the second and third largest in the Philadelphia area market, with the resulting merged firm becoming the largest and its market share exceeding 35% of the market, the merger was disallowed.

Vertical Mergers

A vertical merger transaction acquires the performance of functions, or of resources, from a different market that could otherwise be separately purchased in that market. As we indicated earlier, it is a merger that crosses market lines by way of reaching from one stage of a production process to another stage of the same production process. In essence, a vertical merger could also be considered as a type of conglomerate merger, as the latter is also defined in terms of the involvement of different markets. The vertical merger can be consummated either by outright acquisition, by entry *de novo* into the new market, or by long-term lease arrangement with terms yielding the same benefits to the parties as if they had merged. The first is a concern for Clayton 7, the second could be relevant to Sherman 2 if the new entrant has substantial monopoly power, and the third may of concern to Sherman 1 if restraint of trade (e.g. resale price maintenance) is involved in the contract. Economic terminology also uses "backward" or "upstream" integration if the direction of the transaction is toward early stages of the production process, and "forward" or "downstream" integration with the acquisition occurring in the direction of the consumer stage of the process.

The main concern of public policy in connection with vertical mergers is the *foreclosure effect* on competition. The acquisition of large retailer by an equally large distributor, both with dominant monopoly power in their respective markets, is likely to have the most profound effects: competitors of the acquiring distributor will have no, or only limited, access to sell to the major retailer. In other words, a major portion, or all of competition by way of selling opportunities to the acquired retailer is likely to be foreclosed in the acquiring firm's market. Thus, extent of the foreclosure depends on the market shares, monopoly power, of the firms within their own market. However, it has also been pointed out that vertical integration may actually yield benefits to society, if the transaction lowers production costs and facilitates intermarket transactions[5].

The first vertical merger case, after the 1950 Celler-Kefauver amendment to Clayton 7, involved the issue of duPont's possible policy control at GM by way of the acquisition of a large block of GM stocks. It was held that the block of shares gave duPont an unfair competitive advantage within GM's decision processes as to which paint and synthetic materials to acquire and use for cars[6]. The key factors included the definition of the relevant market in terms of these items, paint and synthetic materials, as they apply to cars only, instead of the broad spectrum of paints and synthetic materials, as it could have easily been. Furthermore, GM's market share in automobile manufacturing at that time being over 50%, the court saw a major foreclosure of duPont's competitors who could have also supplied the same materials to GM. The Brown Shoe case also had vertical dimensions in that the parties to the merger were in both the manufacturing and retailing markets for shoes. The following quote illustrates the court's bi-dimensional concern for the pros and cons of the transaction: "... a significant aspect of this merger is that it creates a large national chain which is integrated with a manufacturing operation. The retail outlets of integrated companies, by eliminating wholesalers and by increasing the volume of purchases from the manufacturing division of the enterprise, can market their own brands at prices below those of competing independent retailers. Of course, some of the results of large integrated or chain operators are beneficial to consumers. Their expansion is not rendered unlawful by the mere fact that small independent stores may be adversely affected. It is competition, not competitors, which the (Clayton) Act protects. But we cannot fail to recognize Congress' desire to promote competition through the protection of viable, small, locally owned business[3].

Economists have gone through stages of transformation in their thinking regarding the social pros and cons of vertical integration. Until about twenty years ago, the dominant view regarding the impact of mergers was negative. They were considered unnecessary for attaining available efficiencies because these efficiencies could be obtained contractually or by internal growth; plus, they foreclosed rival competition, as we noted before. Rivalry in each market, or production stage, was considered essential for providing competitive alternatives to the buyers[7]. In addition, the economic gain possibly sustained by the integrated firm through reducing risks due to economic fluctuations by owning its supplier is offset, from society's point of view, but the increased risk to the foreclosed competitors. At the present time, the preponderance of opinions appears to view vertical integration as a source of production efficiency, and transaction cost savings[5]. Indeed, after the mid-1960, little judicial activity took place against vertical mergers. In a case involving the trucking industry and accessory manufacturing, the country's largest truck and trailer manufacturer, with a 25% market share, acquired a major manufacturer of truck components, the third largest supplier of heavy duty wheels, accounting for 15% of that market, where the top four firms accounted for over 65% of sales, and the top eight for about 95% of sales. The truck manufacturer absorbed about 6% of the heavy duty wheel production. The FTC disapproved of the merger, however, the Court of Appeals reversed. Notwithstanding high market concentration, and prevailing entry barriers, the court considered the foreclosed market small, and finding alternative customers by the foreclosed firms relatively easy[8].

Conglomerate Mergers

We have covered a few basic aspects of conglomerate mergers already. Here, we intend to take a quick look at how some of the opinions treated these acquisitions in terms of their market power dimensions. A conglomerate merger does not fit into horizontal or vertical category. "Pure" conglomerate mergers, that is, acquisitions involving totally unrelated markets, would be those that most people would think of as being typically the conglomeration of primary social concern. Yet, most of the court opinions appear to apply to mergers where the pre-merger parties were in the same market in terms of products but were separated geographically (market extension conglomeration), or were within proximity of each other geographically, but were selling related, if not the same, product (market extension conglomeration).

While there is some question as to whether or not Congress intended the 1950 Amendment to the Clayton Act to reach conglomeration[9], there is little doubt that the common law of cases ensuing the Amendment did. In this connection, competitive injuries were found in general not because of the size *per se* of the firms involved but because of some market relationship between the merging firms, or between the newly emerged firm and its customers and competitors. Furthermore, the remedial considerations of efficiency emanating from horizontal mergers are not as likely to apply to conglomerate mergers as, we noted, they might to horizontal mergers. This is because possibly increased efficiencies between merging firms would normally come about if they produce products with the same or similar production processes, if their products are close substitutes for each other, or if, prior to the merger, they were in vertical relationship with each other - normally entailed by horizontal and vertical merger situations.

Conglomerate mergers may also yield efficiencies. *Product extension* diversification can generate advertising and distribution economies since the involved products are complements and can be advertised as well as distributed together. If one of the parties to the conglomeration has, via persistent and large scale advertising, attained considerable name recognition, that advantage can be passed on to the new product acquired through conglomeration. Since through *market extension* conglomeration two firms produce the same product, although in different regions of the country, they can after the merger coordinate buying and marketing activities with greater economies that individual firms could. In addition, whether market or product extension, a conglomerate merger creates a larger and diversified company. Considerable scale economies may be attained in terms of research and development, and the fruits of R&D may be utilized in the various markets in which the firms affiliates function. The larger firm may have the resources to acquire in-house services of professionals (economists, lawyers, etc) who need to be hired in the open market at prevailing market prices by the smaller firms.

Opportunities and economies attained by way of capital procurement enjoyed by conglomerates are perhaps the most vivid indication of conglomeration generated power. A small or even medium sized individual firm almost always needs to procure its capital from the market, at the prevailing rates. In the procurement process, whether through equities or debentures, it must incur considerable transaction and even nonpecuniary costs through the application and the related mandated information disclosure processes. In addition, the rate of interest it must pay also may reflect its relatively limited pool of resources. On the other hand, large conglomerates, operating in various markets, with substantial internal resources of their own can forego these costs by internal financing either from a larger pool of resources, or simply by allocating resources from highly profitable endeavors to needy ones.

While increased efficiency in horizontal and vertical merger cases has been, especially for the past decade or so, a major point of defense, the courts' attitude to conglomerate generated increased efficiency was less than accommodating. In fact, in some cases essentially the increased efficiency itself that caused alarm. For instance, in a product extension merger case, involving a large household detergent manufacturer and a major player in the household bleach manufacturing market, a decisive point was based on the detergent manufacturer's ability to transfer its substantial advertising economies for the benefit of the bleach manufacturer, and to the detriment of the latter's competitors with no access to those economies[10]. In a later case, a merger was disallowed between two companies whose manufacturing functions almost perfectly complemented each other - thus creating an efficient production unit, by arguing that the new merged unit constitutes a formidable entry barrier[11]. At the present time, efficiency seems to play, one way or another, a much less decisive role in conglomerate merger cases. What appears to have taken its place is a set of direct competitive restraint sources either by way of foreclosing *potential competition* between the parties to a merger, or by the implementation of *direct foreclosure* of those not party to the merger through leverage tie-ins, strategic pricing and entry deterrent practices, and, perhaps most commonly, by reciprocity.

Potential Competition and Direct Conglomerate Restraints

An incumbent firm's market power is constrained mainly by the responsiveness of consumers and that of potential entrant producers to the results of its own price and output actions. If an incumbent firm is aware of the fact that a price increase accompanied by sizable profits will attract new competitors into the market, hence erode its market share with the same essential results as would be generated by its customers switching to its competitor, then conceptual difference between *potential competition* and horizontal competition can be obscure. The only difference is the group of competitors, existing or incumbent, to whom the price raising firm's customers are switching. The conceptual difference becomes artificially magnified only when one views the existence of competition in terms of a large number of existing firms in a market, and a lack of it in terms the presence of a single firm, or a small number of dominant firms. While potential competition may not be a pertinent constraint in the first instance, competition in a single or highly concentrated market may be no more restrained that the firm's or firms' ability to raise price above marginal cost without causing entry. Thus, in essence, *competition* may be defined in this context as a set of market forces that cause the market price to gravitate downward to marginal costs, with the set including the threat of potential entry. Even if, initially, the cross elasticity of *demand* between two sets of firms is low enough to place them into separate antitrust markets, with a high elasticity of *supply* on the part of either set of firms, the market demarcation all but disappears.

Market power in potential entry based conglomerate merger cases has had some significance. In a case, involving the distribution of natural gas in California, one distributor controlled some 50% of the natural gas consumed in the State, and acquired another distributor who has made a number of unsuccessful attempts to sell natural gas in the State[12]. The merger was disallowed because the court viewed unsuccessful bidders just as much of a competition as successful ones, and the larger number of bidders gave buyers a choice. Clearly, there was no distinction drawn in the case between the "horizontal" or "potential" competition caused by the second distributor. In the household detergent case, discussed earlier from another perspective[8], the court viewed the household detergent manufacturer as a likely *de novo* entrant into the household bleach manufacturing market, a possibility that was eliminated by the acquisition of a bleach manufacturer with 50% share in a national market where the two top firms controlled over 65%. A third, brewing industry, case dealt with potential competition much more elaborately[13]. The market extension conglomerate merger involved the nation's fourth largest brewer that made no significant sales in New England, and that region's largest brewer with a 20% share of that market. The national brewer was expected, by the government, to enter into the regional market either *de novo*, or by toe-hold (buying a small brewer), hence increase competition there. The district court rejected the possibility of a *de novo* entry in the case. The final decision of the US Supreme Court, in favor of the government although not subscribing to the government's theory, rested on the perception of the producers in the New England regional market - what counted, in the opinion of the Court, was what the *incumbents believed and perceived* would happen regarding the national brewer's entry, not what it presumably planned to do. The essence of this theory is that in a concentrated market that would likely accommodate pricing substantially above marginal cost, and producing much below the competitive level, the incumbents' pricing and production conduct will be influenced, indeed contained, by the perceived presence of a substantial firm, lurking around the market perimeters, with mouth foaming and salivating for the profits it could earn if entered, and, by perception of the incumbents, it will likely enter if their own profits will warrant it. If, on the other hand, entry is accomplished by acquiring one of the dominant incumbents, the pricing and potential competitive restraints disappear, and price inflating along output restrictive conduct will likely resume. Thus, for potential competition to have impact on market conduct, the market must be concentrated and have the tendency to price and produce monopolistically, the number of potential entrants lurking around market boundries must be one or few enough that the disappearance of one of them will alter the perceived threat on the part of market incumbents, and the perceived threat of entry must be either *de novo,* or toe-hold, and not by acquiring a major incumbent, and, finally, barriers to entry (i.e. the relative cost of entry) must be low enough for the incumbents not to feel protected but to perceive the threat[14].

In addition to the elimination of potential competition, conglomerate mergers have been viewed as posing competitive threats through some direct foreclosures of competition. *Reciprocal deals* have been cited as one of these, which can occur in bilateral or multilateral forms. This restraint is based on the mutually beneficial coercive, instead of voluntary, supply-purchase contracting among firms in the same conglomerate family, and on the exclusion of outsiders. Thus, a food processor required its independent suppliers to purchase their spices from its affiliate spice manufacturer[15]. A conglomerate merger may also facilitate *leveraged tie-in agreements*, especially in product extension mergers where, for instance, a toothpaste manufacturer may purchase a toothbrush manufacturer, and tie the product of the latter to the sale of tooth paste. Finally, *strategic pricing and entry deterrence* entails a multimarket conglomerate engaging in successful predatory pricing in one its markets, thus conveying the threat for the same in his other markets without actually predating there as well, with the final result of being able to charge post-predatory monopoly prices in all of its markets[16].

US Government Merger Guidelines: From 1984 to 1992

The new Guidelines (GLs) appear to be designed to enhance the analysis of the competitive effects of mergers[17]. They evaluate the social desirability of a merger in three major and two relatively minor analytical dimensions. Measurements of monopoly power and concentration in a properly delineated market; the likely competitive effects of the merger; and, entry conditions. Issues of efficiency and failure are dealt with rather briefly. In addition, the 1992 GLs depart from reliance on relatively unscientific opinion polling of customers or competitors, sanctioned by the 1984 Guidelines. Thus, an industry consensus to the effect of a likely or unlikely future entry, or stated intentions by alleged entry candidates to the effect that they do not wish enter, will no longer suffice. Entry in the new GLs is examined in terms of it possibly preventing undesirable mergers, or whether it can reduce or offset the competition constraining effects of a merger. The GLs essentially call for an *analysis* of the potential competitive consequences of a merger, within the context of the specific market conditions and circumstances.

A major structural concern of the GLs remains *concentration* in the relevant market, in order to identify transactions that "potentially raise significant competitive concerns", or further analyses is likely to reveal adverse affects. Thus, a merger is not likely to generate or increase market power, or facilitate the abuse of market power, unless the merger-caused concentration or increase in concentration exceed the levels specified in Section 1.51 of the 1992 GLs. These levels have not changed from the 1984 GLs. In terms of the Herfindhal Index (HI) [see our discussion in Chapter 4], so long as the post merger $HI < 1000$; or, if $1000 < H < 1800$ along with a merger-caused increase of no more than 100; or, if $H > 1800$ along with a merger-caused increase of no more than 50, a merger is viewed within limits of a "safe harbor", and should not cause enforcement concern.

Since concentration is measured within the context of the *relevant market,* the latter and its participants must be delineated and identified.

The 1992 GLs analyses in this area also remain essentially the same as those in 1984, although changes did occur. Central to the market definition model is the response to a "small but significant and nontransitory increase in price" [SNP] persisting for the "foreseeable future" [GLs Section 1.1]. In 1984, this price change was, somewhat problematically, designated to last specifically for one year only, as if consumers were told by sellers, or had reasons to assume, that the price increase was to last for one year only. And, if they did, would they implement changes in their purchasing decisions in response, or simply wait for a year? The duration of "foreseeable future" may be short in industries with frequently recurring product cycles or with rapid technological changes, such as the personal computer manufacturing and distribution markets, and much longer in slowly evolving heavier industries. Thus, the key and fundamental point of analysis focuses on the objectively *observed* consequences of SNP, that is, on the actual behavior, instead of their perception of product demand or supply substitutability, of producers and consumers in response to the implementation of a SNP. Within a given relevant market, the cost incurred by consumers by way of switching from a product to another is low enough to render an SNP by a firm with monopoly power unprofitable. On the other hand, if the cost of switching is high enough to discourage consumers from moving to an alternative product in response to a SNP, then that alternative product is not in the same market.

Important changes have been implemented by the 1992 GLs in terms of analyzing the role of *existing suppliers* and that of *supply switching*. The 1984 GLs market for used consumer durable also included recyclers and reconditioners of those goods. In addition, supply substitution generated goods, in response to an SNP, so long as that substitution occurred with a year from the time the SNP took place, was also included in the market. The 1992 GLs include in the market all existing sellers of the relevant product, as well as vertically integrated firm. If the latter were to withdraw partially or entirely from the market, it is assumed that a proportionate price increase would result. If the market includes used durable goods, their producers and distributors with their inventories are also included as constraints on monopolistic pricing, although recyclers and reconditioners are no longer considered relevant.

The principles, and proponents, of contestable markets, left a notable impact on the 1992 GLs [see our discussion in Chapter 3]. Thus, firms, labeled as "uncommitted entrants", presently outside the relevant market but who can, without having to incur much by way of sunk costs, substantially respond to an SNP within a year, are also included in the market. They are "entrants", but "uncommitted", because they can enter and exit a market without substantial financial commitment, or sunk costs. Conversely, a "committed entrant" would generate a supply response to an SNP only by way of incurring substantial investments, sunk costs, that could not be recouped upon exit. The 1992 GLs define sunk costs as "the acquisition cost of tangible and intangible assets that cannot be recovered through the redeployment of these assets outside the relevant market" [Section 1.32]. Thus, sunk costs are market specific, incurred exclusively for participation in the relevant product and geographic markets. If entry into a market entails the acquisition of tangible assets, *no sunk costs* are incurred if such assets, at their depreciated value, had been or could have been resold, or alternatively used, within a year, and without a loss, outside the relevant market. In the case of resale, sunk costs are equal to the difference between acquisition costs (minus depreciation) and the resale price. With intangible assets, such as R&D, it is the portability, from the relevant market to another market, of the products or inventions, generated by the R&D that determines whether or not the investments involved are sunk costs. A significant sunk cost is "one which would not be recouped within one year of the commencement of the supply response, assuming an SNP [Section 1.32].

Uncommitted entry may fall into three categories. *Production substitution* involves switching production capacity from alternatives to the relevant market without incurring significant amounts of sunk costs at entry or exit, regardless the size of modifications to the existing plants [the 1984 GLs limited this definition to insignificant changes to plant size]. *Product extension* entails using already existing and functioning assets (such as brand names, goodwill, reputation) in other markets in the relevant market, without switching them out of other markets. The third category of uncommitted entry could take place by firms who simply apply *newly acquired assets* to producing and selling in the relevant market, without incurring significant sunk costs upon entry and exit.

Another important structural factor in delineating the relevant market in mergers, *entry*, has been extensively dealt with in Chapter 6.

In the general conduct category, the likely impact of the merger is viewed in terms of its *competitive effects*. The 1992 GLs consider its determination fundamental, regardless of the level of concentration prevailing before or after the merger, and irrespective of the change in concentration caused by the merger. Competitive effects may occur by way of expected post-merger *collusive behavior* ("coordinated interaction" in 1992 GLs terminology), or likely *unilateral* abuse of market power by the newly emerged firm. Coordinated interaction among post-merger firms with dominant market power would normally be expected to occur in terms of price, or reduced output, or both. Furthermore, for such collusion to be effective, deviations from its terms must be detectable, and, readily punishable. Thus, a merger is not likely to harm competition by consequent coordinated interaction if the parties to the collusion may deviate from its terms, their deviation is not likely to be detected, and, even if detected, no easy sanctions are available or applicable. In addition, the 1992 GLs indicate the importance of showing a clear *economic incentive* and ability on the part of the participants to collectively raise price and restrict output. Thus, if the gain from deviating from the terms of collusion is significant enough to be more than offset by the mathematical expectation of loss emanating from being discovered and then fined (i.e. the probability of being discovered times the expected fine), it pays to deviate, and the incentive to remain in a post-merger coordinated interaction, everything else remaining equal, is substantially reduced, or eliminated.

A merger may create a single firm with a market power large enough to abuse in substantial restraint of competition. A merger's *unilateral* conduct effect may be of concern, as outlined in the 1992 GLs, if the new firm's market share is greater than 35%, and the Herfindhal borders are exceeded. In addition, the consumer's perception of close substitutability among the merging firms' products is thought by the current GLs to enhance the conditions for unilateral abuses.

References

1 Sherer, Frederick M., and Ross, David *Industrial Market Structure and Economic Performance*, Third Edition, Houghton Mifflin and Company, Boston MA 1990, Chapter 5.

2 Williamson, Oliver "Economies as an Antitrust Defense: The Welfare Trade-Offs", *American Economic Review*, Vol. 58, p.18, 1968. Williamson, Oliver "Economies as an Antitrust Defense Revisited", *University of Pennsylvania Law Review*, Vol 125, (1977), p.699. See also, Muris John "The Efficiency Defense Under Section 7 of the Clayton Act, *Case Western Reserve Law Review*, Vol. 30, 1980, p. 381.

3 *Brown Shoe Co. v US.* 370 US 307 (1962)

4 *US v. Von's Grocery Co* 384 US 270 (1966)

5 Williamson, Oliver "Vertical Merger Guidelines: Interpreting the 1982 Reforms", *California Law Review*, Vol. 71, (1983), p. 604

6 *US v. E.I. duPont de Nemours & Co.* 353 US 586 (1957)

7 Markham, Jesse "Merger Policy Under the New Section 7: A Six Year Appraisal", *Virginia Law Review*, Vol. 43, (1957), pp.489-97

8 *Fruehauf Corporation* v FTC 603 F.2d 345 (2d Cir 1979)

9 Brodley, Robert "Potential Competition Mergers: A Structural Synthesis", *Yale Law Journal*, Vol. 87, (1977)

10 *FTC v. Procter and Gamble Co* 386 US 568 (1967)

11 *Allis-Chambers Mfg. Co. v. White Consolidated Industries,* 414 F.2d 506 (3rd Cir, 1969)

12 *US v ElPaso Natural Gas,* 376 US 651 (1964)

13 *US v. Falstaff Brewing Co.* 410 US 526 (1973)

14 *US v. Marine Bancorporation* 418 US 602 (1974)

15 *FTC v. Consolidated Food Corp.,* 380 US 592 (1965)

16 Salop, Steven C. "Strategic Entry Deterrence" *American Economic Review* Vol 69, 1979

17 Department of Justice and Federal Trade Commission, *Horizontal Merger Guidelines*, April 2, 1992. Reprinted in Trade Regulation Reporter, Vol 4, #13,104, CCH

PART THREE

HEALTHCARE MARKETS

Chapter 11
THE HEALTHCARE INDUSTRY: AN OVERVIEW

As early as 1927, a committee had been created by the American Medical Association to examine the state of health care delivery in USA. The Committee, at that time, indicated that "The problem of providing satisfactory medical service to all the people of the United States at a cost which they can meet is a pressing one. At the present time, many persons do not receive service which is adequate either in quantity or quality, and the costs of service are inequitably distributed[1]. Many years later, during the 1960s, 1970s, 1980s, and now in thw 1990s, scholars, politicians, businessman, and providers as well as patients speak of "crises" in the US healthcare system. During the mid 1970s, a research body representing a number of major US corporations and banks attributed the crisis in US healthcare to (a) faulty resource allocation causing inadequacies and inequalities in US health services yielding substandard care for a large segment of the population, (b) a private and public insurance system needs to make it possible for all people to cope with the costs of healthcare, and, (c) major alterations are needed in the means of delivering services and paying providers[2]. In 1979, when introducing his National Health Service bill, Congressman Ronald Dellums stated: "We have in this country today a health delivery system where the quality of healthcare received is determined by race, language, national origin, or income level. Health is viewed as commodity to be bought and sold in the market place, it is not viewed as the right of the people; a service to be provided by Government. However, financing is not the only problem facing the people when it comes to the delivery of healthcare. Other, equally important, problems are the maldistribution of health manpower, the unequal access to services, the unreliable quality of care, and the lack of public control over healthcare. No matter how much we guarantee the payment of services to the people, it is of little comfort to them if there is no one around to provide the service"[3]. This thirteen year old statement sums of the problems faced by the US society in connection with healthcare: cost, quality, distribution, equity, and basic availability.

In preparation for examining the application of antitrust statutes to the healthcare field, the chapters in Part Three will take a brief look at the fundamental institutional structure and conduct of healthcare markets. Part Four will examine specifically, and systematically, how the statutes were applied to various structure and conduct problems in the industry, while the Part Five will take a look at if, and how, antitrust enforcement in healthcare may, or may not, have contributed to the alleviation of cost inflation. This chapter will survey some of the most fundamental issues and pertinent concepts.

General Dimensions of the Healthcare Environment

The US is one of the most populous countries in the world, with those over age 65 estimated around 15% of the population. The population composition is diverse in terms of race, ethnic origin, socio-economic and income levels, education, and vocational background. A healthcare delivery system in this Country must possess the magnitude and capacity, flexibility, comparable diversity, appropriate resource allocation, and the necessary resource endowment to accommodate healthcare needs.

The system has a manpower of approximately 10 million employees. It may, somewhat arbitrarily, be divided into three main groups: independent practioners, dependent practitioners, and support staff. These include physicians, dentists, pharmacists, nurses, clerical staff, technicians, and manual workers. The predominant mode, some 75%, of organization by physicians is still entrepreneurial self-employment by way of private practice, a form of organization that is going through transformation at this time[4].

Healthcare is provided in a variety of institutional settings. The most basic and common form is *ambulatory* care, provided in an outpatient environment. Some 75% of ambulatory care is provided in private physician offices, with the rest in hospital emergency rooms, clinics, public health centers, and health maintenance organizations. Care in *institutional* settings normally takes place within about 8,000 hospitals utilizing some 1.2 million beds, some of which are under federal, state and local government ownership, others falling into the voluntary hospital category, with the third category being private proprietory hospitals. Functionally, and somewhat arbitrarily, hospitals may be classified in a variety of ways such as general, mental, tuberculosis, short-term, long-term, and so forth. In general, these categories overlap, and change their characteristics over time as the socio-economic conditions of their markets mandate. In addition, institutional care of one type or another is also provided at hospice centers, and by way of home healthcare programs. Further, there are care institutions that concentrate on medical education and research.

At the present time, the US spends about $700 billion, or 13% of GNP, on various aspects of healthcare, exceeding the total gross national product of most countries. While definition of the ultimate payer for healthcare is simple: the people (though not necessarily only the users), the mechanism whereby the funds are dispensed to the providers can be at times convoluted. Almost half of the payments to providers are made through governments - by way of directly government operated government institutions, and where the government is a third-party payer; one-third is paid through insurance companies; and, a little over 25% is expended directly from user to provider. The private insurance sector is dominated by the not-for-profits (Blue Cross/Blue Shield), and the commercial for-profit insurers. On the receiving end, hospitals get almost half of the moneys, physicians around 20%, dentists about 5%, the drug companies around 10%, and other providers, including nursing homes, the remainder.

The Essence of Medical Markets

A market based economy solves basic resource allocation problems by relying on the dicta of the price system communicated through market forces, yielding a determination of the goods and services to be produced, their quantity, production methods, and how are the fruits of production to be distributed. In Part One, we discussed the functioning of markets, and the consequences of market failures. Medical markets are pervaded by market failures. Yet, the social consequences of spiraling healthcare costs, and the persistence of severe problems in healthcare service distribution, mandates that medical markets be studied and understood carefully, in order to contain costs and reduce social inequities. We will take a careful look at the nature of medical market later in the volume. At this point, a brief overview will serve as the basis for better understanding the rest of this introductory chapter.

We should, even preliminarily, note that in healthcare markets, the price mechanism has traditionally been a poor or no regulator of output and consumption. Buyers cannot make independent purchasing decisions based on price, as they often do not know what product they need, and at times, even if they did know it, they would not be in the position to communicate it. In effect, the healthcare service buyer is a captive of ignorance. The gap is made up by the sellers (the providers). They tell the buyer that he/she has a need for some product in the first place, and what that product should be. In addition, once the needs are communicated, patients rarely have at any one time at their disposal data and information regarding the supply, price, and, importantly, quality choices available to them. In other words, patients are told, ostensibly for their own good, to purchase a product, from a specific source (the hospitals are normally designated by prior staff affiliations), at an unknown price, likely in unknown quantity, and with minimum or no knowledge of quality. The buyer simply does not possess any of the information that would enable him/her to make rational market decisions. All pertinent data and information, as well as the decision to make the sale, is possessed by the seller. Thus, while in a geographic market there may be some competition among providers, (among hospitals, and among physicians), consumers cannot take advantage of it. In many, particularly nonmetropolitan markets, competition even among providers is minimal or none existent; thus, many rural communities and their immediate surroundings are served by one hospital, and a few physicians, all having staff privileges at that same hospital.

Nevertheless, competition of some sort, at least *on the supply side*, has been pervading medical markets, particularly in popular metropolitan areas. The supply of physicians continues to grow. In many areas, hospitals are fighting for survival among themselves, especially in view of the DRG imposed revenue constraints, and the employer efforts to reduce healthcare insurance costs. It was particularly the latter that contributed to the emergence, and relative success, of alternative healthcare delivery systems by way of healthcare intermediation through HMOs (Health Maintenance Organizations), and PPOs (Preferred

Provider Organizations). These, along with other healthcare intermediaries, will be discussed later in this Part. At this point, suffice it to note that HMOs and PPOs in essence contract with large patient pools, normally available through large employers, or concerted groups of small employers, and, particularly in view of the quantity of business involved, are in the position to negotiate reduced healthcare costs with providers.

Competition on the supply side also appears to be enhanced by the emergence of alternatives to traditional inpatient hospital care. Thus, emergi-centers, birthing centers, surgi-centers, various ambulatory clinics with enhanced facilities, operated by physician owners, often in joint venture with nearby hospitals, provide at least components of services which an inpatient would receive in the aggregate at a hospital. In addition, and still on the supply side, the traditional solo medical practitioner is slowly withering away, being replaced by prepaid group practices. Finally, the supply of medical services is now heavily commercialized with the emergence of an increasing number of investor owned for-profit hospital and nursing home chains. Given a state of legal competition, these competitive developments on the supply side may be expected to reduce the cost of healthcare. However, as we will extensively note later in the volume, healthcare costs have continued to increase, apart from the continued inequities in allocation and availability.

Health and the Healthcare Product

Today's medical practice concerns itself almost exclusively with the diagnosis and treatment of disease, already set in, and not necessarily with health as such. Yet, physical cures, even if available and properly applied, is not the only item healthcare consumers demand. They also require caring. Thus, the definition of health, illness, disease and related concepts are interrelated, yet can be different, and at times confusing. Thus, for instance, Webster's Unabridged Dictionary defines health as "physical and mental well-being", only to continue by saying that it is a "freedom from defect, pain or disease". So, health statistics are, if fact, disease statistics, and healthcare is the care for disease. In its Constitution, the World Health Organization defines health as a "state of complete physical, mental and social well-being, and not merely the absence of disease or infirmity"[5]. Subsequently, the definition was modified by a number of writers. For instance, it was suggested that "the ability to function" should be added[6], and the entire dimension of the human being should be emphasized by emphasizing the "well-working of the organism as a whole"[7]. To compound the circular confusion, disease is defined by Webster as "any departure from health". In general, disease has been viewed as a biomedical concept attached to a specific organ, while illness is a state of being, and attaches to the entire human being. Thus, at least theoretically, and without belaboring the point, one can have a disease without feeling ill, and, clearly, vice-versa. More recent developments of health status indices, utilized in cost-benefit analyses of medical care, seem to indicate the increasing importance of "functioning" as an element in defining health[8].

Health has several underlying components. The biological, particularly genetic, component is fundamental. The environmental component, interactively with genetics, is clearly decisive. In fact, epidemiological studies suggest that most cancers are caused by environmental factors. In addition, health's important components include psychological and social. Thus, a physician's negative behavior, and the consequent psychological effects, can have a substantial negative impact on the outcome of a therapy[9]. Socially, illness is endowed with certain rights and obligations. The rights include the exemption from performing certain duties or from participating in certain activities. The obligation entails cooperating with prescribed treatments, and, financially, may involve mitigating some to the costs involved; thus, a smoker may be charged a higher health insurance premium. In addition, social networks appear to have mitigated at least the stress factors involved with certain health problems, thus, mitigating the healing or pain toleration process itself[10].

In terms of individual rights, the economic and healthcare distribution systems determine who already has, and who should have, rights to health and healthcare. From an ethical point of view, it can be stated that every one is entitled to health, and, therefore, healthcare. Perhaps, the same thing can be said about any commodity of positive utility - with the degree of entitlement diminishing in some proportion to the degree of necessity involved in the commodity or service. In actual practice, correctly or incorrectly, presently the market determines who shall and who shall not have access to health, including the quality distribution of health, via the healthcare process, by allocating access to insurance opportunities, or simply by wealth allocation. Those few with unlimited financial resources can be said to be "self-insured", hence require no outside support. Most people with limited financial resources purchase risk coverage of some sort or another, and from some source or another (including government sources). There are some 40 million people who have no health insurance at all, hence are exposed to sustaining the financial risks, and the possibly resulting financial catastrophe, of illness themselves. This latter problem, along with inadequacies in existing coverage, generated a perennial political issue: health insurance, and therefore, the financial (as distinct from the moral) right to healthcare for everyone. The scarcity of resources, and prohibitive costs, will under any circumstances preclude the availability of all healthcare to everyone, at all times. Thus, the solution of the problem will rest with an allocative or rationing mechanism in order to stay within the economic means of society as whole. For most standard commodities and services, other than healthcare, we have allowed the "dollar vote" of the consumer through the market mechanism to determine what, how much, how, and for whom the production process will perform. As we will extensively note shortly, healthcare is not a standard commodity, nor are the necessary resource allocation and cost related problem solutions.

Healthcare Providers

Healthcare delivery is intrinsically labor intensive. The education, composition, and distribution of personnel heavily impacts on costs, availability, efficiency and quality. Until the mid-1970, there was a steady inflow of professional personnel into medicine, due to the continuous expansion of the industry, and the seemingly limitless availability of private and public funding. Efficiency and costs were rarely a concern, as payment systems were based on retrospective cost estimates, instead of preset prospective rates. New technology, personnel, and host of services were consistently added. With the highly labor intensive nature of the industry, the influx of new services was accompanied by a further influx people. In addition, the physicians' and other healthcare workers' alleged ability to create their own demand[11] accelerated the cost spiral by creating and promoting additional services, which, in turn, may promote demand for those services (an issue to be dealt with in greater detail later on in this part of the book).

Functionally, and traditionally, the healthcare labor force may be divided into three rather broad, and somewhat arbitrary, categories. A group of *independent practitioners* in private practice, is licensed to

deliver a specific range of services to anyone, without outside interference
(the latter prompted the "traditional" caveat), such as physicians, dentists,
and other private practitioners. *Dependent practitioners* essentially do
the same, however, function by the authority of independent practitioners,
such as nurses, pharmacists, therapists, and so forth. Thirdly, the so called
support staff, functions under the direct supervision of dependent and
independent practitioners; the range is broad extending from technicians,
nurses' aids to clerical members of the office staff.

In 1990, there were some 640,000 physicians in the US [Health
United States, 1991], with most of them engaged in private office patient
care, specifically in the practice of family and general care. An issue of
some notoriety has been the *geographical distribution* of physicians,
both throughout the US among states, and within certain states, or even
cities. Thus, Mississippi with the lowest physician/100,000 ratio (120),
has only a little more than one-third of the number of physicians
practicing in Massachusetts (320)[12]. Maldistribution of this type has a
direct bearing upon the cost of healthcare (higher physician concentration
generates higher costs), and on the quality of care due mainly, though
by no means exclusively, to the apparent correlation between physician
concentration and the presence of ample tertiary care facilities. In
addition, and not unlike other professionals, physicians are generally
attracted to favorable markets, population centers with their amenities,
geographical locations, and climate zones. Incidentally, intra-state
physician distribution can be just as uneven as inter-state. Thus, in New
York State, physician over-supply is 1% if New York City is not included
in the calculation, but becomes 12% when it is. Similarly, intra-state
Maryland comparisons showed a thousand percent variation between
metropolitan and non-metropolitan counties (from 30/100,000 to over
300/100,000)[13]. Maldistribution within metropolitan areas is also
indicated by a comparison between the Central Park South and the South
Bronx areas of New York City.

Factors that contribute to lopsided manpower distribution include
the site of clinical training after graduation, geographical roots of the
students, climate and other geographical amenities contributing to the
quality of life, and the availability of peers particularly in university
affiliated medical centers[14].

The supply of an average commodity, or that of an average service,
is normally determined through the price mechanism in the market by
the interaction of demand and supply. However, the supply of medical
services, particularly those of physicians, is not sensitive to market forces

for a variety of reasons that include a lack of adequate consumer information regarding the product, legal barriers to entry by way of licensing, provider capability to shift the demand curve, and a dynamic technological environment[15]. Thus, along with an uneven distribution of physician supply, the *aggregate supply of physician services* has substantially increased, over and beyond what could be construed as market warranted. What the proper level of physician supply should be is another complex question. As indicated before, supply stimulates demand. In addition, need and demand are very difficult to evaluate in medicine because of differing physician practice patterns, and because of the complexities associated with identifying precise product and service identities. The consumer usually does not know what service is required, how many units of it, and for how long[16]. The oversupply, in turn, brings with it conflicts, controversies, and, indeed, dog-eat-dog type of competitive environment in some medical circles and communities. Antitrust litigation in medicine increased to an extent because of this over-supply. In particular, hospitals, having closed their doors to additional staff, along with exclusive contracting with a selected groups, were exposed a variety of law suits. We will deal with these extensively later in the volume.

This predicament is seen as contributing to major changes in the practice of medicine. These changes are expected to include an increase in the number of salaried physicians, a decrease in the number of hours worked, a decline in physician real income, limited physician service diversification, a decline in the utilization of foreign medical graduates ("FMGs"), and possibly even unemployment of less competent, frequently sued, physicians in the less trained categories[17].

FMGs, and American medical students studying abroad, while served to fill gaps in the past, have come under closer scrutiny in the more recent past. One concern was undue US dependence on FMGs, although it was found that, at least some years ago, they tended to gravitate towards shortage areas[18]. The trend in US students studying abroad has taken an apparently disturbing turn in the mid-1970s. Until that time, US students attended university affiliated established medical schools along the country's nationals. More recently, private profit-motivated medical schools, located mostly in the Caribbean, Mexico, and Puerto Rico, were set up specifically to cater to students from the USA, apparently without much regard for the quality of undergraduate preparations and the abilities involved [19].

Working closely with physicians, a major proportion of provider manpower is *nursing*. It is the largest single category, encompassing a wide range of healthcare workers. This category includes mostly licensed practical nurses with one year training, and registered nurses with a variety of training backgrounds ranging from a 2-years associate degree from a junior college to a PhD in the field. California and New York have the largest concentration of nursing personnel, while the New England states have the highest nurse/population ratio, and the south-central states the lowest.

Financing Healthcare

In 1993, this country spent over $800 billion on healthcare, some 14% of GNP. The *destination of funds* can be divided into two categories: some three-fourth goes to payments for health services and supplies, and about one-fourth to research and medical facilities, including capital expenditures. The former cover hospitals, physicians, nursing home care, drugs, and dentists - with the proportions approximately in that order. As to the source of the funds, ultimately it is the general population, although most of the moneys take a variety of routes, such as via governments, private insurance companies, and independent plans.

A major portion of government channeled funds into healthcare is routed through the *medicare* system of payments, initiated in July 1966. Part A of the program covers institutional care (hospitals, extended care facilities, or home care) and is financed by Social Security payroll deductions. The voluntary Part B of the program covers largely ambulatory care, and is financed mostly by general tax revenue. Both plans are subject to deductibles and copayments, as well as to limits of coverage as to the number of days or visits. The quality and cost of care delivered under medicare has been under scrutiny for some time. The PSROs (Professional Standards Review Organizations), set up in 1972 to police the quality and quantity of care under the public programs, were replaced in 1982 by TEFRA's (Tax Equity and Fiscal Responsibility Act) so called PROs (Peer Review Organizations) which, under contract to the Health Care Financing Administration, monitor quality and utilization. TEFRA, along with the 1983 Amendments to it [Title VI of PL-98-21], also gave birth to the Prospective Payment System by way of DRGs (Diagnostic Related Groups). Prior to TEFRA, largely a cost-based retrospective payment system was the basis for medicare reimbursements. DRGs provide set rates of reimbursement for each hospital based transaction, prompting hospitals to minimize cost under the constraints of those rates, and limiting hospital revenue increases.

Along with the federal government, state governments also contribute to the channeling process of healthcare funds. The joint federal-state *Medicaid* programs, as diverse as the 50 states' pertinent policies are, is designed to provide care for the poor. Federal funds, allocated to states according to per capita income, contribute to the states' burden of program implementation by way of inpatient and ambulatory care, skilled nursing care, and laboratory or x-ray services. In addition to medicaid, governments also channel healthcare funds to providers through the care of veterans, military personnel and their dependents, medical benefits through workmen's compensation programs, and through other related efforts.

Apart from the direct fee-for-service payments by the patient to the provider, the *private sector* channels healthcare moneys from the population to providers largely through non-profit and profit motivated insurance plans. After some sporadic hospital-specific plans, the AHA and AMA sponsored *Blue-Cross and Blue-Shield* (BC/BS), respectively, "non-profit" plans were the first in the US to act as payment intermediary between the aggregate of healthcare users and individual providers. BC/BS are established under specific state statutes. Their non-profit status exempts them from the need to maintain cash reserves and pay taxes, and their operations are, or supposed to be, closely monitored by each state's commissioner of insurance. Their rates have traditionally been based on community rating, that is, a uniform rate for the community, representing some average of the various risks there. However, following the example of more recently appeared profit oriented commercial insurers, who have always charged "experience rates", that is, individual or group premiums commensurate to applicable risks, BC/BS have gradually shifted to that pricing structure[20].

For-profit insurers entered into the health insurance market earnestly after the second World War when the Supreme Court recognized fringe benefits as a legitimate collective bargaining item. The market for health insurance opened up. Policies have been sold to groups as part of fringe benefit packages, with usually much higher premiums and more limited coverage accorded to individuals. In addition to the voluntary (not-for-profit) and commercial plans, other channels for healthcare payments opened up by way of independent insurers. These included major plans like Kaiser Permanente, Health Insurance Plan of Greater New York, and several others[21].

Physician providers are paid in two major ways. *Fee-for-service,* in contrast to capitation and salary, has been a dominant way for physicians to receive compensation. The provider is directly paid by the user, or by third parties, according to, and at the time or shortly after, the performed service. *Salary* is the predominant form of provider compensation, outside the physician sector, although a substantial proportion of physicians is also compensated in this manner. These physicians have been shown to generate lower utilization of costly diagnostic and treatment procedures than those compensated by fee-for-service[22]. *Capitation* form of compensation involves a set annual fee per patient, regardless of visit frequencies.

The payment of *hospitals,* on the other hand, has historically taken two standard forms: restrospective and prospective. The former has been set after the performance of the service either by way of charges or cost. Charges are hospital set prices for room and board plus services and the extent to which they cover costs depends on the proportion of free care provided. Cost based retrospective payments, used when patients receive service instead of dollar reimbursement, have been contractually set between the hospital and third-party payers. Reimbursed costs were calculated by the payers on a per-patient-day basis.

The latter, applied to inpatient care of Medicare patients, as indicated above, is based on DRGs, and the hospitals are paid a set amount per case, depending on the type of case. It is based on the principles (a) that a hospital's output can best be measured in terms of substantive diagnoses, i.e. clinically meaningful and reasonably homogenous cases treated, instead of the number of individual services, routine inputs, or length of stay; and, (b) the rate of reimbursement is predetermined and fixed. Patients are classified into 23 MDCs (Major Diagnostic Categories) based on major biological function categories, which, in turn, are divided into 470 DRGs based on diagnoses, procedure, gender, age, and other patient dimensions[23]. Some States (e.g. New Jersey, Maryland) have their own versions of DRG payment systems, hence do not exactly apply the federal standards. In addition, hospital costs like direct medical education and the cost of capital, are still reimbursed on their individual cost basis, instead of being included in the bases for DRGs. A DRG based payment to a hospital for a Medicare case is calculated by multiplying a standardized (allows for differences in wages and teaching intensity) average Medicare patient cost factor with DRG set cost-based weights. Annual adjustments ("update factors") allow for changes in the cost of hospital acquired goods and services, and a DAF (discretionary adjustment factor), with a maximum of one-quarter percent, allows for productivity and technological changes[24].

The Quality of Care

The ultimate evaluation of quality for standard goods and services is through the market and consumer accommodation in the light of price (at a low enough - including zero, price, anything can be sold). The market's toleration of a product or service based on quality assumes that consumers possess the information, and opportunity, to assess a product's or service's quality. As we pointed out earlier, that is not the case in medicine.

A fundamental premise pertaining to the prudent practice of medicine is *premium non nocere* ("primarily, do not harm") is incorporated in the Hippocratic Oath. Yet, at this time, a major portion of delivered healthcare is of less than superior quality; indeed, given the total volume, and the nature, of medical malpractice litigation, checking into some hospitals may constitute a further hazard to a patient's health. Thus, the evaluation of the quality of healthcare services delivered is important. However, the techniques available for such measurements are far from perfect or even settled.

Even during during the 19th century, the practice of medicine was considered an *art*, as medical treatments were largely unreliable, and the success of surgery was dependent more upon the speed than on available technology. Physicians were trained only by way of apprenticeship programs. With moral support playing a predominant part in medical practice, the evaluation of quality was virtually impossible. However, as the precision of diagnostic tests and treatment procedures increased, science has, to a large extent, replaced art, and quality measurements became more feasible. This is so, in spite of the relative slowness with which provider professionals were ready accept the fact that the quality of their work could, or should, be assessed. Physicians have traditionally viewed quality control efforts as an infringement on their professional autonomy, their status and control over the patients, certainly political power, and on their financial rewards, especially since the latter was viewed as a function of their knowledge unshared with others, and of the myth that medical judgments were infallible[25].

The first effort to measure the quality of healthcare delivery were the so called "outcome studies" which relied on the end-results to make judgment about the quality of care delivered[26]. Shortly afterward, the so called "tracer method" of quality assessment gained attention that relied on the patient's progress at various stages of the treatment, instead of only the final outcome[27]. By the mid 1970s, with substantial increases in the influx of government funds into healthcare, the quality of healthcare delivery came under consistent assessment.

The methods of presently prevailing quality control and measurements in US healthcare delivery are diverse. In general, and briefly, we have *licensing, accreditation,* and *certification* of physicians, healthcare delivery institutions, and allied health professionals, respectively. More specifically, hospital *medical staff review committees* and *peer review organizations* oversee the functioning of physicians in their specific environment. These are enhanced by *patient satisfaction* interviews and surveys, and close observation of *medical malpractice* litigations. The general target areas include health care facilities, the administrative organization, personnel qualifications, physician and healthcare staff evaluation, survey of outcome in terms of health or well-being attained, and patient satisfaction[28].

Medical Technology

A major portion of healthcare costs has been attributed to the applied technology in medicine. Galbraith refers to technology in a generic sense as a "...systematic application of scientific or other organized knowledge to practical tasks"[29]. More specifically, technology in medicine has been defined as "the drugs, devices, and medical and surgical procedures used in medical care, and the organizational and supportive system within which such care is provided"[30].

The contribution of technology to healthcare costs has long been a major concern to academics and policy makers. In general, its estimated share (ranging from about 30% to 80%) depends, among other factors, on the definition of technology for purpose of the study, the time period involved, and the method of calculation[31]. The level of costs, in turn, drew attention to the need for technology; specifically, whether or not technology is being overapplied in particular situations, and if the benefits derived from technological applications in medicine in fact, at least, offset the applicable costs. The answers have often been unclear, due largely not so much to measurement problems of costs, but rather to those of benefits[32]. In addition to explicit and opportunity costs, on the cost side, application specific risks need also be taken into consideration. This has been done to a limited extent. In the case of some drugs, (e.g. thalidomide) the severity of the problems have been discovered in hindsight, after much dramatic damage has been done. In other cases, such as surgery, the risks are relatively well known in advance. In addition, there is a host of situations, drugs, and procedures, where the risks are less dramatic, but may not be know until after application[33].

In addition to explicit, implicit, and risk related costs, technological applications in medicine also have social consequences. One problem is allocative equity, and lack access. Another is that technologically intensive medical practice "depersonalizes" healthcare [Office of Technological Assessment, 1976, and 1984]. The printed and broadcast news media are replete with the ethical and legal questions relating to when, to whom, and for how long, to apply life-sustaining technology.

References

1   Committee on the Costs of Medical Care. *Medical Care for the American People*. University of Chicago Press, Chicago, 1932, p.2

2   Research and Policy Committee, *Building a National Healthcare System*, Committee for Economic Development, 1973, p.17

3   Dellums, Robert "The Health Service Act H.R. 2969, *Congressional Record* 125, 1979 p.33

4   *Statistical Abstract* of the United States, 1992, and US Department of Health and Human Services, *Health United States 1991*

5   WHO "The Constitution of the World Health Organization" *WHO Chronicle*, No. 1, p.29, 1944

6   Terris, M. "The Approaches to an Epidemiology of Health", *American Journal of Public Health*, Vol. 65, 1975, p.107

7   Kass, L. "Regarding the End of Medicine and the Pursuit of Health", in Caplan, A. et. al. *Concepts of Health and Disease*, Addision Wesley, Reading MA. 1981, pp.3-30

8   Deyo R. and Inui, T. "Toward Clinical Applications of Health Status Measures: Sensitivity of Scales to to Clinically Important Changes" *Health Services Research*, Vol. 19, 1984, p.275. Also see McPeek, B. Gilbert, J. and Mosteller, F. "The End Result: Quality of Life", in Bunker, J., Barnes, B. & Mosteller, F. (eds) *Costs, Risks, and Benefits of Surgery*, Oxford University Press, New York, NY 1977, pp.170-75

9   Engel, G. "The Need for a New Medical Model: A Challenge for Biomedicine" in Caplan, A. et.al. (eds). *Concepts of Health and Disease* Addision-Wesley, Reading MA. 1981, pp.589-607

10 Szasz, T. *The Manufacture of Madness*, Harper & Row, New York, 1970. See also Asher, C. "The Impact of Social Support Networks on Adult Health" *Medical Care*, Vol. 22, 1984, p.349.

11 Maloney J. V. and Reemtsa, K. "Cot Containment by A Naval Armada", *New England Journal of Medicine*, Vol. 312 1985, p.1713. See also Fuchs, V. and Kramer, M.J. "Determinant of Expenditures for Physicians' Services in the United States, 1948-68" USDPTHEW, Pub# 73-3013, US Government Printing Office, Washington, DC 1972

12 Culler, S.D. & Daigle, A. The American Healthcare System, AMA, Chicago, 1984. Also see Wennberg, J.E. "Dealing With Medical Practice Variation: A Proposal For Action", *Health Affairs*, Vol. 3, 1984, p. 6., amd Hudson, J.I. and Nourse, E.S. "Perspectives in Primary Care Education", *Journal of Medical Education*, Vol. 50, *December* 1975, Part 2.

13 Alexander, C.A. Boweden, G.R. *Physician Manpower in Maryland*, University of Maryland Press, Baltimore, 1973

14 Sloan, F. *Economic Models of Physician Supply*, PhD Dissertation, Harvard University, 1968. See also, Balinsky, W.L. "Distribution of Yound Medical Specialists from Western New York", *Medical Care*, Vol. 12, 1974, p.437, and Mason, R. "Medical School, Residency, and Eventual Practice Location: Toward a Rationale for State Support of Medical Education" *JAMA*, Vol. 223, 1975, p. 49

15 Fuchs, V. *Who Shall Live? Health Economics and Social Change*, Basic Books, New York, 1974, and Reinhardt, U.E. *Physician Productivity and the Demand for Health Manpower*, Ballinger, Cambridge MA. 1975

16 Bailey, B.J. "Manpower Issues for Surgical Specialty: The Impact of Oversupply" *JAMA* Vol. 253 1985, p.1025. See also, Wennberg, J.E. "Dealing With Medical Practice Varioations: A Proposal for Action" *Health Affairs*, Vol. 3, 1984, p.6.

17 Freedman, S.A. "Megacorporate Healthcare" *New England Journal of Medicine*, Vol. 312, 1985, p.579. Ginzberg, E. "What Lies Ahead for American Physicians: One Economist's Views", *JAMA*, Vol. 253, 1985, p.1878. Igelhart, J.K. "Difficult Times Ahead for Graduate Medical Examination" *New England Journal of Medicine*, Vol. 312, 1985, p.1400]

18 Butter, I. *Foreign Medical Graduates: A Comparative Study of State Licensure Policies*, DHEW, Pub#77-3166, Rockville MD. 1976. Saywell, R.M. et al "A Performance Comparison: USMG-FMG Attending Physicians", *American Journal of Public Health*, Vol. 69, 1979, p.57. Stevens, R. et al. *The Alien Doctors*, John Wiley, New York, 1978. Mick S.S. & Worobey, J.L. "Foreign Medical Graduates in the 1980s: Trends in Specialization" *American Journal of Public Health*, Vol. 74, 1984, p.698

19 Bloom, M. "The 'Other' Medical Schools", and "Coming Home", Medical World News, May 28, 1979. Imperato, P.J. "The Offshore Medical Schools" *New York State Journal of Medicine*, Vol. 84, 1984 pp. 337-71

20 Sommers, H. & Sommers, A.R. Doctors, Patients and Health Insurance, The Brookings Institution, Washington DC 1961. See also, Krizay and Wilson, A. *The Patient as Consumer,* D.C. Heath, Lexington MA. 1974

21 Arnett, R. and Trapnell, G. "Private Health Insurance: New Measures of Complex and Changing Industry" *Health Care Financing Review*, Vol. 6, Winter 1984, p.2.

22 Roemer, M. I. et al "On Paying the Doctor and Implications of Different Methods", *Journal of Health and Human Behavior*, Vol. 3, Spring 1964, p.4. Also see, Manning, W. "A Controlled Trial of the Effects of a Prepaid Group Practice on Use of Services", *New England Journal of Medicine*, Vol 310, June 1984, p.23

23 Grimaldi, P. and Micheletti, J. *Diagnosis Related Groups: A Practinioner's Guide*, Pluribus Press, Chicago, IL. 1982

24 Hellinger, F. "Recent Evidence on Case-Based Systems for Setting Hospital Rates", *Inquiry*, Vol. 22, Spring 1985, p.1. See also, Horn, S. "The Severity of Illness Index as a Severity Adjustment to DRGs", *Health Care Financing Review*, 1984, Annual Supplement

25 Starr, P. *The Social Transformation of American Medicine*, Basic Books, New York, 1982. See also Jonas, S. *Medical Mystery: The Training of Doctors in the United States*, W.W. Norton, New York, 1978

26 Lewis, C.E. "The State of the Art of Quality Assessment" *Medical Care*, Vol. 12, 1974, p.999

27 Brook, R.H. "Critical Issues in the Assesment of Quality of Care and their Relationship to HMOs" *Journal of Medical Education*, Vol. 48, 1973, p. 114. Also see, by the same author, "Assessing the Quality of Medical Care Using Outcome Measures: An Overview of the Method", *Medical Care*, Vol. 15, 1977, Supplement; Brook, R.H. and Williams, K.N. "Quality of Healthcare for the Disadvantaged" *Journal of Community Health*, Vol. 11975, p.132

28 Ellwood, P.M., Jr. et al. "Assessing the Quality of Health Services", in Ellwood et al (eds) *Assuring the Quality of Healthcare*, Interstudy, Minneapolis MN 1973. Also see Roemer, M.I. "Controlling and Promoting Quality in Medical Care", Havinghurst, C.C. and Weistart, J.C. (eds) *Health Care from the Library of Law and Contemporary Problems*, Oceania Publications, Dobbs Ferry NY 1972.

29 Galbraith, J. *The New Industrial State*, New American Library, New York, 1977

30 Office of Technology Assessment, *Assessing the Efficacy and Safety of Medical Technologies*, Pub. No. OTA-h-75. Government Printing Office, Washington DC., 1978

31 Klarman, H. "Application of Cost-Benefit Analysis to the Health Services and the Special Case of Technology" *International Journal of Health Services*, Vol. 4, 1974, p.325. See also, Feldstain, M. and Taylor, A. *The Rapid Rise of Hospital Costs*, President's Council of Wage and Price Stability, 1977. Waldman, S. *The Effect of Changing Technology on Hospital Costs* USDHEW, Pub#72-11701, US Government Printing Office, Washington DC 1972. Office of Technology Assessment, *Intensive Care Units (ICUs) - Clinical Outcomes, Costs, and Decisionmaking*. Pub No. BP-HCS-28, GPO Washington DC 1984.

32 Chalmers, I. and Richards, M. "Intervention and Causal Inference in Obstetric Practice", in Chard T. and Richards, M. (eds) *Benefits and Hazards of the New Obstetrics*, Heinemann Books, London 1977. Banta, D. and Thacker, S. "Assessing the Costs and Benefits of Electronic Fetal Monitoring" *Obstetrical and Gynecological Survey*, Vol.34, 1979, p. 627

33 Dowling, H. *Medicines for Man*, A.A. Knopf, New York, NY 1970

Chapter 12
HOSPITAL MARKETS

The hospital, as we know it today, is a relatively young entity; it is less than a hundred years old. Its evolution, as traced in the next section of this chapter, has gone through various stages, both functionally and financially. Today, many hospitals possess a concentration of technology and equipment which, along with the various forms of collaboration with physicians (also to be discussed later in the volume), constitutes the nucleus of medical care in their communities and even the region of the country.

Evolution of the Hospital

During the 19th century, hospitals were nonmedical institutions, caring not for the sick but for the outcasts of society and the very poor. They were essentially shelters for the unprivileged, the poor, the homeless. Medicine, such as it was, was practiced by physicians largely within people's homes, for the those who could afford it[1] Thus, not being able to treat the body, hospitals attempted to treat the soul, the mind, and morality. Privately run hospitals of the last century were financed by public contributions, with municipal hospitals also getting some tax revenues. All hospitals relied on charities, particularly for funding from the church.

The end of the 19th century and the beginning of the 20th witnessed the emergence of the more modern hospital, increasingly implementing medical care, as we tend to perceive it today. This hospital development was generated by three main groups of factors. First, the increasing acceptance of the physiologically based, *bacterial organism caused, view of disease* [initially enunciated by Louis Pasteur in 1870]. This, in turn, spurred the development of various drugs, particularly antitoxins (the predecessors of modern antibiotics) [2]. The application of drugs, due to poorly researched and often fatal side effects, in turn, precipitated the arrival of drug regulation. Thus, the death of several children as a result of the administration of contaminated diphtheria antitoxins provoked the passing of the Biologics Control Act of 1902[3]. The increasing acceptance of the bacterial based disease theory brought about the establishment of clinical laboratories, mostly within hospitals, and increased their recognition as indispensable for the practice of effective, scientifically based, diagnostic medicine. Other similar developments at about this time, such as the introduction of general anesthesia by way of ether, facilitated therapeutic medicine by way of surgery, although the incidence of infections remained very high because of the slow acceptance of antiseptics and various disinfectants.

A second major factor contributing to hospital development, particularly in the field of diagnostics, is *technological*. X-ray was introduced around the turn of the century, improving diagnostic techniques. Since, at least initially, they were acquired, and maintained, at hospitals, X-rays contributed to the concentration of diagnostic and technological capital equipment at those institutions, increasing the hospital's importance in medical practice, and the need to support them. The third factor contributing to the development of the modern hospital was *demographical*, namely, the increase in the number of people who moved to the cities for career opportunities. When ill, these people were treated not in the traditional home environment, but only in hospitals. Thus, the hospital was transformed from an institution caring for the homeless, to one that administered medical care, in an improved technological and transportation environment, to the middle-class [2]. As the hospital became the scene of care for the masses of the middle class, instead of primarily for the indigent, its position in the medical care market, particularly from an economic point of view, increased correspondingly. The need and source of financing has also changed. The hospital, and hospital based physicians, became a competitors to care alternatives outside the hospital. Private donations began to wither. The market responded with the opening of some private hospitals under physician operation and ownership. In response, public hospitals opened wings caring for the middle class of paying patients. Hospitals began marketing their efforts and care toward the paying patient. In 1917

Massachusetts General (Boston) opened a branch designed rather luxuriously to accommodate paying patients, with similar efforts noted on the part of major new York hospitals[4].

An initial form of health *insurance*, by way of workmen's compensation, first introduced in Massachusetts back in 1911, also contributed to the changing financial scene at hospitals. Instead being a matter of charity, the state, in fulfilling its obligation to the voters, began to pay for injured workers' hospital care, although, at least initially, not for the services of attending doctors. Furthermore, as the market for insured care increased, hospitals found themselves in the position to replace charity with insurance as their main source of income. This, in turn, shifted the position of political power away from the trustees, whose earlier role in procuring philanthropy was critical, to physicians in the position to draw patients to the hospital. *Doctors* became the center of hospital power structure[5]. This brought about an integration between major hospitals and medical education; in the past, the latter was largely independent of the former. With the emphases of medical training shifting to science and clinical training, and to the utilization of laboratory based tests, collaboration between medical schools and hospitals became a focus of medical education. By 1910, with the Flexner Report concentrating on related issues, the predecessors of the modern teaching hospitals, and medical internship came into existence[6].

Direct payments from patients became an important source of income for hospitals by the Great Depression of the 1930s. Thus, the onset of the Depression also caused a financial crisis for hospitals, and some sort of insurance program became essential for the industry. The patient's ability to pay their hospital bills had to be increased. As indicated in the previous chapter, the Blue Cross Plans were established under the sponsorship of the American Hospital Association, and, after health insurance became pertinent for collective bargaining, they were also supported by the unions. It is essential to note, however, that Blue Cross plans were not designed to monitor hospital functions, costs, efficiency, or expenses. They were simply meant to facilitate the flow of funds from the patients to hospitals, regardless of the costs of operation. As hospital plants were aging, the Federal Government stepped in, by way of the Hill-Burton Act (1946), to provide funds for facility renewal, under certain conditions, and mainly with the cooperation of states by way of controlling the planning and creation of hospital facilities within their boundaries, and licensing hospitals[7]. In addition, the passage of the Medicare and Medicaid programs received full support from the AHA and Blue Cross.

The Cost of Hospital Care

Hospital planning, necessitated by the Hill-Burton Act, was enhanced by the passage of the 1966 Comprehensive Health Planning Act, only to be replaced by the National Health Planning and Resource Development Act of 1974, establishing a national network of Health System Agencies. The target was to control hospital costs. The means to that end were envisioned by way of *Certificate of Need* (CON) programs, designed to control the expansion, and avoid undue duplication, of hospital facilities. Whether the programs have indeed reduced costs were questioned, particularly since only certain kinds of hospital expenditures, and only over set minimums, were scrutinized, and because of the sizable transaction costs of the program itself[8].

Some significant attempts were made to explain the high rate of increase in hospital costs[9]. It was observed that both the *cost of hospital care*, and its *insurance* covered share, have increased substantially since the Second World War. Between 1950 and 1975, the average per patient-day hospital cost increased from $16 to $152, with public and private insurance covering about half in 1950, and some 88% in 1975. Thus, the patient's direct cost of care increased from $8 in 1950 to only about $18 in 1975. In fact, once adjusted for inflation of about 50% during that same time period, the real direct cost of hospital care to patients hardly rose at all.

Not surprisingly, Feldstein found a close relationship between increases in hospital costs and hospital insurance. Higher hospital costs stimulate demand for hospital insurance, and higher levels of insurance stimulate costs by reducing the direct cost of hospital care to the patient. The important bilateral relationship between insurance and cost is, in terms of the direction of causation, by no means uniform and consistent, with the impact of insurance on costs being substantially greater than that of cost on insurance. The underlying model is based on three basic functional relationships. (a) Demand, as a function of price, for hospital care is negatively slopped, with the price elasticity of demand being very low; the conditions under which patients choose hospital care are not conducive for price shopping, and, in any case, the physician normally chooses the hospital. (b) There may be a functional relationship between hospital costs and the quality of care. The question is: does quality increase with costs? Can all past increases in costs be attributed to quality increases? At least a substantial portion of them must be; hospital profits have not increased enough to account for a major portion of hospital cost increases, nor has the efficiency of hospital operations declined enough to account for the excessive cost increases. Thus, increases in hospital care, in the quality and composition of care, must account for a major portion of cost increases. When combining the two functions, demand for hospital care and the cost of hospital quality, a constraint may be derived by way of a trade-off between the quantity of care (measured by the number of beds) and the quality of care (measured by cost). The physical location of the constraint, the trade-off curve, is directly determined by people's willingness to pay for hospital care, that is, by the demand curve. On that continuous curve, there are an infinitely large number of quantity-quality combinations available, at least in theory. However, they are not sufficient to determine the ultimate quantity of social choice for hospital care. (c) The third function, giving expression to the preferences of the hospitals themselves, will ultimately provide society with a specific point on the trade-off curve. The three function model allows hospitals to decide on the number of beds and the quantity of care provided. If hospital insurance increases, the demand curve for care shifts to the right, causing an outward shift in the quantity-quality trade-off curve, correspondingly raising the trade-offs. Thus, an increase in hospital insurance increases both the quality and quantity of hospital care, that is, the number of hospital beds and their cost. The impact of insurance on costs and quality, via the shift of the demand curve, could be traced because of the existence of some, though not high, price elasticity of demand for hospital care. As insurance coverage increases, the direct cost of hospital care to the patient decreases, causing the patient to positively react, at least to some extent, to the lower effective price of care [9, p.187]. Patients react to their net (direct) cost of care, and not to the total cost of care, when the burden for most of the latter is born by society as whole. In other words, a large proportion of healthcare, the cost of which being covered by insurance, is viewed by the consumer essentially as a free good, at least to the extent that major portions of deductibles and co-payments do not offset this perception.

Some Elements of Hospital Cost Control

Hospitals are in the position to control at least some of their cost elements. A source of excess cost is related to *capacity utilization*, which, in turn, appears to vary directly with hospital size. In fact, occupancy rates ranged from about 40% in the smallest (6-24 bed) rural hospitals to some 80% in large nongovernment urban general hospitals[10]. Although excess capacity tends to concentrate in smaller non-urban hospitals, they still constitute a source of excess costs. A key issue appears to center on the extent to which costs are in fact reduced by eliminating excess capacity appearing in the form of unused beds. Unused beds may consume, under less than optimum plant construction configuration, some resources in the form of heating, electricity, cleaning and maintenance. On the other hand, assignable variable costs, such as nursing services, drugs, food, linen and direct medical support services, are not needed for unused beds. Other fixed cost items, such as diagnostic equipment and the needed maintenance personnel must be retained for sustaining the hospital's functioning. Thus, eliminating some excess capacity, along with a proportionately less number and amount of related cost elements, would necessitate spreading a given level of total costs over a somewhat reduced number of beds, yielding an increase in average total costs.

The increased participation of the government in healthcare finance raises not only financial but also social issues. Governments now channel large amounts of tax dollars into financing hospital operations. For instance, society needs to cope with the difficult question of which surgical procedures (such as electives versus necessities) at hospitals to finance. If this issue is examined within the context of capacity utilization, then the pertinent questions asked extend from what to finance to actually what to perform at all, that is, whether or not hospital capacity should be accorded to some procedures while not to others. From that point, it is only a short jump to raising the issue of whether or not a free society can control individual rights to the extent of controlling personal income disposal for legal purposes.

Government initiated cost controls through peer review functions, such as *PSROs*, later *PROs*, and through the capital expansion program of *CONs* have already been discussed. Hospital compliance with these programs may have, and could likely, contribute to cost control. A source of cost control that appears to be more directly within the hospitals', as well as physician providers', purview is reducing the number of *surgical procedures*. Frequent questions are raised regarding the performance of a number of unnecessary coronary bypass procedures, mastectomies, hysterectomies, particularly in the light of data showing that similar procedures in Britain and Canada, where national health insurance prevails, are performed at a much lower rate[11].

Unnecessary surgery has been defined as any surgical procedure performed for "asymptomatic, nonpathologic, nonthreatening disorders", or, "where no pathologic tissue is removed", or, "where indications are a matter of difference in judgment and opinions among experts", or, to "alleviate endurable or tolerable symptoms", or "outdated, obsolete, or discredited", or, "done primarily for personal gain of the surgeon, wherein the weight of informed opinion would deny any indication to the present"[12]. Unnecessary surgery, itself performed in good faith pursuant to incompetent diagnosis, while possible, is no longer a frequent occurrence in view of the various quality control, accreditation and peer review functions, along with the availability of second and even third opinion options, in existence.

The length of patient *hospital stay* has long been, in the past, a source of major cost elements, although recent trends point to shorter stays. Longer hospital stays were a means available to hospital management to overcome capacity utilization problems. The DRG system of fixed payment per case for Medicare patients eliminated much of the incentive for prolonging patient stay. Besides lengthy stays, another source of hospital costs involved *unnecessary hospital admissions*. A common form of this occurrence was when physicians wanted to perform diagnostic tests for their patients but let the insurance company bear the cost: since insurance company normally do not cover diagnostic tests in an ambulatory environment, doctors would have those tests performed in an inpatient environment, more likely covered by policies. Effective utilization review procedures seem to have reduced the frequency of unnecessary admissions.

Technological progress in medicine gives rise to newer and more effective equipment for diagnosis and treatment. The presence of the newest major item of equipment within a hospital environment, in turn, gives the hospital, and its staff, the prestige necessary to attract the most competent physicians, and patient flow. Hence, the acquisition of the most advanced technology has often been conducted in a competitive environment of its own among hospitals. However, the technological marvels of medicine are very expensive to purchase, as well as to maintain. While they are, although by no means undisputed, of essence for quality care, they substantially contribute to the cost hospital operations. Thus, questions as to how to deal with these costs have often been raised. In particular, the incidence of duplication, and related, presumably unnecessary, costs have been of concern. While theoretically appealing, equipment sharing brought with it other problems that virtually offset the financial advantages of cost sharing[13]. In addition, possessing the most modern equipment, and related medical/surgical programs, such as a well equipped cardiac surgery unit, yields financial and nonpecuniary benefits to the other clinical departments of the hospital not only in terms of prestige, but also in terms of derivative patient flow.

Hospital Categories

The hospital is a major economic and competitive factor on the healthcare scene. Many litigated issues regarding competition, or lack thereof, in healthcare involved hospitals. Let us take a quick look at the major types of hospitals that function in the US today, and, in the next section, at the fundamental organizational structure of hospitals. The most common form of hospital entity is the *general* hospital, often thought of as a short-term (30 days or less) acute care providing institution. While in the past, they were categorized on a functional basis (TB, mental, so forth), today the main dimensions for grouping them include technological factors, such as the ability to perform complex medical procedures with relatively minimum risks. That, in turn, depends on the size of the hospital, patient volume in the specialties, and on the thereby acquired proficiency, competence, and, for cost reasons, efficiency. General hospitals are owned or sponsored by a church, a community, some level of government, a university, physician(s), or other groups of investors. A *community general hospital* is normally a voluntary/nonprofit organization. Its *voluntary* nature emanates from the fact that its development and financial support is arranged voluntarily by private persons, or institutions, instead of the government; it is *nonprofit* because it does not distribute any surplus as profit, and it pays no income or property taxes. Management and policy making responsibility rests with an elected board of trustees. Depending on the size of the community served, range of services provided, and the extent of referrals, a community general hospital may be of any size, teaching or nonteaching. The latter is one with the presence of an approved residency program. This brief description also applies, in general, to *church general hospitals.*

Government (general) hospitals refer to a multitude of government owned and operated institutions designed largely to serve government related personnel. On the *federal* scene, the army, navy, air force have their own hospitals, largely general in nature, although some with a degree of specialization. The Veterans Administration operates a number of largely general hospitals throughout the country. The US Department of Health and Human Services' Indian Health Service operates close to fifty hospitals on reservations, and the US Department of Justice operates healthcare facilities for federal prison inmates. At the *state* level, the most prominent hospitals are usually within the state university system, operated by the university. Others include facilities operated within the penal system, or general hospitals designed to serve the indigent. *Cities and counties* also operate healthcare facilities, traditionally for the indigents, but in recent years, with the infusion of federal moneys into the healthcare system through Medicaid and Medicare, and the increasing role of the private health insurance sector, they started treating private patients. In fact, in major metropolitan centers, they also function as medical school affiliated teaching hospitals of some stature (e.g. Cook County in Chicago, Bellevue in New York, and Boston City).

Proprietary (private), *for profit*, hospitals are investor owned. The investor may be a private person, a group of partners, or a corporation. In recent years, their numbers and size (in terms of beds) have increased to about 15% and 10%, respectively, of nonfederal facilities[14], although, in general, they are still smaller than voluntary nonprofit institutions. Some of the corporate owned proprietary hospital firms are quite large. They own, or manage, general and specialized institutions in the US, and even abroad. For instance, the Hospital Corporation of America (Nashville, TN.) has, at least in recent years, been operating over 200 hospitals, and Humana Inc.(Louisville Ky) close to 100[15]. Efforts were made to contrast nonprofit with investors owned institutions in terms of the quality of care provided, efficiency and cost of operation. The self-proclaimed virtues of for-profit hospitals, in contrast to nonprofits, included quality care along with efficiency, low cost, and a positive profit. Nonprofits attribute any success of investor owned institutions in this regard to the latter's smaller size and the generally simpler cases they take on, allowing them to keep their costs down, while voluntary hospitals take on the major high-cost patients. Empirical studies appear to indicate no marked difference in efficiency between the two hospital types, in fact, for directly paying patients, for-profits tend to be more expensive. If investor owned hospitals generated higher profits for their owners, it was because of their higher charges rather than higher efficiency. It was found that for-profit hospitals administered more tests and traditionally used more supplies, at a higher price, per admission than did voluntary healthcare institutions[16].

Hospital Organization and Management

A typical hospital has a fundamental policy setting governing board ("Board of Trustees") that also retains a hospital administrator and other key administrative and medical personnel. The generic term, "hospital administrator", applies to the top administrative person under the Board; often designated as "president", "CEO", "executive director", or, in mental hospitals, the "superintendent". The medical staff, while ultimately accountable to the Board, functionally responds to the Administrator. The largest medical personnel in the hospital, nursing, works under the immediate supervision of the medical personnel, although ultimately answers to the administrator. A lack of managerial clarity, and, in particular, of a corporate style management system in hospitals, has given rise in the past to damaging intra-hospital rivalries within the administrative channels, within medical personnel, and between the administrative and medical channels of managerial communications (in addition to the time honored conflicts between the nursing and medical staffs). The trend in solution, particularly motivated by increased financial constraints by some competition and the increased role of government in hospital finances, is toward the corporate style hospital management systems. Thus, physicians are often appointed to Boards, the administrator is the President, and hospitals establish profit-making affiliates (e.g. free-standing clinics, surgi-centers, emergi-centers, medical office complexes), which turn "donate" the profits to "nonprofit" hospitals. Furthermore, the frequent mergers and acquisitions in the hospital industry of the past decade prompted hospital management to develop multi-unit management systems to accommodate expansion, particularly by way of diversification.

A physician, once admitted, may use the hospital's facilities by way of one of several levels of privileges. The scope ranges through "active medical staff", "associate medical staff", "courtesy medical staff", and "consulting medical staff", designating a downward graduated intensity of staff privileges from the first category to the last one. The medical staff in headed by a "chief of staff", or "medical director", with direct line responsibilities to the Board. Depending on the size (in terms bed count) of the hospital, the medical staff functions in specialized departments, with the number and functional diversity of these departments varying directly with increases in the absolute size and patient mix of the institution. In addition, recent years witnessed the increased significance of hospital related ambulatory (one day service) care facilities, such as emergency room services, and outpatient clinics. In most major medical institutions, the diagnostic and clinical departments are supported by service departments, such as pathology, radiology, and anesthesiology, with a full-time salaried staff. Additional support services include nursing, medical records, pharmacy, dietary, various therapeutics, and medical social work. Finally, recent cost considerations prompted hospitals to share laundry, supply procurement, and other non-medical functions with other institutions[17].

Hospital Regulation

While hospitals are fundamentally state licensed organizations, most states' direct regulatory function does not extend beyond controlling the physical dimensions of hospital operation, particularly by way of the Certificate of Need Programs. In general, states do not directly involve themselves with the hospitals' quality of care related issues. Much of that function is performed by the *Joint Commission on Accreditation of Hospitals* (JCAH), a private not-for-profit corporation, founded initially as a joint effort of the American College of Physicians, American College of Surgeons, the AHA and AMA. The JCAH responds to the hospital's *voluntary* request to be reviewed, pursuant to a very important self-evaluation, in terms of its individual and particular functions as to performance level.

The norm is "optimal achievable standards of quality of care and services"[18]. While its determination *per se* is not tantamount to licensing or certification, the JCAH's report is often relied upon by licensing and regulatory agencies, insurance companies and even Medicare in response to payment claims, professionals seeking employment, and individuals seeking care. The evaluation is conducted by a JCAH recruited survey team of several people, including a physician, a nurse, and an administrator, and is culminated by a report to the Accreditation Committee of the JCAH Board of Commissioners. The accreditation is granted for three years.

The work of the JCAH has been subject to criticism. The main one appears to be based on the sponsorship of JCAH by the medical organizations themselves, such as the AMA and the AHA, which may not view a serious quality enforcement effort in the interest of its members. In fact, at one point a government study found that some 65% of the accredited hospitals did not meet Medicare reimbursement conditions[19].

Hospital utilization performance has been monitored by the *Commission on Professional and Hospital Activities* (CPHA), established in 1955, and, once again, sponsored by the medical associations such as the American College of Physicians, American College of Surgeons, and the AHA. It has been preparing periodic utilization reports to hospitals, based on a review of in-house hospital patient records. This effort, along with another major one, *Hospital Utilization Project* (HUP), was designed to deal with frequent state insurance commissioner complaints regarding unnecessary hospital utilization, and related excessive costs which the then dominant Blue Cross programs (originally, also founded by the AHA) unscrutinizing covered.

With the influx of government funds into the healthcare delivery system, particularly through the Medicare and Medicaid programs, resulting in substantial and perennial increases in healthcare costs, government mandated utilization programs were initiated. A 1971 amendment to the Social Security Act brought about the *Professional Standards Review Organizations* (PSROs), to oversee that Medicare and Medicaid payments were made for services that were necessary, of adequate quality, provided at reasonable costs, that is to "limit the cost of care while assuring the proper quality of care"[20]. Due to Congressional dissatisfaction with their performance, in 1981 the PSROs were replaced with the presently functioning *Professional Review Organizations* (PRO), aimed at a more vigorous implementation of cost and quality control efforts.

It is further pertinent to note that, after having enjoyed an exemption until then, as of 1967, the healthcare industry became subject to the provisions of the *Fair Labor Standards Act*, subjecting it to the legal minimum hourly wage constraints. In addition, as of 1974, Congress subjected hospitals to the provisions of the *Taft-Hartley Act* which empowers the *National Labor Relations Board* (NLRB) to investigate and adjudicate employers, or unions, for alleged unfair labor practices, thus leading to increased unionization in the healthcare sector. It is fair to say, that while Congress has, at least during the past four decades, attempted to control healthcare costs via the various control methods we just discussed, these latter two Congressional Acts may have clearly contributed to substantial increases in those costs.

There are other Congressional Acts which can also be viewed as contributing to spiraling healthcare costs, although the quantitative dimensions of their contribution are by no means clear. These include the Equal Employment Opportunity Laws (Title VII of the Civil Rights Act of 1964, The Equal Pay Act of 1963, and other related statutes) that increased the size of employee record keeping; The Federal Unemployment Compensation Amendment of 1970 providing coverage for hospital employees; The Employee Retirement Income Security Act of 1974 which increased benefits cost to hospitals; Occupational Safety and Health Act of 1970; and, Life Safety Code (1973) requirements under titles XVIII and XIX of the Social Security Act. It is doubtful that the complex task of ascertaining and resolving the causes of healthcare cost spiraling during the past two decades or so can be reliably completed unless some weights can be given to the transaction costs, compliance and compliance monitoring costs, and other financial consequences of the Congressional Acts themselves.

Hospital Costs in Retrospect

Hospital costs have increased much faster than inflation between 1970 and 1989. In fact, the positive changes in hospital costs were greater than inflation every year during that time period, and peaked out in 1976 at 9% in real terms. Growth in cost per admission also exceeded the rate of inflation, so greater patient volume does not appear to be the only reason for the large increases in hospital cost.

Hospital cost increases were slowed somewhat by the introduction of the Prospective Payment System (DRG) of reimbursements, presumably because it prompted hospitals to function more efficiently than they did under the traditional cost-based reimbursement. Hence, hospital costs, in real terms of average annual rate of increase, grew at a slower rate after 1983: 5% during 1983-89, in contrast to 8%. during 1946-83, although by 1988 the rate of increase reached 7%, suggesting a petering out of DRG's initial impact. The post 1983 cost slow-down was attributed mainly to decreases in hospital capacity, and to shorter stays.

In fact, hospital capacity dropped by 8% between 1983-89, and the average length of hospital stay (ALS) decreased from 7.6 days to 7.1 days par admission in 1986. By the late 1980s, however, ALS began to increase[21]. Hospital costs would have likely declined faster due to reduced capacity and lower ALS if they had not been accompanied by increases in outpatient visits. Many traditionally inpatient, simpler, services were shifted into an outpatient environment. While outpatient visits increased at an average annual rate of 1.1% during 1980-83, it increased at 5.1% per year between 1983 and 1989 [21, p.13].

The impact of hospital input costs may also be noted. Increases in various forms of compensation, wages and fringe benefits, contributed substantially to hospital cost increases. In 1989, 53% of hospital operating costs were made up of labor costs. Along with additional recruitment for newly established outpatient services, the skill level of more complex inpatient care required better educated employees. The need for, and the shortage of, RNs intensified. Inter-hospital competition bid up RN salaries substantially, particularly in major metropolitan areas, further escalating healthcare costs. Thus, while in 1985 the hourly rate for LPNs was 75% of that for RNs, this proportion declined to about 66% by 1989 [USGAO, 1992, p.15]. In addition, nonlabor inputs augmented hospital costs. Increases in the level of technology, meeting CDC precautionary requirements, and the higher cost of prescription drugs, have all contributed to healthcare costs[22].

The impact of medical technology on costs merits further attention. Technological progress in most industries normally yields cost reductions. However, in medicine, particularly in acute care hospital setting, the opposite is true. New medical technology generates new medical services, with correspondingly higher medical costs. It may be argued, however, that the increase in the private pecuniary cost of medicine caused by improved technology is to a large extent, if not entirely, offset by consequent increases in pecuniary and nonpecuniary private and social benefits emanating from the life-improving, even life-saving, medical devices. On the same vain, the cost increase for a particular procedure over, say, a twenty-five year period would include the higher cost of inputs utilized in the procedure as practiced at the beginning of the time period, plus the sum of marginal costs associated with the incrementally improved methods and equipment utilized by the end of the time period.

Hospitals use technology as a tool for competition with other hospitals. With price competition being of secondary importance, hospitals attempt to attract new patients by way of attracting new staff, or attending, physicians along with their patients. The latter, in turn, are attracted by new equipment, the most modern physical facilities, and new services, yielding increasing costs for hospitals, and for the entire healthcare scene.

Medical malpractice liability is normally assessed by the courts in terms of whether the provider has utilized or applied medical care of at least conventional standard for the community. That standard often includes the most modern methods of care, requiring the latest diagnostic techniques and equipment. Furthermore, in case of malpractice liability claims, medical charts indicating that all pertinent tests and procedures were performed, with the most modern equipment ("defensive medicine" - to be discussed more extensively in chapter 15), may often mean the difference between a plaintiff and defendant's verdict. Thus, while the direct cost of medical malpractice premiums constitutes a small proportion of hospital operating costs, substantial indirect costs may be attributed to the practice of defensive medicine. However, the line between what is clearly "defensive" medicine and what could be viewed as merely prudent medicine is rather fine, unclear, and difficult to delineate. Thus, it may be argued that at least some of the additional private costs associated with the practice of so called "defensive medicine" are offset by the private and social benefits generated by the beneficial results that can be attributed to prudence, rather than defense.

Finally, third-party payer systems likely have an impact on hospital capital expenditures. If the reimbursement is cost based, as has long been the case for capital expenditures even under Medicare until 1991, hospitals have little incentive to control investments in the most modern equipment and methods of treatment. Some states attempted to control capital investment projects by Certificate of Needs programs (CONs), but only major ones. This was discussed earlier.

References

1   Rosenberg, C.E. "And Health the Sick: The Hospital and Patient in 19th Century America" *Journal of Social History*, Vol. 10, 1977, pp.483-97. Also see Rosenberg, "The Therapeutic Revolution: Medicine, meaning, and Social Change in Nineteenth Century America" in Vogel M.J. and Rosenberg (eds) *The Therapeutic Revolution: Essays in the History of American Medicine*, University of Pennsylvania Press, Phila. PA. 1979].

2   Vogel. M.J. *The Invention of the Modern Hospital: Boston, 1870-1930*, University of Chicago Press, Chicago, IL 1980, pp.97-119.

3   Kondratas, R.A. "The Biologics Control Act of 1902" in *The Early Years of Federal Food and Drug Control*, American Institute of the History of Pharmacy, Madison WI, 1982

4   Rosner, D. *Once Charitable Enterprise: Hospitals and Medical Care in Brooklyn and New York, 1885-1915*, Cambridge University Press, New York, NY 1982, pp.77-80

5   Starr, P. *The Social Transformation of American Medicine*, Basic Books, New York, 1982, pp. 161-62. See also Rosner, pp. 103-108, and Stevens, R. "A Poor Sort of Memory: Voluntary Hospitals and Government Before Depression" *Milbank Memorial Fund Quarterly*, Vol. 60, 1982, pp.551-84

6   Ludmere, K.M. "Reform at Harvard Medical School, 1869-1909" *Bulletin of the History of Medicine*, Vol. 55, 1980, pp.343-70

7   Lave, J. and Lave L. B. *The Hospital Construction Act: An Evaluation of the Hill-Burton Program*, 1948-73, American Enterprise Institute, Washington DC 1974, p.13. Also see, Somers, A.R. *Hospital Regulation: The Dilemma of Public Policy*, Princeton University Press, Princeton, N.J. 1969, p.105

8   Schwartz, W.B. and Joskow. P.L. "Duplicated Hospital Facilities - How Much Can We Save by Consolidating Them", *New England Journal of Medicine*, Vol. 303, 1980, pp.1449-57. See also, Salkever, D.C. and Bice, T.W. The Impact of Certificate-of-Need Controls on Hospital Investment", *Milbank Memorial Fund Quarterly*, Vol. 54, 1976, pp.185-214, and Joskow, P.L. *Controlling Hospital Costs: The Role Government Regulation*, MIT Press, Cambridge, MA 1981.

9   Feldstein, M. S. *The Rising Cost of Hospital Care*, Information Resources Press, Washington DC. 1971. See also *Hospital Costs and Health Insurance*, Harvard University Press, Cambridge MA 1981

10 AHA, *Hospital Statistics*, Chicago, 1990

11 Bunker, J.P. Barnes, B.A. and Mosteller, F. Costs, Risks and Benefits of Surgery, *Oxford University Press*, New York, NY 1977. Also see, Dyck, F.J. "Effect of Surveillance on the Number of Hysterectomies in the Province of Saskatchewan" *The New England Journal of Medicine*, Vol 296, 1977

12 Barcklay, W.R. "Unnecessary Surgery", *JAMA*, Vol. 236, 1976, pp. 387-88

13 Brust, J.C. Taylor, D. et. al. Failure of CT Sharing a Large Municipal Hospital" *The New England Journal of Medicine*, Vol. 304, 1981. See also, Schwartz, W.B. and Joskow, P.L. "Duplicated Hospital Facilities: How Much Can we Save by Consolidating Them?" *The New England Journal of Medicine*, Vol. 303, 1980].

14 American Hospital Association, *Guide to the Healthcare Field*, 1990

15 Federation of American Hospitals, *Directory*, Washington, DC. 1990

16 Lewin, L.S. Derzon, R.A. Margulies, R. "Investor Owned and Nonprofits Differ in Economic Performance" *Hospitals*, July 1, 1981. Also see Pattison and Katz, H.M. "Investor Owned and Nonprofit Hospitals" *The New England Journal of Medicine*, Vol. 309, 1983, pp. 370-2, and Relman, A.S. "Investor Owned Hospitals and Healthcare Costs" *The New England Journal of Medicine*, Vol. 309, 1983, pp.370-2.

17 Harris, J. "The Internal Organization of Hospitals: Some Economic Implications" *The Bell Journal of Economics*, Vol. 8, 1977, pp.476-82

18 JCHA, *Joint Commission on Accreditation of Hospitals*, Chicago, IL. 1976

19 Comptroller General of the United States, General Accounting Office. *Report to Congress: The Medicare Hospital Certification System Needs Reform*. HRD 79-37, Washington DC 1979

20 USHHS, *Professional Standards Review Organization 1979 Program Evaluation*. Healthcare Financing Research Report No. 03041, Washington DC 1980, p.ii

21 US General Accounting Office, *Hospital Costs*, September 1992, pp.10-15

22 Ashby J.L., Jr. and Lisk, C.K. "Why Do Hospital Costs Continue to Increase", *Health Affairs*, Summer 1992, pp. 134-47

Chapter 13
PRICING HOSPITAL SERVICES

In view of the perennial concern for the cost of healthcare, it should be noted that the largest expenditure component still goes to the hospital sector, in particular to short-term general hospitals. The prospective reimbursement (DRG) schemes initiated for Medicare and Medicaid patients, and discussed earlier, were designed to cope with cost increases in this sector of the healthcare industry. Another method envisioned to control costs in the hospital sector was through promoting competition. Thus, hospitals were encouraged to join preferred provider organizations (to be discussed later in this Part) in order to foster price competition: physicians and hospitals individually contract, on a discounted fee-for-service basis with third party payers and employers to provide comprehensive care to participating patients[1]

In a standard market environment, an important, often the most important, competitive variable is price. Because of the nonstandard complexities of the healthcare product, and of the environment in which it is produced and distributed, the study of pricing in the hospital sector, in contrast to standard product or service markets, is fraught with analytical problems. These problems are compounded by the fact that the sector is substantially populated by *not-for-profit* institutions, whose prescribed conduct is not in line with the *dicta* of neo-classical price theory. As indicated earlier, nonprofits do not distribute excess earnings to the owners (whether public or private), and they are not taxed. Thus, while members of the growing for-profit hospital sector may at least be assumed to maximize profits, there are some questions as to the operating motives of nonprofits. Their behavior has been viewed as rational in terms of output maximization, administrators' utility maximization, quality maximization, and the utility maximization of the trustees and even of the physicians with staff privileges (we will look at these at some detail in this chapter). Further complications are inserted into the pricing analysis of hospitals by the predominant presence of third-party payers on the entire hospital scene. Medicare reimburses based on DRGs. Medicaid pays on a state-by-state basis. Blue Cross pays on costs, minus a discount if market share permits. Commercial insurers pay on reasonable charges. Thus, pricing may be manipulated among third-party payer alternatives so as to maximize patient revenue. Prior to the introduction of the DRGs, Medicaid patients were subsidized by commercial insurers by way of well documented "cost shifting" mechanisms. Similar cost shifting occurs today between *fixed rate* third-party payers, and indigent nonpayers, on the one hand, and *flexible rate* third-party payers, direct out-of-pocket payers, or self-insured payers, on the other hand, clearly on the expense of the latter categories. All of the above must be viewed in addition to some standard pricing issues that may apply to hospitals, such as price discrimination among intra-hospital departments with significantly varying price elasticities, or by hospital service category with substantial monopoly power within the relevant markets[2].

Hospital Pricing Theories

The multitude of dimensions, possibilities, and uncertainties in hospital pricing behavior gave rise to a number of pricing models. Given the historical dominance of nonprofits on the hospital scene, and, at least in principle, the inapplicability of profit maximizing behavior to them, alternative theories as to the target of their "rational behavior" were developed.

Some of the earlier models concentrated on *output maximization* as a possible nonprofit operating target. It was assumed that hospitals would price increase patient load as much as they could subject to an operating deficit or break-even constraint, with the former covered by government subsidies or donations[3]. Another group of models hypothesized pricing at what the market would bear, that is, *elasticity based pricing*, both at single product (with price lowered to attract additional patients to the breakeven point level), and at multiple product (with elasticity based system of third degree price discrimination financing cross subsidization) institutions[4].

Another group of nonprofit pricing models was based on the notion of *quality maximization*, or quantity maximization subject to quality constraints. Quality proxies included staff-patient and equipment-patient ratios. Since increased quality would increase patient flow as well as costs, the quantity-quality maximizing institution would ultimately serve fewer patients than the quantity maximizing one, yielding a quality-quantity trade-off. The choice of exact location on the quality-quantity constraint line would be a presumably nonarbitrary administrative one, since the administrator will want to maximize his total utility. Since donations are attracted by quality instead of quantity, the administrative choice is more likely to serve the utility maximization goal of the administrator than that of society; quantity and efficiency would be sacrificed in favor of higher quality[5]. A similar model, discussed in Chapter 12, was developed by Feldstein.

Another, *net revenue maximization,* model postulated that administrator utility maximization is a function of the hospital's prestige, which depends on the quality of equipment and the number and quality of affiliated physicians. The latter, in turn, depends on the former, and the former on the amount of net revenues available for equipment acquisition[6]. All of the above, particularly the quality and prestige of medical staff, contribute to the ultimate volume of patient flow through the hospital. In a profit maximizing setting, the neoclassical model would suggest new equipment acquisitions up to the point where the marginal cost of the newly acquired equipment reaches the marginal revenue yielded by it.

Yet another model envisions a nonprofit hospital as a *physician's cooperative*, and emphasizes the physician's role it its governance. Instead of an institutional target variable, rational behavior entails the maximization of the physicians' average income[7]. Hospitals would simply attempt to break even, including any donations. *Utility maximization* models centered on rational behavior by hospital administrators, specifically attaining optimal levels of personal satisfaction, income, prestige, office comfort, and power. These in turn were a function of the quality and moderness of hospital equipment which, as we noted earlier, drew quality medical staff, yielding higher patient flow and increased hospital size, completing the utility maximization circle back to the administrator's higher indifference curve[8.]

Perhaps the most pervasive theoretical view of the nonprofits' pricing policy is reflected by the *break-even model* that postulates pricing at the average total cost level. In practice, this translated into varying markups above costs depending on the elasticity of service demand, with prices being closer to costs for better understood and more discernible services such as room and board, and higher for less measurable services such as laboratory and radiology[9].

Hospital Pricing Practices and Constraints

Prior to 1965, the enactment of the Medicare and Medicaid programs, hospital pricing practices centered on all inclusive per diem rates (covering all services rendered to the patient), modified per diem rates (per diem rates adjusted for the severity of cases), and so called "a la carte" rates (matching charges to the specific case). The latter were preponderant just before the commencement of the so called retrospective payment system in 1965, brought in with the Medicare and Medicaid programs. Between 1965 and 1982 (the year when prospective payment systems were initiated for Medicare and Medicaid patients), the emphases were placed on establishing cost bases for reimbursement.

The *pre-1982* government payment system was based on incurred costs, as determined by the hospital. Any reasonable cost would be reimbursed. Thus, hospitals engaged in cost and utilization maximization efforts, particularly through increasing their older patient census. Sharply increased costs, necessitating correspondingly increased reimbursements, in turn, prompted the government to begin to clamp down. Cost control measures were implemented (limiting routine services and capital expenditures, and program utilization reviews - see our earlier discussion). Hospitals alleged the existence of unreimbursed costs, and began to shift those costs to non-reimbursed fee-for-service patients with commercial, Blue Cross, or self-insurance. The pre-1982 cost frenzy was also made possible by a lack of an adequate number of alternative delivery systems, and the absence of large employer based purchasing power.

Since 1983, with the enactment of the DRG based Prospective Pricing System (PPS), hospitals are reimbursed for Medicare patients by the government on a case category determined discharge basis, and by commercial insurers on a negotiated flat per diem rate or discounted charge basis. However, in spite of the predetermined case based reimbursement rate, hospital discretionary price determination is still called for in some areas. Thus, hospital pricing is still fundamental in setting many categories of Medicare Part B (ambulatory care) reimbursements. This becomes particularly significant since the stringent application of DRGs to inpatient care has prompted increased transfers of that care into more ambulatory outpatient environments. Since Medicaid reimbursements are normally not to exceed Medicare levels, pricing in the former category is largely congruent with Medicare.

Other pricing constraints emanate from states, Blue Cross Plans, Commercial Insurance Vendors, major employer coalitions, Alternative Delivery Systems, and direct competition from Physicians. *State* operated pricing and revenue control agencies. Operating much like public service commissions, they set patient service revenue ceilings, rates of increases, and hospital utilization goals. A notable exception is New Jersey. Exempt from Medicare's PPS provisions, the State has an all-payer state specific DRG-based one price system. With no opportunity to manipulate revenue sources, New Jersey hospitals are constrained to concentrate on costs. The dominant market power of *Blue Cross* plans, secured largely through early entrance into the field, places a constraint on hospital pricing practices. Operating a large variety of plans, including Preferred Provider(PPOs) and Health Maintenance Organizations (HMOs), and often functioning as a Medicare intermediary, Blue Cross has attained considerable success in discount contracting with hospitals to whom the plans supply a major proportion of patient flow. *Commercial* sources of health insurance, often targets of cost shifting, have also been parting with fee-for-service and charge-based payment systems in favor of HMO and PPO types of arrangement. *Employer coalition* of a group of smaller firms together constitute purchasing market power that may yield desirable results in terms of reduced costs by way of direct discount contracting with providers or through sponsoring alternative delivery systems, such as HMOs and PPOs. Finally, *physicians* have been attempting to increase their income, hence competition to hospitals, by performing ambulatory functions (through minor surgical procedures, walk-in clinics, and emergency centers) that, in the past, were performed exclusively by hospitals.

Strategic Pricing

While traditionally hospital marketing efforts were largely inpatient volume and composition oriented, modern healthcare marketing efforts also target pricing for inpatient and ambulatory care. Standard competitive considerations, applied to the hospital sector, include rivalry among existing competitors, potential entrants with substitute services (such as emergi centers with ambulatory surgery facilities), buyers' market power (e.g. employer coalitions), the physician supply sector bargaining power, market power on the part of other suppliers, and competition from substitutes[10].

In view of these competitive dimensions, a hospital may have at its disposal a number of pricing strategies, depending upon its objectives within the market in relation to competitors, and in relation to the service/ product itself. One or more of these pricing strategies may replace traditional hospital-wide pricing techniques. These traditional policies often involved across the board uniform average cost markups, preventing the utilization of market dictated cross-subsidization opportunities, such as allowing lucrative high markup reconstructive surgery subsidizing less profitable preventive procedures; or, with negative results, they prevented the implementation of product target price policies such as aggressive new product introduction, or the closing of less popular product lines by excessive markups.

Without changing product character, a hospital, with zero market share, may engage in aggressive short-run *predatory pricing* aimed at market penetration and quick growth potentials. Once the market is successfully penetrated, market share may be increased or solidified by substantial *long-run price reductions*, along with improved product image promotion. On other hand, if the product has not gained market acceptance, it may be closed out with *phase-out pricing*. If a service, or group of services, is perceived to be of unusually high quality (e.g.the Mayo Clinic), with correspondingly low price elasticities of demand, long-run *premium pricing* will allow the institution to attract a steady flow of well financed patients. In other instances, sliding scale *price discrimination* may allow the hospital to extract maximum income from various social groups, in the same time performing a social service for the poor; for instance, preventive prostate cancer checks may be administered and charged for in different communities in accordance with prevailing socio-economic status, provided that a limited form of service arbitrage (members of the high price community consuming in low price regions) can be prevented. Finally, without meaning to imply the absence of other pricing schemes, a hospital may engage in *loss leadership*, charging barely above average cost for some services if the practice will yield an increased patient flow for the hospital in other areas; e.g. underpriced neonatal services may attract adult relatives into the hospital to procure other care.

Major Hospital Income Sources

Hospital revenue sources in general fall into two major categories: (a) private insurance such as Blue Cross, HMOs, and commercial intermediation, as well as self-insured programs and out-of-pocket coverage; (b) Public plans such as Medicare, Medicaid, Workers' Compensation, and other government based plans. The proportion of private sourced patients dropped between 1979 and 1990 from about 19 million (52%) to 12 million (39%). The corresponding public coverage was 15 million (40%) in 1979, having increased to over 15 million (49%) by 1990. Thus, there appears to be some shift of the healthcare burden from the private to the public sector, possibly due to the increasing proportion of the patient population reaching Medicare age. There were some 3 million self-paying patients both in 1979 and 1990, but with an increased corresponding proportion from 7% to 9%, respectively[11].

Similar declines were registered in terms of the number of patient days, instead of patients. Some 43% of all days care was covered by private insurance in 1979, while 30% in 1990. While there was also a decrease in the number of publicly funded patient days from 1979 through 1990 (135 million to 120 million, respectively), the corresponding proportions increased from 51% to 60%. PPS installed DRG Medicare payment system was often thought of as a catalyst for increasing patient turnover, and reducing the length of hospital stays; yet, publicly funded patients had consistently longer average lengths of stays (ALS) than privately funded ones (7.8 days versus 4.9), although the ALS for both decreased between 1979 and 1990. Once again, this may be attributed to the increased Medicare intensity of the patient population [11, p.3].

In terms of patient characteristics, private insurance accounted for at least half of the under-65 patient population, and some 90% of the over-65 population was financed by medicare in 1990. Medicaid was found more prevalent among those under age 45 than those over that age. In terms of gender, some 50% more female patients used Medicaid than male. Based on race, over 40% of white patients used private insurance, while only 29% of blacks, in 1990. During the same year some 38% of whites, but only 24% of blacks, used Medicare. On the other hand, Medicaid was used by three times as many blacks as whites in 1990 [11, p.3].

Finally, in terms of inpatient procedure utilization, private insurance covered some 41% in 1990 for both sexes, 37% for males and 44% for females. For the overall 45-64 age group, private insurance financed almost two-thirds of all procedures performed. Medicare covered some 33% of all procedures in 1990, and 41% for males, while 29% for females. Once again, the high Medicare intensity of patient population is indicated by 90% of all procedures performed on those over age 65 having been covered by Medicare [CDC, 1992, p.4-5]. Medicaid covered 11% of inpatient procedures in 1990, with some 25% of the procedures performed on patients under age 15. Among specific surgical procedures, some 70% of the often controversial hysterectomies, and about half of obstetrical procedures, were covered by private insurance. Medicare covered some 30% of all surgical procedures, but almost 75% of cardiac and prostate related procedures, as would be expected due to pertinent age distribution for these diseases. Medicaid covered no more than about 10% of all surgical procedures, with some obstetrical procedures specifically covered by Medicaid to the extent of about 30% [11, p.5-6].

References

1   American College of Surgeons, *Socioeconomic Factbook of Surgery*, Chicago, 1985

2   Kaitz, E.M. *Pricing Behavior and Cost Behavior in the Hospital Industry*, Prager Publishers, New York, 1968. Also see White, W.D. "Regulating Competition in a Nonprofit Industry: The Problem of For Profit Hospitals", *Inquiry*, Vol. 16, 1979, pp.50-61

3   Klarman, H.E. *The Economics of Health*, Columbia University Press, New York, 1965. Also see Long, M.F. "Efficient Use of Hospitals", in the *Economics of Medical Care*, University of Michigan Press, Ann Arbor, 1964

4   Davis, K. "Economic Theories of Behavior of Nonprofit Provate Hospitals" *Economic and Business Bulletin*, Vol. 24, 1974, pp. 1-13. See also, Rice, R.G. "Analysis of the Hospital as an Economic Organism" *The Modern Hospital*, Vol. 106, 1966, pp. 87-91. Clemens, E.. "Price Discrimination and the Multiple Product Firm" *The Review of Economic Studies*, Vol. 19, 1951, pp. 262-76.

5   Newhouse, J.P. "Toward a Theory of Nonprofit Institutions: An Economic Model of a Hospital" *The American Economic Review*, Vol. 60, 1970, pp.64-74.

6   Davis, K. "Relationship of Hospital Prices to Costs" *Applied Economics*, Vol. 4, 1971

7   Pauly, M. and Redisch, M. "the Not-for-Profit Hospital as a Physicians' Cooperative" *The American Economic Review*, Vol. 63, 1973

8   Reder, M. "Some Problems in the Economics of Hospitals", *The American Economic Review*, Vol. 55, 1965, 472-480. Also see Joseph, H. "On the Interdepartment Pricing for Not-for-Profit Hospitals", *Quarterly Review of Economics and Business*, Vol. 16, 1976, pp.33-44. Lee, M.L. "A Conspicuous Production Theory of Hospital Behavior", *Southern Economic Journal*, Vol. 38, 1971, pp.48-58

9   Ingbar, M.L. and Taylor, L.D. *Hospital Costs in Massachusetts*, Harvard University Press, Cambridge MA, 1968

10 Porter, M. *Competitive Strategy: Techniques for Analyzing Industries and Competitors* Free Press, New York, 1980

11 CDC, National Center for Health Statistics, *Vital and Health Statistics*, #220, November 1992, p. 3-21.

Chapter 14
HEALTHCARE
INTERMEDIATION

People live in the midst of real and perceived risks that pervade their lives. These risks involve persons and property. To mitigate the financial consequences of these risks, insurance policies are purchased. Most people tend to be risk averse. They pay premiums to insurance companies that are, on the average, far in excess of their feared financial loss. On the other hand, people's risk aversion is hard to reconcile with their proclivities to gamble in masses, both in terms of the number of participants and the amount of moneys wagered, in the nation's casinos.

In most instances, the acquisition of insurance coverage has no further direct economic impact on the insured, nor calls for further action on the part of the insured, until, or if, the risk is realized, that is, the feared event occurs. In the medical industry, health insurance coverage seems to generate a *derivative demand* for another product: healthcare. Thus, the insurers and third-party payers in healthcare marketing become *intermediaries* between the ultimate consumers, the patients, and the suppliers/providers, the hospitals and physicians. While health insurance cannot insure against the risk of poor health itself, it entirely (or at least largely) shifts the financial risk from the insured to the healthcare intermediaries, who in turn spread that risk among their customers.

Public and private healthcare intermediaries have evolved in various institutional and ownership forms. At the federal level, Medicare, and Medicaid with state participation, dominated for almost three decades. In the private sector, not for profit organizations, initially sponsored by hospital, medical, and dental associations, have been dominating healthcare intermediation through Blue Cross and Blue Shield, and Delta

Dental plans, with commercial insurers sharing smaller segments of the market. Relatively recently, spurred on by healthcare cost control drives, so called managed healthcare plans gained momentum with, as we shall see later, less than expected positive results for healthcare costs.

The Blues, Commercial Plans and the Cost of Healthcare

Some of the basic institutional elements of the nonprofit Blue plans have already been discussed. Here, I will contrast their competitive role with commercial insurers. In addition to other regulatory exemptions, such as reduced payments to hospitals, the nonprofits normally enjoy freedom from a type of state sales tax ("premium tax"), which is levied on commercial insurers, yielding a distinct competitive advantage. It should also be noted that the Blues have normally covered 100% of the relevant service costs, while the commercials have been applying deductibles and copayments.

While some writers, closely affiliated with the development of the Blue Plans movement, emphasized their designed benefit for society, the benefits of nonprofit status for the Blues have been questioned, particularly in terms of the ultimate distribution of surplus funds. Some experts argued that the Blues have come under physician domination, thus, indirectly, diverting premium generated funds back to providers[1] Others felt that the financial benefits of the nonprofit status finance utility maximization efforts by the Blue Plan administrators themselves[2].

Questions have also been raised as to the competitive impact of the *premium tax*, levied on commercials, but not on the Blues, however, no consensus appear to have emerged. Some writers opined to the effect that the lack of premium tax on the Blues gives them a competitive edge, indicated by their larger market shares[3]. Others could not find a significant relationship between the Blue's larger market share and the premium tax[4].

The Blues' share in the under age 65 healthcare market ranges from at about 50% to, in some geographical markets, as high as 80% (although, some states have no Blue plans at all). This market share leverage has been used to contractually extract discounts from hospitals, although the rationale presented was based upon the Blues' full service benefit system not generating any bad debts for the hospitals, hence not wanting to pay them (self-insured patients and commercial insurers under traditional plans normally pay full price, with partial service coverage). This arrangement, along with the lack of premium tax, presents a potent scenario of the Blues' self-reinforcing economic pricing structure. If the lack of premium tax on the Blues indeed increases their market share, the latter can be used to extract lower contracted hospital prices, yielding lower insured patient premiums, a larger insured patient pool, with the consequent larger market share, and so forth. In fact, even without the tax advantage, the historically sustained larger market share by the Blues could give them the leverage to extract lower hospital costs, generating a similar self-reinforcing power scenario.

It may also be noted that the profit-seeking *commercials*, and mutual insurers, compete, both in terms of price and service output, among themselves. Entry into that sector has traditionally been easy, and concentration relatively low. Their customers are largely employer groups, possessing considerable product information and cost consciousness. The Blue Plans system, on the other hand, is largely void of intra-system competition. Implemented largely through national associations, they function in a cartel like manner in designated geographical areas. Plans that insure hospital expenses (Blue-Cross) are separate from those that insure physicians services (Blue-Shield). Their board of directors has traditionally been dominated by hospitals and physicians.

It was indicated earlier that Blue Plans, with substantial market power, tend to generate more complete insurance, causing a rightward shift in the demand curve, higher care prices, an increased ability on the part of the hospitals to select their patients, along with sophisticated technology, all of which may culminate in higher healthcare costs[5]. However, it was also argued that the Blue Plans' greater market power may also contribute to higher healthcare costs by way of *inefficiencies*[6]. These inefficiencies, relative to commercial and mutual (policy holder owned) insurers, most likely manifest themselves in higher administration costs. Thus, Medicaid claims have been found to be processed by Blue Shield plans by about 40% slower than by commercial insurers, without regard to their market power or extent of physician domination.

Another study found a somewhat indicative but less convincing negative comparison between Blue Cross and commercial performance in terms of Medicare A claim (per bill regardless of size, rather than per dollar) processing[7]. Another investigator found convincing evidence in favor of private sector efficiency by comparing even voluntary Blue

Plans with the then United States Department of Health, Education and Welfare in terms health insurance implementation[8]. This result may be viewed as a powerful omen of costs and inefficiencies that will likely emerge under a national health insurance regime.

Health Maintenance Organizations (HMOs)

The generic predecessors of today's HMOs are by no means new. As so called Prepaid Group Practice Plans, they have been around since the late 1920s (the Ross-Loos Clinic was founded in 1929)[9]. The modern HMO movement appears to have gained momentum in 1973 with the passage of Public Law 93-222, providing funding for HMO development, protection from some state regulatory provisions, and securing market access for the HMOs by requiring employers to make HMO as an option available to their employees[10]. HMOs, in turn, were required to accept community premium rating based on the average of the high and low risk groups, to practice open enrollment without discriminating in favor of low risk groups and against high risk groups, and to prove a minimum set of basic and necessary benefits. These requirements were somewhat relaxed by way of the 1976 Public Law 94-460 in order to prompt an acceleration in HMO growth rates. HMOs continued to benefit from available federal funding and a legislatively secured market, in return for being subjected to federal regulations. A 1978 amendment to the Act provided for construction loans, and managerial training, although the loan programs were discontinued by 1982.

Even before the federal government entered the HMO scene, a number of large prepaid plans were already in existence. Thus, plans like Group Health of Puget Sound, Kaiser Permanente, Health Insurance Plan of Greater New York, and the Harvard Community Health Plan, have been going strong for a number of years. Congressional support implemented during the early 1970s, amounting to some $400 million in less than ten subsequent years, simply increased the momentum of their growth, having also brought in some heavy players, such as Blue Cross, CIGNA, and Prudential, as first time sponsors of HMO plans. In 1985, contracts for Medicare related HMO business were released, giving rise to unprecedented revenue potentials, along with the closer ties to government regulators. The traditional HMO, within the spirit of initial federal HMO regulations, was a nonprofit organization. After the cessation of federal grants to HMOs in 1982, many became profit motivated, and, in fact, publicly owned corporations. For instance, US Health Care of New Jersey and Pennsylvania with over 300,000 members went public in 1983, followed by impressive market performance, at least for a short while.

HMOs models may be grouped into four basic categories. The *staff* model retains physicians as salaried employees [e.g Group Health Cooperative of Puget Sound, Seattle; or ANCHOR Health Plan in Chicago, and Group Health of DC]. The HMO assumes risk for virtually all care, including hospitalization. Primary care is typically provided in an HMO hospital attached multi-specialty clinic setting. As expected, to some extent, with other HMO models, this model was designed to minimize the frequency of hospitalization and the number of surgeries, and emphasize preventive care. In a *group* model, physicians either function in a group practice by way of a partnership or corporate organization that contracts with the HMO ("dual group") [e.g. Kaiser Health Plan with Permanente Clinic physicians, or Peak Health Plan with Colorado Springs Medical Center], or the group creates its own HMO, health or insurance plan, as separate provider products ("single entity group") [Western Clinic in Tacoma, WA.]. The *Independent Practice Association* (IPA) is a legal entity, separate from the HMO itself, that contractually engage practitioners who otherwise function in their own office environment. The traditional pre-1981 IPA version provided physician services to HMOs on a fee-for-service basis by way of contracts. In a more recently developed scenario, promoted since 1981 by the federal office of HMOs (now the Office of Prepaid Group Plans), the IPA maintains and controls its own but separate HMO (e.g. Crossroads IPA in East Orange, N.J.). Both types of IPA generate a holdback risk pool (about 20% of the charges) in order to cover over utilization contingencies; the funds are largely redistributed at year-end if no significant over utilization occurs. In coping with various, from the physicians' point of view, less desirable managed care alternatives, the structure of IPAs allows participating physicians to use that form of organization as a competitive tool against the possible spreading of less desired, group or staff, model HMOs in the region. Indeed, most of the existing IPAs were initiated by local medical societies in order to cope with patient migration to emerging local HMOs.

Finally, a *network* HMO model, often favored by multistate employers, entails prepaid health care delivery by way of franchised partnerships with local providers, staff HMOs, and IPAs, in order to compete with local or regional independent HMOs (e.g. the contract between the Voluntary Hospitals of America, VHA (with its over 500 affiliated institutional providers), and Aetna Life Insurance on the one hand, and the Teamsters on the other, to provide care for some 300,000 union members through a network of HMOs.

The proliferation of IPAs was facilitated by some distinct advantages for the practitioners. There are no large start-up costs involved, as providers continue to practice in the same environment. Furthermore, reimbursement to physicians is more appealing since it is done on a per-unit of service basis. They can endure utilization controls usually without close panels, and benefit from some scale economies without having to practice outside their offices.

Recent HMO Developments

While in 1987, the number of HMOs nationally was 662, largely mergers and acquisitions reduced their number to 550 by December 31, 1991, with a total enrollment of some 38 million people, about 18% of the insured population. Furthermore, the last six years witnessed a 100% increase in HMO enrollment, with 2.2 million having been added in 1991 alone. Of the existing HMOs at the end of 1991, the IPA types dominated the field to extent of some 61% of the total, followed by network, group, and staff models in that order, and in roughly with the same proportion (10%-15%) for the latter three. In terms of enrollment distribution among the four major models, as of December 31, 1991, once again IPAs lead the way with some 46% of the enrollees, followed by group models with about 27%, network with 15%, and staff with some 12%.

The *regional distribution* of HMOs seems to concentrate somewhat in the Midwest with about 30% of the total, followed by the South Atlantic region (15.8%), Pacific (13.8%), Mid Atlantic (12.7%), with rest of the regions following with around 10% or less. New England appears to have the lowest frequency of the national HMO distribution. Yet, in terms of enrollment, the regional distribution appears to present a somewhat different picture, with the Pacific having over 31% of the enrollees, followed by the Midwest (22%), Middle Atlantic (15%), and South Atlantic (12%), and the other regions under 10%, pointing to a regional concentration of the larger HMOs in the Pacific region, and many small ones in the Midwest.

By the end of 1991, over two-thirds of the US HMOs were for-profit organizations, but with roughly equal enrollment proportions. The largest proportion of HMOs (some 58%) were neither Blue Cross/Blue Shield nor commercial insurer affiliated; they were independents. Some 14% were affiliated with Blue Plans, and about 30% with commercials. Some 73% of the enrollees were in independent in HMOs, with only 12.3% in Blue Plan sponsored ones, and the rest with those sponsored by commercial insurers[11].

HMO *market penetration* has substantially increased in 1991. HMO enrolled of populations increased in 36 states during 1991, while dropped in 9 states. Nationally, HMO penetration reached 15.9%, a 1.2 point increase since the end of 1990. The 10 states with the greatest HMO penetration proportions, CA. (32.5%), MN (30.6%), MA (30.6%), AZ (30.1%), OR (26.1%), MD (23.1), RI (22.9%), CO (22.5%), WI (21.9%), and HI (21.5%), also registered increases in 1991. In fact, HMOs enrolled at least 25% of the population in the first five states. The largest enrollment increases were reported in AR (59.8% to a 3.9% penetration level), MT (53.4% to a 1.2% penetration level), AZ (49.5% to the already noted 30.1% penetration), KY (31.7% to a 7.2% penetration level), and LA (25.1 % to a 7.9% penetration level).

In terms of *market structure*, HMOs with more than 100,000 enrollees made up some 18% of the entire HMO industry in 1991, up from 15% in 1990. Some 52% of these were IPA model HMOs. Large group models accounted for about 20% of the biggest plans, while network and staff models accounted for 17% and 11%, respectively of the largest HMO organizations. Over one-third of all HMOs reported at least 50,000 enrollees in 1991, with over 50% of the group models fitting into this category, but only 28% of the IPAs does. Although only 18% of all HMOs had 100,000 members or more in 1991, these very large HMOs accounted for 64% of all HMO enrollees in 1991, a 1 point increase since 1990. The market share of the smallest HMOs (enrollment under 25,000) dropped one point to 8% in 1991, indicating a notable growth in the average size of an HMO on the national scale.

The *age distribution* of HMOs indicates a strong IPA youth bias. Of the IPA models, about half were less than six years old in 1991. Only about 33% of networks and groups, and about 10% of staff models fell into this category in 1991. Yet, entry into the industry does not seem to be gaining momentum. In 1990, only four plans were in the development stage, as were in 1991. Only nine of the existing plans were under two years old in 1991 (contrast with 18 in 1990, and 37 in 1989). Fewer than

65% of all HMOs were more than five years old in 1991, accounting, nevertheless, for over 80% of all HMO enrollees throughout the country. Enrollment in plans less than two years old were kept under 1% of total enrollment, suggesting relatively strong competitive currents in the HMO arena, although, these smaller HMOs represented only 2% of the total number of plans.

The number of *government beneficiaries* among HMO members rose by 13% in 1991, with specifically Medicare members increasing by 15%, Medicaid members by 33%. The number of states having more than 10% of their total HMO enrollees as government beneficiaries rose to 24, or by 4 in 1991, with 12 of them having more than 15%. The largest increase in the number of Medicare beneficiaries enrolled in HMOs was in Florida, registering a 53% increase to almost 300,000 members. California registered the biggest HMO membership increase in Medicaid beneficiaries, over 150%, from about 95,000 to 260,000. The proportion of government enrollees to total HMO membership rose to 13% in 1991, from 12% 1990, with their actual numbers being at about the 5.1 million level. California's HMOs government enrollees of about 1.5 million was the largest in terms of absolute numbers, representing about 15% of the states total HMO enrollment, while the District of Columbia had the highest proportion (28%) of government enrollees, of its total HMO membership. The largest increase (113%) in the number of federal government enrollees was reported by Texas. As indicated earlier, the proportion of government members relative to total membership increased in 24 states, with 13 states experiencing a decline (DC having the greatest decline to 28% in 1991 from 36% in 1990), and 10 states remaining constant[12].

HMO Cost Control by Constrained Utilization

There are several broad methods used by HMOs to restrain hospital utilization. These include physicians practice style, physician behavior constraints, patient incentives, and physician incentives. Specifically, in non-IPA models, these methods involve prior approval for elective admissions, ambulatory care incentives for providers, and annual utilization related bonus schemes[13].

These utilization constraints appeared to have yielded some results. It has been found that HMO patients pay on the average about 25% less for premiums and out-of-pocket expenses than conventionally insured patients do, although the rate of increase in the HMO per-unit cost of service has been about the same as in alternative forms of insurance. The frequency of ambulatory visits appears to be determined mainly by socio-economic backgrounds rather than form of insurance. Since HMOs experience ambulatory visit frequencies similar to those of non-HMO members, much of healthcare cost savings experienced by HMOs are generated by controlled hospitalization rates, some 30% lower than in conventionally insured population segments. The latter is due largely to lower admission rates, with no significant difference in lengths of stay[14]. Arguments to the effect that HMOs offer inferior care do not, thus far, appear to be empirically substantiated[15].

Preferred Provider Organizations (PPOs)

While it exists in many different varieties and under several different sponsorships, a PPO may generically be defined as an arrangement or technique whereby healthcare providers contract to supply services to specified groups of people on a contracted fee-for-service basis. In other words, a PPO integrates health services for sale to bulk purchasers, normally self-funded employers The PPO organizes various types of healthcare providers, such as physicians and hospitals, into "preferred" vendor groups of healthcare services, and, in return for contracted reduced fees, refers its enrollees to them as "preferred (but not required) providers". The group of contracted providers are often referred to as the "provider panel". Thus, the basic difference between a PPO and an HMO is that the latter assumes the actuarial risk of paying for care while the former leaves the risk with the employer or insurer. Like and HMO, a PPO uses utilization control to control costs. However, unlike an HMO's prepaid capitation, per diem, payment or DRG based system, a PPO's payment system is fee-for-service based. In terms of marketing, and in contract to an HMO, a PPO has the advantage of promoting freedom of choice, though usually at a premium outside the provider panel. Normally, the fee-for-service based advantage for the physicians is also accompanied by prompt reimbursements.

The PPO organization may be sponsored by a hospital or a group of hospitals, group of physicians, third-party payers, employee benefit consultants, and any persons with entrepreneurial talents. PPOs sponsored by hospitals often rely on cooperating staff physicians supplemented by nonstaff practitioners, and other institutions to increase the portfolio of services provided under the plan. Physician sponsored PPOs are primary care based plans, often accompanied by the participation of solicited hospitals based on contract which the hospitals themselves make with the payers, or with the PPO itself. Third party sponsored PPOs simply contract with individual and institutional provider groups.

The obvious benefit that providers derive from a PPO is by way of a contractually secured and predictable patient flow. In addition, the initiation of a PPO requires relatively small capital investment, compared to the initial capital requirements of some HMO models. Nor is there a need for large reserves, as the risk remains with the purchaser instead of the provider. The preservation of the fee-for-service environment suits physicians, and the PPO's suitability for hospital-physician joint ventures enhances the opportunity for cooperation between the two provider groups. There are risks as well. While the relatively limited initial investment limits sponsor financial risks, a potential PPO failure compromises future provider credibility with third party payers, bulk purchasers, and particularly with employer groups. Finally, in the case of hospital sponsored PPOs, physicians left out of, or removed from, the panel for any reasons, may cause intra-hospital functional disruptions. Employers can create the incentive to use PPOs by reduced or waived copayments or deductibles. For employees, the available choice between provider panel member and non-member physicians may also be important.

Functionally, a PPO is not unlike an IPA HMO model, except that the PPO does not assume any actuarial risks. The IPA assumes such risks by committing itself to pay all contracted providers for the services they render to the patients, in return for the patients' fixed monthly premium. The PPO avoids actuarial risks by normally contracting with a self-insured employer, where the latter pays the provider (contractually reduced) charges; the PPO merely arranges for a panel of institutional and individual providers who are willing to implement and maintain a utilization control program aimed at reducing the employer's actuarial risk. Thus, a PPO is an intermediary between the purchaser (employer) and the providers. In Part IV, we will examine the competitive implications\of PPOs functioning within the healthcare market place, particularly the manner whereby a PPO arranges pricing among otherwise independent healthcare provider competitors.

Recent PPO Developments

The number of corporate PPOs increased by 2% in 1991, to 584. They operated some 980 individual medical/surgical PPOs, a 19% increase from 1990. Some 36% of PPOs were owned by insurers in 1991, up by two percentage points since 1990. In contrast, 22% of PPOs were owned by investors in 1991, a 5 percentage point increase since 1990. The extent to which wellness programs were offered by PPOs in 1991 has been reduced substantially, 52% in 1990 to 34% of them in 1991. On the other hand, the proportion of PPOs offering of other services has increases from 1990 to 1991, such as psychiatry (67% to 78%), chiropractic (35% to 51%), and dental care (20% to 30%). Exclusive Provider Organizations (EPO), arrangements similar to HMOs, gained popularity in 1991. Only 33% of PPOs offered EPO arrangements in 1989, with 42% in 1990, and 45% in 1991.

The largest forty PPO plans experienced a 19% increase in enrollees, compared with 27% in 1990, with the number of enrollees reaching 12,124,579 in 1991. Blue Cross and Blue Shield plans had in 1991 a 37% share of the forty largest plans' eligible enrollees, and some 12% of all PPO enrollees. US Healthnet owned four among the forty largest PPO plans in 1991, covering some 2.3 million enrollees. Twenty-seven of the largest forty plans experienced enrollment increases, four reported no increases, and five reported decreases. The largest enrollment increase, some 475%, was at the Blue Cross Blue/Shield Preferred Provider Plan in Washington DC. Large increases were also reported by Consumer Health Network, So. Plainfield NJ (250%), First Choice Health Network, Seattle (196%), and Primary Health Services, Chagrin Falls, OH (115%).

The top ten PPOs in 1991 were as follows [enrollment]: USA Healthnet-Network/TX [1,217,431], Blue Cross Prudent Buyer Plan/CA [830,392], Preferred Provider Network/PA [750,000], Community Care Network/CA [626,000], Blue Cross & Blue Shield Preferred Care/AL [600,630], Blue Cross and Blue Shield of Florida/FL [465,649], USA Healthnet-Network/FL [405,043], USA Healthnet-Network/CA [398,470], Participating Provider Option/IL [369,104], and PO Alliance/CA [345,476]. These largest ten represented some 16% of total PPO enrollment in 1991.

Geographically, PPOs could be found in every state, including DC. California, with a total of 104, had the largest number of PPO plans in 1991; Hawaii, with 18, had the fewest. Other heavily endowed PPO states were Texas, 85), Florida (83), Illinois (83), and Pennsylvania

(81). In terms of organization, in 1991 there were 49 corporate PPO chains, operating 679 plans, with 24.7 million enrollees, not including dependents. The Blue Cross/Blue Shield Association members covered some 6.5 million enrollees, or over 25% of the total. Aetna Health Plans of Hartford, CT operated the largest number of plants (113) in 1991, but ranked only eighth in terms of the number of enrollees (784,848). Private Healthcare Systems Ltd of Lexington MA followed with 106 plans enrolling some 861,000 members, and the Blue Cross/Blue Shield Association members with the already indicated 6.5 members enrolled in 60 plans. Each of the 49 largest PPO chains operated in more than one state, and accounted for over two-thirds of total PPO membership. A year earlier, the 35 largest chains operated 568 plans with 57% of total PPO membership, and in 1989 421 [plans with 60% of the membership.

During 1991, a 25% increase in PPO administrative revenues (gross sales) were attained, or some $2.2 million per plan, compared with $1.8 million in 1990. The older PPOs, established before 1989, showed a gross per-plan revenue of $2.3. The total PPO industry generated revenue is estimated about $1.6 billion. PPOs that started operation before 1989 experienced an 18% decline in per-plan administrative revenues in 1991. Those that started in 1989 had a $1.5 million per-plan revenue in 1991. Investor owned PPOs generated much higher per-plant revenues than other PPOs, with an average of $4.9 per plan, including an increase of 51% from 1990. Insurance company owned PPOs generated an average of $3 million revenues per plant, down 40% from 1990.

Based on reported data, overall industry profitability is difficult to determine. Only about 20% of operating PPOs report complete financial data. Of those, some 80% reported breaking even or positive net profit. Based on ownership categories, more than half of the PPOs reported breaking even, or profitability. Specifically, this success rate was 100% among HMO and third party administrator operated PPOs. Based on the same sample, 85% of hospital operated PPOs, 65% of hospital-physician PPO joint-ventures, and 88% of physician-medical group PPOs were successful.

The contracting patterns for PPO enrollee procurement suggest that over half of the members of employer, employer coalition, HMO, hospital, and physician operated PPOs came through group health insurance companies, with about 25% through third party administrators, and just over 20% through self-insured employers. Some 20 million members were covered through workman compensation programs.

Over 70% of PPOs conducted in-house utilization reviews, 11% contracted it to outside reviewers, and 13% requested providers to perform the task. Hospital admission precertification by PPOs in 1991 dropped by 45% compared to the previous year, and the average number of precertification per 1,000 members was 3.6, an 18% decrease.

Almost half of all PPOs had managed pharmacy programs, specifically with 80% of insurance company plans, and only 5% of physician managed plans offering this program. Larger PPOs were much more inclined to offer this type of program than smaller ones, with more than 70% of those with over 500,000 members offering them.

The number of physicians under contract by the average PPO was 4,100 in 1991, a 30% increase from 1990; of these, some 2,000 were primary care practitioners, with the rest being specialists. Insurance company managed PPOs had some 50% more doctors under contract than the industry average.

Over 80% of PPO plans capped physician fees, but the trend appears to be toward negotiated discount fees along with capping. The average discount procured from individual providers was 20% in 1991, compared with 17% in 1990. The largest PPOs were more likely to apply fee-capping than smaller ones. In fact, a 100% of PPOs (in contrast to 80% in 1990) with over a million membership used fee capping. The use of package prices per episode (PPPE) was present only at 4% of the PPOs, a drop from 5% in 1990, and from 15% in 1988. The average hospital discount was 17% in 1991, compared to 16% in 1990. The most frequent single hospital reimbursement method in 1991 was through discounted charges, although most PPOs use a combination of reimbursement systems, including fee caps, PPPE, and discounted fees[16].

The Rand Study on Healthcare Intermediation

The Rand Health Insurance study was designed, during a little over seven year period ending in early 1982, to estimate the impact of cost-sharing on consumer demand for healthcare, based on randomly selected family units with various insurance plans. The sample size of sub-62 aged people of average income level was about 7,700, assigned to fourteen experimental insurance plans. The plans contained four basic dares of coinsurance: 95%, 50%, 25%, and 0%. The maximum family expenditure was generally capped at $1,000.

With respect to hospital and ambulatory care, an inverse relationship was found between the level of cost sharing and healthcare expenditures. After hospital admission, however, cost sharing had no effect on hospital expenditures. Increased cost sharing for ambulatory care had no apparent impact on hospital inpatient service utilization. The former was shown to be neither a substitute nor a preventive factor for the latter. In addition, no significant relationship was found between cost sharing and lab test frequency, or between the former and the amount of time physicians spent with their patients. Nor did the coverage appear to impact upon the unit cost of ambulatory care[17].

It was further reported that healthcare expenditures on children were much less affected by cost-sharing than those on adults, suggesting the perception of indispensability of healthcare expenditures on children while the same viewed with less intensity for adults. In addition, even for healthcare expenditures for adults, no evidence of comparison shopping was revealed[18]. Finally, it was also noted that responsiveness to cost sharing did not vary with family income.

The Rand Study had some shortcomings. For instance, the participants faced no financial risks due to a high coinsurance factor, for if the Rand related coverage was lower than their actual "real life" coverage, they were reimbursed for the difference with funds that could be spent anywhere, not just on healthcare. The fact that there was a net participant attrition of some 40% from the study raises some questions regarding the extent to which the samples were indeed random. Finally, it did not appear to take into consideration possible provider reactions to the introduction (or increases) in coinsurance, by way of, for instance, physician attempts to generate more visits if the number of patient visits was otherwise reduced due to the coinsurance.

Employer Based Healthcare Intermediation

Rising healthcare costs preoccupy all segments of our society. The US leads the world both in terms of per capita healthcare costs and in terms of the proportion that healthcare costs represent of gross domestic product. During the past ten years, the average annual rate of increase in healthcare was almost 100% higher than that in the Consumer Price Index. We have already noted the reasons, which, in general, fall into three main categories: (a) developments in medical technology, advancing not only the quality of care but also the cost of care; (b) moral hazard, namely the protection of the patient from the full cost of increasingly utilized care by way of various healthcare intermediation programs; and, (c) increases in the cost of input along with relatively slow advances in healthcare productivity.

Healthcare costs in the US are basically shared by three major groups of payers: household, the public sector, and business, by covering 39%, 33% and 28% of the costs in 1980, and 36%, 34%, and 30% in 1990, respectively. Thus, at this stage, business still carries the lowest proportion of the direct cost burden, although a slight shift appears to have occurred from household to business, and even to government.

Employer healthcare expenditures increased during 1987-1990 by 12%, compared to 5% in the Consumer Price Index. In fact, healthcare coverage was the fastest growing component of employee remuneration, representing some 6% of total employee remuneration in 1980, and almost 9% in 1990. Since during this period real wages have declined, health benefits have apparently been substituted for direct wage and salary receipts[19].

Health insurance premiums constitute by far the largest proportion of employer based healthcare expenditures (75%), followed by Medicare hospital insurance trust fund contributions for employees (16%), medical segment of workers' compensation (8%), and corporate on-site health clinics (1%) [19, p.22].

A major concern among employers is the inter-employer adverse shifting of healthcare costs. Normally, employee coverage extends to dependent family members. If covered family members work for another employer who does not provide healthcare coverage, or provides only partial coverage, the effective cost of dependent coverage is shifted to employer of the head of the family. Thus, inter-employer healthcare cost shifting, or what could be called "healthcare free-riding", constitutes a redistribution of income from the insurance providing employer to the one that do not provide insurance.

The uninsured segment of the US population, some 37 million people, often receives political and some policy attention. Much of that lack of insurance may be traced to employers' insurance coverage practices. In fact, some 50% of the uninsured in 1990 were made up of either full-time or part-time employees, and another 30% were the dependents of these employees [19, p.23]. Thus, four-fifths, an overwhelming majority, of the uninsured population may be found among those who are either employed, or are members of an employed family head, and not among those normally considered indigent. Some employees do not offer healthcare coverage all, while others offer limited or minimal coverage. In addition, even with some of those employers that offer coverage, the plans involve copayments substantial enough not to be afforded by employees, hence the latter stay out of the plan. Finally, some employees cannot receive coverage because of health risks. This point will be dealt with in somewhat greater detail in the following section of this chapter.

Healthcare costs are not uniform across industry lines. Some industries and member firms are exposed to greater health care costs than others. In fact, in 1991, healthcare contribution per employee and employer ranged from $1,500 to $5,000, depending on the industry and the firm, and the expected risks involved [19, p.25]. Factors such as age, occupation, and income appear to impact on industry or firm-specific health insurance premium determination. Firm characteristics in terms nature of business, size, location, and health plan design also appear to have played some role. A study by the US Research Chamber Center suggests that in 1991, the average healthcare costs per covered employee, for both employees and employers, ranged from just under $3,000 in the wholesale/retail sector to over $4,500 at public utilities, with the dominant manufacturing sector at the $3,800 level. The employer's share of that cost in 1990 ranged from about $1,500 in wholesale/retail to some $4,800 in the utilities sector, with the manufacturing sector at over $4,000.

Considerable variations in average healthcare costs may be traced to firms within industries. Thus, within the US wholesale/retail industry, the modal class of $2,500-$2,900 included some 20% of the firms, the $2,000-$2,499 class some 19%, with only 4% of the firms experiencing under $1,500, and some 3% incurring $5,000 or above. In manufacturing, the distribution was weighted heavily toward the high end. The modal class was $3,000-$3,499 with 19%, the $3,500-$3,999 with 17%, the $5,000 or above class with 16%, and only 1% of the firms experienced under $1,500[20].

Failures in Healthcare Intermediation

The number of potential and actual patients completely without health insurance in this country is about 37 million. Additionally, some 20 million people have coverage that would likely prove inadequate in case of catastrophic illness. Policies that require large co-payments, basically under-insure the patient. In fact, some 13% of the under-65 population, some 20 million people, fell into the inadequate coverage category, namely having to spend over 10% of their income in case of a serious illness, in 1987[21]. Some 15% of health insurance plans cap-out at $250,000, while almost 70% at $1 million. The cost of many automobile accidents exceed this amount[22]. Furthermore, a 1991 federal court decision limits the liability cap for self-insured employers to their employees at $5,000 for AIDS patients[23].

Some three-fourth of group plans required *deductibles and copayments* for physicians services in 1987[24]. Non-PPO and non-HMO based plans included on the average a $170 deductible in 1990[25]. In fact, some 95% of employers surveyed in 1990 plan to increase deductibles and copayments[26]. While *Medicare* covers only about half of medical expenses, and about 25% of the covered elderly have no medigap (Medicaid or other supplemental private) coverage. Even with the latter, some 25% of healthcare costs incurred by the elderly is covered out-of-pocket. As evidence of under-coverage, some 20% of Medicare patients in 1986 needed about 15% of their income to cover medical bills addressed directly to them. In the absence of supplemental coverage, Medicare patients need to cover $628 hospital deductibles, $78 co-payment from day 21 through day 80 in a nursing facility, and $100 deductible for physician services. In addition, Medicare covers less than 2% of nursing home bills, with private insurance picking up only another 1%. For most elderly, the choice is to live alone, or enter a nursing home and qualify for Medicaid by becoming impoverished within one year[27].

While nine months is the typical waiting period before getting coverage for *pre-existing* conditions by a newly insured person, it can last up to seven years. Some 60% of existing illnesses in 1990 were not covered at the time of coverage commencement. Economic conditions, not only causing employment losses but also employment changes, can augment restrictions in the scope of coverage of pre-existing conditions. It has been estimated that over 80 million people in this country have pre-existing conditions (e.g. diabetes, asthma) not considered coverable by insurance companies. In 1990, some 6% of the population was denied partial or entire health insurance coverage because of pre-existing conditions[28].

A number of procedures and medical needs are simple *left out of coverage*. In 1986, some 20% of physician office visits were not covered by employment based plans. Nor were basic child vaccinations. Almost two-thirds of the plans in 1989 did not cover prenatal care and related physical examinations. Nine percent of women with private insurance are not covered for maternity benefits.[29]

In addition to an explicit lack of insurance, or the prevalence of under-insurance, there appears to be a pervasive lack of psychological comfort even when some or adequate coverage exists. This lack emanates from the fear of losing the coverage, for whatever reasons. Indeed, during 1986 through 1988, some 65 million people, almost twice as many as those not having insurance on any given day, had no insurance for at least one month[30]. In addition, a 1991 New York Times/CBS survey revealed that about one-third of the people, or a relatives, remained in an unwanted job only because of the health insurance coverage[31]. Thus, the actual and anticipated problems with obtaining coverage, or even adequate coverage, directly bears upon various other aspects of peoples' lives, and prompt people to make decisions which, on their face, would otherwise appear to be, and would likely be, completely irrational.

References

1   Frech, H.E. "Market Power in Health Insurance, Effects on Insurance and Medical Markets" *Journal of Industrial Economics*, Vol. 28, 1979, pp. 55-72. See also Kass, D.I. and Paulter, P.A. "Physician Control of Blue Shield Plans", FTC, Washington 1979

2   Blair, R.G. Ginsburg P.B. and Vogel, R.J. "Blue Cross Blue Shield Administrative Costs: A Study of Nonprofit Health Insurers", *Economic Inquiry*, Vol. 13, No.2, 1975, pp. 55-70.

3   Frech, H.E. and Ginsburg, P.B. "Competition Among Health Insurers" in Greenberg, W. (ed) *Competition in the Healthcare Sector*, Aspen Systems, Germantown, MD.1978. Also see Sindelar, J.L. "State Taxation of Health Insurance: Preferential Treatment", *Yale Working Papers*, July 1987

4   Adamanche, K.W. and Sloan, F.A. "Competition Between Nonprofit and For-Profit Insurers" *Journal of Health Economics*, Vol. 2, No. 3, 1983, pp.225-43

5   Frech, H.E. "The Regulation of Health Insurance", and "Market Power in Health Insurance, Effects on Insurance and Medical Markets", *Journal of Industrial Economics*, Vol. 27, 1979

6   Frech, H.E. "The Property Rights Theory of the Firm" *Journal of Political Economy*, Vol 84, No.1, 1976

7   Kuo-Cheng Tseng "Administrative Costs of Medicare Contractors: Blue Cross Plans Versus Commercial Intermediaries" *Economic Inquiry*, Vol. 15, December 1978, pp.371-8

8   Hsiao, W. "Public Versus Private Administration of Health Insurance: A Study in Relative Economic Efficiency" *Economic Inquiry* Vol. 15, December 1978, pp.379-87

9   Meyers, S. "Growth in Health Maintenance Organizations" in *Health United States*, 1981, DHHS Publication 82-1232, DHHS, Hyattsville MD 1981

10 Benyak, J.M. *A Digest of State Laws Affecting Prepayment of Medical Care Group Practice and HMOs* Apsen Co, Rockville MD, 1973, pp. 383-86

11 Group Health Association of America, *Patterns in HMO Enrollment*, 1992 Edition, Washington, DC. 1992, pp.3-36

12 Marion Dow, *Managed Care Digest*, HMO Edition. 1992

13 Homer, C. "Methods of Hospital Use Control in HMOs", *Health Care Management Review*, Vol. 11, Spring, 1986, pp.15-24

14 Luft, H. "How Do Health Maintenance Organizations Achieve Their 'Savings'? Rhetoric and Evidence", *New England Journal of Medicine*, Vol. 298, June 15, 1978, pp.1336-43. Also see Luft, H. "HMOs and the Medical Care Market", in Hough D. and Misek, G. (eds) *Socioeconomic Issues of Health*, AMA, Chigaco Il, 1980, pp.85-102

15   Cunnigham, F. and Williamson, J. "How Does the Quality of Health in HMOs Compare to that In Other Settings? An Analytic Literature Review, 1958-79", *Group Health Journal*, Vol. 1, Winter 1980, pp.4-25. Wolensky, F. "The Performance of HMOs: An Analytical Review" *Milbank Memorial Fund Quarterly*, No. 57, Fall 1980, pp.537-87. Retchin, S.H. and Brown, B. "The Quality of Ambulatory Care in Medicare HMOs", *American Journal of Public Health*, Vol. 80, No. 4, 1990, pp. 411-414

16   Marion Dow, *Managed Care Digest, PPO Edition*, 1992

17   Newhouse. J. et al. "Some Interim Results from a Controlled Trial of Cost Sharing in Health Insurance" *New England Journal of Medicine*, Vol. 305, No. 23, 1981, pp.1501-15-7. Also see, Danzon, P. et al. "Factors Affecting Laboratory Test Use and Prices", *Health Care Financing Review* Vol. 5, No. 4, 1984, pp.21-32

18   Marquis, M. "Cost Sharing and Provider Choice", *Journal of Health Economics*, Vol. 4, No. 2, 1985, pp. 137-57

1^   USGAO, *Employer Based Health Insurance*, September 1992, pp. 18-30

20   Foster Higgins & Co. *Health Care Benefit Survey: Indemnity Plans*, Cost Design and Funding, 1992

21   Pepper Commission, *Bipartisan Commission on Comprehensive Healthcare*. A Call for Action. Government Printing Office, Washington, DC 1990

22   Citizens Fund, *The Seven Warnings Signs*, Washington DC 1991

23   Freudenheim, M. "Employers Winning the Right to Cut Back Medical Insurance" *New York Times*, March 29, 1992, p.1

24   DiCarlo, S. and Gael, J. "Conventional Health Insurance: A Decade Later" *Health Care Finance Review* Vol. 10, No.3, 1989, pp.77-89

25   Sullivan, C.B. Rice, T. "The Health Insurance Picture in 1990" Health Affairs, Vol. 10, No. 2 1991, pp.104-15

26   Foster Higgins, *Health Benefit Survey*, Princeton NJ 1990

27   Rice, T. Gabel, J. "Protecting the Elderly Against High Healthcare Costs" *Health Affairs*, Vol. 5, No. 3, 1986, pp. 5-21. Also see, Feder J. et al "Medicare Reform: Nibbling at Catastrophic Costs", *Health Affairs*, Vol. 6, No. 4, 1987, pp.5-19. Social Security Administration, *Publication No. 05-10043*, Department of Health and Human Services, Baltimore MD 1991. Christensen, S. et al "Acute Healthcare Costs for the Aged Medicare Population: Overview and Policy Options" *Milbank Quarterly*, Vol. 65, 1987, pp.397-425.

28   Cotton, P. "Preexisting Conditions 'Hold Americans Hostage' to Employers and Insurance", *JAMA*, Vol. 265, 1991, pp.2451-3. See also, Citizens Fund, and Blendon, R.J. et al. "The Health Insurance Industry in the Year 2001: One Scenario", *Health Affairs*, Vol. 10, No. 4, 1991, pp.170-7

29   Skolnick, A. "Should Insurance Cover Routine Immunization?", *JAMA* Vol. 265, 1991, pp.2453-4. See also, Braveman, P. et al "Women Without Health Insurance: Links Between Access, Poverty, Ethnicity, and Wealth" *Western Journal of Medicine*, Vol. 149, 1988, pp. 708-11, and Foster Higgins.

30 Friedman, E. " The Uninsured: From Dilemma to Crisis", *JAMA* Vol. 265, 1991, pp.2491-5
31 Eckholm, E. "Health Benefits Found to Deter Job Switching", *New York Times*, September 26, 1991, pp.1

Chapter 15
THE PHYSICIAN
MARKET PLACE

The physicians are the first hand core providers of healthcare. They are also agents for institutional healthcare delivery. Essentially, they stand in the center of healthcare trafficing between providers and users. They constitute input into healthcare production, function as entrepreneurs in their own rights and in joint ventures with hospitals and other institutional providers, and, they generate healthcare products in a variety of forms.

In traditional practice, the physician is the entrepreneur, as well as constitutes the human-capital and labor input. Physician labor input is normally augmented by nursing and allied health professional, as well as clerical service inputs. The product output of the physician firm may be viewed as "treatment". It entails a variety of training based activities aimed at improving the patient's health. Output may be generated in the physician's office, by telephone, or in a hospital room by way of consultations or procedure performance. Treatment, as a unit of output, may pose some measurement problems. This may be overcome by using variables such office visits, or hospital visits, as a unit of physician output. This is particularly important when measuring the impact of factor-proportions on output. The healthcare production process in the physician's office, particularly in capacities requiring minimum or no medical training, allows for some factor substitution. As the required medical training-based technical competence increases towards diagnosis and surgical procedure performance, the degree of factor substitution is reduced. A number of statistical studies attempted to show the impact of factor substitution on physician output, and utility function (income and leisure) maximization[1]

Physician income may be dissected into two components: opportunity cost and a return on entrepreneurship. The former is simply income foregone by not pursuing alternatives such as group practice, or institutional employment as in a hospital, or drug company. The latter may be viewed as the physician's organizational and managerial reward. Much information will be provided later in this chapter on physician income levels and trends in various specialties.

In addition to the single practitioner, physician firms may function in a group and interactive environments. *A group practice* may be of a single specialty (e.g. neurology), or multi-specialty, possibly with an emphases on one or two specialties among the others. The economic justification for the functioning of such groups rests with the existence, and extent, of scale and scope economies, while their functioning in excessive size may be hampered by scale and scope diseconomies. Positive economies initially are generated by an increasing base upon which performance overhead (administrative, clerical and maintenance) can be spread. Negative economies (diseconomies) often emanate from efficiency, communication and cost control problems. Whether or not physicians have an incentive to control costs, and function efficiently, depends on their own financial incentives. Thus, salaried doctors are less likely to observe the principles of efficient functioning than those paid by capitation.

Multispecialty group form of practice (MSGP) has been increasing in frequency, containing a number of physicians with various specialties. Its advantage from the patient's point of view is to find various specialties under one roof, reducing travel time and expense in cases involving cross-specialty referrals, while members of the group also benefit from established sources of ready referrals. The practitioners function interdependently in a common location, sharing medical records, and personnel.

Patient flow is fundamental for the survival of the group. Consequently, many groups contract with various alternative delivery systems, HMOs and PPOs, to secure a steady supply of patients. In some areas the groups are located within the proximity of hospitals, where members of the group also enjoy staff privileges at the neighboring hospital. The latter, in turn, may constitute additional source of patient flow.

The proximity of a multi-specialty group practice to a hospital may also be a source of problems, if the hospital perceives the group as a competitor in some healthcare product lines. For instance, if the group contains a cardiac surgeon with an affiliation at a hospital that competes with the group's neighboring hospital for cardiac surgery patients, the neighboring hospital may view the presence of the group, with its cardiac surgeon, as a competitive threat and take steps to either divert cardiac patients to itself by offering staff privileges to the cardiac surgeon, or to eliminate the group by denying staff privileges to all or most members of the group. The antitrust implications in such situations are obvious, and can be a source of litigation. This "diversion scenario" may be pertinent to various other specialties where neighboring multispecialty groups divert patients away from local hospitals to other competing, or even geographically noncompeting, institutions.

Historically, multispecialty groups may be traced back to the early part of the century. The Mayo Clinic was founded in 1913, and the Los Angeles based Ross-Loos Clinic in 1919. In fact, the latter was also one of the forerunners of the delivery of prepaid care.

During past two decades, group practices appeared to be growing in number and size. In 1969, single specialty groups represented about half of all groups, but by 1984 the proportion reached about 70% . Multispecialty groups, on the other hand, appear to have been growing mostly in size. The average size of a multispecialty group practice increased from 10 members in 1969 to 27 members in 1984[2].

There are factors, however, which may limit the profitability of MSGPs. For instance, those organized as partnerships cannot retain earnings to finance future growth since excess revenues need to be annually distributed to physicians. Similar dilemmas face professional corporations due to physicians' tendency to retrieve income from the organization. In addition, the labor intensive nature of the work involving doctor-patient personal and telephone interactions, and the large diversity among the diseases treated, prevent the emergence of significant production scale economies. Furthermore, reimbursement practices predetermine physician income patters and, unless it can be offset by vertical integration, discretionary operating margins need to be set aside by the hospital, the HMO, and the physician, all subject to the constraints of cost control methods[3]. Finally, while hospitals have relatively ready access to financial markets, for instance through issuing tax-exempt bonds, no such access is available to a group practice.

In the case of solo practices, the possession of specialized unshared knowledge and information by a primary care practitioner enables him to make decisions as to whether to treat the patient for a specific ailment, or refer the case to a specialist. The economic rationale in general with such referral may rest with possible efficiencies, and even competence, possessed by the specialist and not possessed by the primary care practitioner, thus yielding a diversification of treatment risks. From the patient's point of view, referral means receiving possibly more reliable care for a specific ailment, although likely at a higher cost; assuming that the patient would, by his or her choice, decide to seek such treatment in view of the higher cost, rather than go with the treatment accorded by the general practitioner, if possible, at a lower fee. At any rate, given the normal state of patient information, the decision is not likely to rest with the patient, but rather with the physician. If the physician's motive also includes *fee-splitting* (partial fee kickback to the primary care practitioner from the chosen specialist in return for the referral - viewed as highly unethical, and even illegal, practice by state and county medical societies and disciplinary boards), then the referral will more likely be made without the patient's consent, and for the economic motive of the referring doctor.

Theories that describe *physician behavior* may, in general, be grouped into two categories. One is based on utility maximization[4], and the other on profit maximization[5]. In addition, standard two element utility functions, based on profit and leisure, have been used to depict physician behavior[6]. At any rate, profit maximization is included in most physician utility functions. Profit, in general, is defined as earnings minus overhead costs and imputed profession-wide basic earnings. The later allows for a consideration of leisure-income trade-off by the physician. Thus, a typical physician utility function includes, among other variables, profit, leisure, professional status, professional challenge, case mix, ability to keep up-to-date in the literature, allied health, administrative and clerical support staff.

Supply Creates its Own Demand: Fact or Fiction?

It has traditionally been thought that limited physician supply in given geographical areas is conducive to fee increases. Yet, it has also been found that in spite of increased physician supply, fees have increased or have been maintained[7]. The circumstances under which physicians can maintain, or even increase, their income, in spite of their apparent over-supply in a particular region, have been given considerable thought.

One theory suggested what could be called the *treatment intensity effect*. Namely, an increase in physician supply is accompanied by increased treatment intensity, whereby even minor ailments that otherwise, with a shortage of physician-time supply, would simply go untreated, are accepted and charged for; thus maintaining a patient demand level commensurate with any physician supply[8]. In fact, any increase in physician supply could be managed to generate excess, medically necessary or otherwise, demand for their services. A more aggressive offspring of the Feldstein theory suggests that, instead of just rendering medically unnecessary treatments, there is brand new *physician generated demand* for their services[9]. While these two theories are premised on the assumption that physicians can manipulate patient demand for their services, a third one, an *income maintenance hypothesis*, suggest that even if they do not, or cannot, generate or sustain new demand for their services, physicians can adhere to certain income goals, and simply adjust their fees accordingly to meet changing market or demand conditions[10]. Finally, these physician income and pricing related practices are probably in need of shelter from competition.

In a more competitive environment, such as may be found among family or general practitioners, these apparently manipulative implementations are less likely because treatment slacks may be absorbed by other physicians, and the scope of new treatment options are much more limited. In a traditional competitive environment, most sellers tend to act as price-takers, with, in a more modern competitive setting, little leverage over price. This predicament may be counter-acted by physicians becoming members, and following the pricing dictum, of various (trade)associations, at least until the 1975 Goldfarb decision, that rendered the professions vulnerable to antitrust sanctions. As we will see in the next Part of the book, this has now become a dangerous way of doing business, and in recent years has been largely avoided. Furthermore, organized third party payers have become a major force in physician pricing. In addition, and in order to avoid the price controlling impact of peer competition, physicians have started significant trends of geographic dispersions shortly after the Goldfarb decision[11].

Whether or not there is significant supply-induced demand in actual medical markets has been questioned. At least one study found, on the aggregate, some relationship between surgeon density and a per-capita increase in surgical procedures, although data per practice does not appear to confirm this relationship[12]. Other studies, however, dispute the notion entirely. For instance, a study of primary care services markets in some

100 large urban areas, using 1975 AMA data, found little or no evidence of supply-induced demand[13]. If demand is not induced, physicians may attempt to maintain a desirable income level by "unbundling" their services, and thereby increase billing volume and frequency. In recent years, however, such attempts have been controlled with relative effectiveness through peer and claim reviews efforts.

It is likely, however, that an increase in the number of physicians has imposed sufficient competitive pressures on a large enough number of practitioners to render them vulnerable to cost containment measures, particularly by way of managed care delivery systems. Furthermore, intensified competitive pressures brought about by increased physician supply, and controlled physician income trends, will increase competition for the healthcare dollar, likely to the detriment of allied health professional, and physician assistants since latter often function at the pleasure of the doctor. This latter trend may, however, be countervailed by the inclination on the part of managed care organizations to use, whenever possible, allied health professional and physician assistant types in order to control costs.

Pricing Physician Services: Theoretical Issues

For some two decades, economists have attempted to devise a model that would most likely reflect on the pricing environment in the physicians office. Of the various models and theories postulated, two major trends appear to have emerged. One group, that may be labeled as *monopoly based price-maker models*, is based on the assumption that the physician has adequate freedom, even in the presence of third-party payers and some minimum competitive forces, to set prices. The second group, *competition based price-taker models*, is predicated on the assumption that doctors are, to a decisive extent, at the mercy of market forces that compel them to accept some market determined price.

A price-maker model, largely in the absence of third-party payer dominance, assumed that doctors engage in perfect, or 1st degree, price discrimination based on the patient's estimated income; it entails capturing the patient's entire consumer surplus (total area under a nonshifting demand curve) by charging the patient's reservation price at which ultimately a market equilibrium is generated[14].

Another price-maker model allowed for shifting demand functions along with market clearing equilibrium due to the physician's assumed market power. The doctor, benefiting from consumer ignorance regarding the quality of the medical care product, is assumed to create demand for its services, shift the demand curve to the right, and then, perceiving himself as a virtual monopolist satisfy that demand at a discretionary price.[15]. A third type of price maker model also perceives the physician as a monopolist who set prices in a discretionary manner, irrespective of the demand function, leaving substantial market segments unserved and excess demand unsatisfied[16]. In general, these three models have not received firm empirical supported.

Price-taker models are based on a competitive environment where physicians are assumed to be a small part of the market, without any significant control over price. Since this situation normally fits only the relatively heavily populated general and family practice segments of geographical medical markets, their application to specialist medical product markets is tentative at best. Empirically, this situation would be depicted by a negative relationship between service supply and price. Some studies addressed this issue within the context of specialists. For instance, negative relationships of various magnitude were found between the supply of general practitioners and their fees on the one hand, and between the supply of general surgeons and their fees, on the other[17]. Other studies, however, found a positive relationship between provider supply and their fees, amounting to a refutation of the competitive pricing theory[18].

Some theories postulated physician pricing behavior aimed at income-specific goal attainment, mainly by manipulating the demand function in response to income reduction due to cost increases or due to an exogenous downward trend in demand itself[19]. If externally imposed price controls exist (e.g. by insurance companies, or government regulation), then supply will likely fall short of demand, without a market clearing equilibrium ever occurring. Other studies depicted this type of situation where physicians, simply accepting the regulation set price, limit output to the level where the marginal cost of production just reaches the exogeneously set price level, leaving excess demand as a chronic syndrome[20].

Physician Pricing:
Resource Based Relative Value Scale

The Resource Based Relative Value Scale (RBRVS) is a new Medicare physician payment system covering physicians' services under Part B of the Medicare program. Its conception and subsequent development was inspired, if not prompted, largely by the 1983 introduction of the Medicare prospective pricing system (DRGs) covering payments for inpatient hospital services and nursing home care [discussed earlier in this volume]. Indeed, this system may be viewed as the most significant improvement in Medicare Part B, since its inception in 1966.

Typically, some 80% of payments under Medicare Part B has gone for physician services, with the rest of the program absorbed by clinical laboratory services, durable medical equipment, hospital outpatient services, drugs, home health services, and other Medicare benefits[21]. For over a quarter of a century since 1966, physicians were paid "customary, prevailing, and reasonable" (CPR) fees, not unlike the "usual, customary, and reasonable" (UCR) fee schedule used by private commercial carriers. In effect, Medicare payments were in the approximate range of the 90th percentile of all pertinent fee structures. However, CPR allowed for considerable variation among Medicare reimbursed physician fees, causing some concern among providers, with the latter reaching its peak during the second half of the 1970s and the first half of the 1980s when Medicare placed a series of limits on CPR reimbursement levels, along with wage and price controls extended to physicians services. Subsequently, physician fees were adjusted according to a Medicare Economic Index that reflected provider practice cost growth since 1973, and changes in general income trends throughout the economy. Thus, Medicare basic reimbursement patterns of the early 1970s were engraved in stone for many years to come, certainly until 1992. Reimbursements for new capital intensive procedures were adjusted to costs, but payment for other basic physician services were perceived to be outdated and lagging behind costs. A second round of fee caps introduced in the 1980s, making the CPR payment system complex to a degree barely manageable, provided the impetus to call for change and reforms. The courts' affirmation of congressional authority to limit physician fees augmented the campaign for change[22].

The options for change included several possibilities, such as improving on an already unmanageable CPR system, extending the 1983

DRG system to physicians, a broader application of capitation based fee structures, such as HMOs, to Part B, and, finally, the introduction of a *relative value scale* (RVS) system. The latter ranks for provider services on a value basis. Two versions of RVS were considered: charge-based, and resource-based. The former ranks the relative value for services according to some representative fee basis, such as Medicare payments, or some average fee per service category. However, it thus also retains the problems that were inherent in a CPR related system discussed earlier. The latter ranks services based on relative costs needed to provide them. The cost basis for ranking may include the time factor, a difficulty factor, overhead intensity, and the like, as well as their geographical dimensions, to determine the RBRVS ratios. A dollar conversion factor translates the RVS system into payment formulas. In 1985, by way of the Consolidated Omnibus Budget Reconciliation Act (COBRA), Congress ordered the Department of Health and Human Services to develop an RBRVS by July 1, 1987 [at the same time, major hospital based physician services, such as radiology, anesthesiology, and pathology, were brought under a DRG payment system]. In 1985, HCFA, with AMA participation, funded a Harvard study on resource-based relative value scales for physician services. COBRA also created a thirteen member Physician Payment Review Commission (PPRC) to assess the various payment reform options. The completion deadline was subsequently extended to July 1, 1989.

Initially, the Harvard Study was to develop RBRVS for twelve physician specialties (anesthesiology, family practice, general surgery, internal medicine, OB/GYN, ophthalmology, orthopedics, otolaryngology, pathology, radiology, cardiac surgery, and urology), with additional ones (allergy an immunology, dermatology, oral surgery, pediatrics, psychiatry, and rheumatology) having been added subsequently. Although similar studies have already been undertaken earlier by the principals, in particular William C. Hsiao of the Harvard School of Public Health, this study turned out to be much broader, aiming not only at developing RBRVS scales for each of the 18 specialty but also at combining the field-specific scales into a comprehensive cross-specialty scale [a subsequent phase 2 of the study included 15 additional specialties].

After the four-year Harvard Study, Congress enacted in 1989, for a 1992 implementation, a new Medicare physician payment system based on RBRVS principles. The fundamental principles of the new system included (a) an RBRVS-based payment system for physicians that narrowed geographical and specialty differences among rates; (b) permitting balance billing of patients, essentially amounting to the difference between the provider's reasonable fee and the Medicare reimbursement, and, (c) a close scrutiny of increases in government outlays to physicians[23].

Pursuant to the new payment system, 1992 already appears to witness some fundamental changes. The CPR system appears to have been eliminated. Specialty differentials are expected to be minimized, and geographical differences substantially reduced. Over 15% of the services are moved under the new system. In fact, the estimated percent changes from 1991 to 1992 in average Medicare payments *per service* and by specialty are estimated to turn out to be quite significant. For all physicians (-4%); general/family practice 16%; internal medicine 1%; ophthalmology (-15%); nuclear medicine (-21%); thoratic surgery (-13%); gastroenterology, neuro-surgery, anesthesiology, pathology, (-10% each); and non physician providers (9%). On a geographical, *state-by-state*, basis, per service, the larger estimated percent changes from 1991 to 1992 in average Medicare payments suggest Alaska (-10%); Nevada (-9%); Florida (-8%); Hawaii, California, and Arizona (-7% each)[24].

Cost Containment by Medical Gatekeeping

Medical gatekeeping is a technique implemented at the individual patient clinical level. It is a care coordinating and possibly even rationing strategy, designed to keep, subject to competently recognized life threatening health constraints, patient care at the primary care ambulatory stage. Gatekeeping tools include the solicitation of second opinions, and cost-benefit review of tests and procedures, directed at financial efficiency. Thus, for better or worse, and in the interest of financial expediency, decisions regarding patient care beyond the primary care level remains within the purview of one person, his financial concerns, his competence, and ethical conscience. Given the amount of published, and the likely larger amount of unpublished data on medical malpractice, in some cases, gatekeeping's pecuniary cost savings may far be outweighed by nonpecuniary costs in terms of human suffering and even loss of life.

Gatekeeping may take on different characteristics under different institutional settings. In some setting, such as in a traditional IPA/HMO environment, gatekeeping simply means a reluctance to hospitalize, which may, indeed, be viewed as being not only in the financial interest of the HMO, but also in the interest of the patient's welfare. In situations where the physician is a salaried employee of the HMO, and is designated as a gatekeeper, a conflict of interest may arise between protecting the financial interests of the doctor's employer, on the one hand, and personal welfare of the patient, on the other. There appear to be no generally accepted standards governing conduct involved in such conflicting dual roles[25]. In fact, the conflict of interest predicament may take on intolerable proportions, and the jeopardy to the patient's welfare multiplies, if the gatekeeping physician receives a bonus commensurate with the reduction of nonprimary care services. In an investor-owned multi-institutional healthcare setting, with constant pressures to maintain a favorable financial profile toward the security markets, similar conflict of interest predicaments were found[26]. Thus, it appears that while physician gatekeeping may contribute to healthcare cost reduction, it does so on the likely expense of patient welfare due to varying degrees of applied physician competence, and on the added expense of diluting even competent physician practice into quasi administrative financially and underutilization motivated work, distracting from primary concern for the patient's welfare.

Managed Care and Managed Income

HMO incentive arrangements, (e.g. capitation fees, risk sharing and incentive pools and payments) for physicians are as varied and numerous as the types and numbers of HMOs themselves. However, they share one common purpose; namely, to induce doctors to make cost-effective medical decisions. The source of risk sharing and incentive pools vary by the type of HMO. In IPAs, the participating members make up the pool. In individual contract based HMOs, the pool is made up of a network of doctors either by hospital affiliation or by geography. They risks and the incentive for cost-effective practice under some type of quality constraints. The pool if funded from a percentage of the capitation payments or from discounted fees withheld by the HMO.

Reimbursement from financial pools is contingent upon the target performance of the involved group of doctors in terms of the preservation of hospital, specialists, and ancillary service budgets. Specifically, the risk pool may be made up of a certain percentage of income withheld. Along with that, a target budget of a certain amount is set up for the year to cover hospital, specialist referral, and ancillary services. If, at the end of the year, expenditures fall short of the budgetary ceiling, the risk pool will likely be reimbursed according some formula based on initial contribution. Any budgetary excesses are covered from the risk pool, leaving a reduced, or zero, amount for physician reimbursement. Depending on prevailing contracts, doctors may even be held responsible for utilization costs that exceed the sum of the budget plus the risk pool. In addition to group utilization performance, individual practitioners are also scrutinized for acceptable utilization standards.

A recent study reviewed the nature of physician involvement in various incentive programs. Some 70% of the responding sample with capitation-based payment arrangements, and 80% of plans with fee-for-service arrangements, withhold a percentage of physician income against potential deficits; only 20% of plans with salaried physicians do so. Thirty percent of the plans had penalties in addition to withholding. Some 20% of the plans base the return of withheld amounts on the experience of individual doctors, instead of the collective experience of the relevant group. Investor owned HMOs tend to be more aggressive in the utilization of incentive based physician payment systems. They are less likely to employ a salary-based payment, are more inclined to withhold a percentage of physician income, and to utilize individual practitioner experience when deciding on reimbursements[27].

Once again, the emphases are on savings, presumably subject to some patient care quality constraints. However, since the latter is much more difficult to define, and, in particular, measure, than the former, any flexibility that needs to be exercised will likely be found in terms of patient care quality rather than financial expediency. This needs to be kept in mind later when we will examine physician malpractice trends, and their various costs to society.

Physician Earnings During the Past Decade

The environment of medical practice has been changing for a number of years now. Managed care delivery systems, utilization reviews, preoccupation with healthcare costs and accessibility, and clamoring for healthcare reforms have all condition medical practitioners for change and accommodation. Although the new RBRVS Medicare fee schedule has not gone into effect until the beginning of 1992, constraints on physician income growth trends have already become noticeable by 1990.

The annual rates of increase, (year-to-year percentage change in median net income after expenses but before taxes, for office and hospital based practitioners, not including residents, and other physicians who spent at least 20 hours per week in patient care, and whose primary activities were administration or research), in physician income peaked out in 1988 at 11.1% (6.6% in 1981 dollars). By 1989 it has gone down to 4.2% (-0.6%), and in 1990 to 4% (-1.3%). The 1989 and 1990 data reverses the upward trend between 1985 through 1988 where annual increases jumped from 2.2% (-1.2%) in 1985 to the indicated peak in 1988.

During the decade of the eighties (1981-1990), the average annual increase in all physician income was 6.5% (2.1% in real terms, with pathologists and surgeons having experienced the highest increase at 8% (3.7%), and general/family practitioners at 5% (0.8%). By census division, the West South Central region grew the fastest at 7.2% (3%), and the West North Central the slowest at 5.5% (1.4%). It may be noted that during the 1981-1990 period, median family income, adjusted for inflation, grew at an average annual rate of 1%.

By specialty in 1990, surgeons, radiologists, and anesthesiologists earned the highest median net income level at $200,000 ($139,000 in 1981 dollars), while general and family practitioners earned the lowest at $93,000 ($65,000). By census region, physicians in the West South Central earned the highest medium net income in 1990 at $150,000 ($104,000), with the lowest having been in New England at $120,000 ($83,000).

In terms of averages (standard error of the mean), all physicians had a 1990 mean income of $164,300 ($2,200), with surgeons being the highest at $236,400 ($6,700), and, once again, family practitioners the lowest at $102,700 ($2,700). Regionally, the New England census divisions had the lowest mean earnings for all physicians at $142,500 ($7,100), and the West South Central region the highest at $178,800 ($7,900).

The highest earnings variation within specialties was noted for radiologists and pathologists (at around $9,000 standard error of the mean), with the lowest for general and family practitioners ($2,700). Regionally, the Mountain census division indicated the highest standard error of the mean ($11,300), and the Middle and South Atlantic regions the lowest ($5,200).

It is obvious that physician income is high relative to other occupations. One reason may be the typically much larger number of hours that physicians put in during an average week, almost 60 in 1990, some 50% higher than the average work-week. Many practitioners experience continuous stress, even after leaving the office or the hospital. In many specialties, the margin of error can be small, and the threat of a malpractice suit is often perceived to be, or actually is, present. If one makes the assumption that an average practitioner keeps up with the medical literature, hence with the latest research, then the additional time spent on that effort would further justify the earnings differential for some physicians. Finally, the demographics of physician population is such that most are still on the rising phase of their life-time earnings curve, giving an upward bias to income statistics[28].

Medical Malpractice and Healthcare Costs

Physicians' practices have long been scrutinized my by some of their patients through the legal system. While there have been many claims of questionable merit, and, indeed, even today, litigating and winning a medical malpractice suit is a major and unpredictable task, there have been many major aberrations, and instances of recognized gross negligence on the part of practitioners. While there are databases maintained of those physicians against whom claims have been filed in the past, the general public is not likely to learn of the problem, in particular the essential details of the problem, and indeed the dangers, unless the victim happens to be of some public notoriety[29].

Medical malpractice and the claims arising from it are costly in various ways. This treatise is not equipped to deal with the emotional and other nonpecuniary aspects of the process, for claimants and the objects of claims alike. Our main interest here is an objective examination of the contribution of medical malpractice claims to healthcare costs. Nor are we prepared at this stage to assess whether or not the incurred claim-related expenditures are morally justified, socially warranted, or that increases in healthcare costs due to the pecuniary costs of medical malpractice claims are, in fact, economically unjustified, hence should be curbed. One line of argument could clearly be that the various pecuniary costs, the size of the awards, lawyers' and related derived incomes, are excessive and should be curbed. As a matter of fact, some states have already enacted rules of tort reforms limiting the size of medical malpractice awards, legal fees, and the filing of claims. Another line of argument could assert that the medical profession does not police, or police adequately, the conduct and competence of its own members.

Practitioner malfeasors appear rarely disciplined adequately within the profession, and often are allowed, and possibly even encouraged, to merely relocate and resume their pattern of practice elsewhere. A general lack of product and supplier information on the part of the consuming public appears to be conducive to this practice. Hence, it appears necessary to police medical practice, and protect the well-being of unsuspecting and vulnerable patients, by means available from outside the medical profession. State health departments do impose some sanctions, but rarely provide remedies to the victims, or survivors. Enters the judicial system. Normally for a generous fee, lawyers are prepared to pick up the torch and seek remedy for their clients. Thus, it may be argued that medical malpractice claims are necessary, although costly. There may be an authentic "med-mal cost trade-off" in existence, one that is socially and morally justified, and possibly even necessary: the total pecuniary cost of legally pursuing medical malpractice may fall far short of the aggregate social costs of medical-malpractice by way of patient welfare depreciation, suffering, damage to wellness and life, and even to the family structure. This may be true even if we consider only those cases, a relatively small proportion of the total, which are legally pursued. If filed medical malpractice claims have a derivative effect upon non-targeted practitioners by prompting them to practice more prudent and conscientious medicine, then the social benefits of reducing the instances medical malpractice, whether claimed or the many that may remain unclaimed, may far outweigh the pecuniary costs of medmal litigation. An argument that may, to an extent, counter the above may refer to the explicit costs incurred by the excessive number of tests and diagnostic procedures that practitioners may order to practice "defensive medicine", and, indeed, there may be a fine line between the practice of "defensive medicine" and that of prudent medicine.

Between 1975 and 1984, claims per physician increased by over 10%, and claim frequency per 100 doctors increased from 13.5 to 17.2 per year during the five year period preceding 1986. The average amount of paid claim increased some 100% faster than the CPI during the ten year period preceding 1984, and the average claim resolution amount was about $80,000 in 1984. As we will note later on, considerable differences may be found in this regard among geographical areas and practice specialties. Similar increases could be found for coverage premiums, with a total increase registered during 1977-84 for the relatively low risk general practice without surgery of some 110%, and 180%-190% increase for the higher risk fields of surgery and obstetrics specialties[30].

Whether medical malpractice insurance is a significant element in total healthcare costs (at about 2% of total healthcare expenditures) is debatable. It may be of concern if physicians can pass on the cost of liability insurance to patients without any constraint. In some remaining segments of payment system, such as in traditional fee-for-service practices, it is still possible. However, third-party payment constraints, particularly under managed care, normally set predetermined fees, making premium pass-throughs on a fee basis, as distinct from patient volume basis, rather difficult. This may also explain to an extent the liability induced departure of many practitioners from higher risk practices, such as obstetrics.

Notwithstanding the above, recent years did witness some moderation in the increase in the number of claims and premium costs. The average annual rate of liability claims *per 100 doctors*, profession-wide, increased only to 7.7 in 1990 from 7.4 in 1989, in contrast to the sharp increases during the first half of the 1980s, and has declined by an average annual rate of some 9% since 1985. Although a substantial rate of 1985-90 decline was experienced in the field of obstetrics/gynecology (22.7%), this group continues to experience the highest per 100 claim frequency (11.9) in 1990. Geographically, the New England census division experienced by far the steepest 1985-90 decline (31.9%) in claims per 100 physicians, compared with the decline in the West north Central region (15.5%), and a 12.4% increase in the mountain states.

The proportion of all practitioners experiencing malpractice claims during 1985-90 period also appeared have declined, largely along the same lines as the decline experienced per 100 physicians. On the other hand, the proportion of all doctors who were the subject of claims throughout their careers, up to and including 1990, has substantially increased. Among those surveys by the AMA, over half (57%) of the OB/GYN specialists, and of the general surgeons (52%) experienced claims. About one third of practitioners in other major fields of endeavor such as family practice, internal medicine, pediatrics, radiology, and anesthesiology, experienced malpractice claims. At least until 1990, psychiatrists experienced the lowest career proportion (19.3%). Geographically, the West South Central, Middle Atlantic, Pacific, and East North Central census areas report the highest career ratios.

On a specialty basis, in 1990, the highest average professional liability premium has been paid by OB/GYN practitioners ($34,300), with surgeons and anesthesiologists having paid the seconds highest (about $20,000), and psychiatrists the lowest at $4,500. It may further be noted that the traditionally three highest risk specialties, surgery, OB/GYN and anesthesiology have all experienced a decline in average premium costs between 1989 and 1990, following consistent increases between 1985 and 1989.

Professional liability insurance premiums have often been cited as significant sources of healthcare cost increases, particularly for self-employed physicians. The average premium rose from $5,800 in 1982 to $14,500 in 1990, with an average annual increase of 12.1% per year, and 8% in 1982 dollars. Yet, medical malpractice insurance premium as a percent of total practice revenue for self-employed physicians averaged a little over 4% annually during 1982-90, suggesting that in general it does not constitute a major expense item for physicians, possibly because much of the premiums may have been passed on to their patients. On the other hand, if subject to third-party payer constraints, pass-throughs may not be readily implemented, suggesting that even without pass-throughs, these costs may be viewed as relatively insignificant. In addition, annual increases in professional liability insurance costs for all specialties have consistently declined since 1984-85, and the absolute levels of the premium itself have declined since 1988 [28, 23-105].

The Current and Future State of Practice Environment

There appear to be some fundamental issues and questions that can be raised regarding current developments and future situations in medical practice. A concern could relate to the apparent *over-supply* of doctors. The number of doctors practicing in the US has increased from a little over 300,000 in 1970 to over 512,000 by 1987. Physician-to-population ratio increased by 40% during the same time period. Only a small proportion of this increase may be attributed to an increase in the number of foreign medical graduates. In addition, given the long road to medical graduation, physician supply for the time being has already been determined by the number of those who have already been accepted. Another 30% increase in physician supply, and a 20% increase in physician-to-population ratio may be expected by the year 2000[31]. Future physician manpower growth will be somewhat mitigated by attrition for a variety of reasons.

What adverse consequences may be attributed to an oversupply of individual healthcare providers? The additional number of physicians will need to be paid at a level commensurate with their skills, and will likely require expensive equipment. Thus, they will contribute to the absolute increase in healthcare costs. Secondly, there may be a concern for the quality of the care. Unnecessary care frequency, and utilization intensity, will likely increase as the larger number of doctors will attempt to occupy themselves. Furthermore, increased competition for patients in various specialty groups may prevent practitioners to accumulate experience and the derivative skills necessary for a socially desirable competence level. It has been shown that in most specialties, high risk surgery in particular, practitioner competence is directly related to performance frequency[32]. Finally, physician labor market imperfections, and, increasing third-party payer dominance, will likely prevent the price system for physicians to clear the market, as would be the case in standard product markets.

Another concern may be the *changing environment* for medical practice. "It's not what it used to be". Indeed, it is not. One type of change that appears to take hold to an increasing extent is the transformation of the traditional solo-practitioner into an employee. By 1985, over one-quarter of nonfederal patient care physicians were employees, and of those under 36 years of age, almost half practiced in employment, instead of solo practice, circumstances[33]. Practice setting changes were enhanced by the emerging prominence of managed care organizations. By 1986, over one third of practitioners received their income from HMOs of some form or another, and almost 40% of practitioners had contracts with PPOs[34]. These trends appeared to have reduced patient autonomy in their physician choice, and, as discussed earlier, transformed, not necessarily to the benefit of patient care, the financial incentives faced by the doctors.

Healthcare *quality* became an issue. Hospital specific mortality statistics, of some value, are published, and similar data may soon become available regarding individual practitioners. While peer review functions, or their likes, have existed to an extent for some time, their objective external use has intensified in recent years. "Quality assurance" and "risk management" have become staple topics within the hospital environment. Thus, for instance, physicians have become keenly aware of the potential consequences in court of keeping an infant patient alive with the risk of creating a disabled survivor, versus having to deal with the consequences of the patient's death. Furthermore, the public's increased awareness of healthcare quality related issues created a receptive market for journalistic accounts of various types medical malfeasance, and their morbid consequences[29].

Physician *payment practices* have drastically changed during the past decade, and even during the past year. During the earlier years of Medicare, the system was relatively simple and its payments predictable for both the practitioner and the patient, involving a small amount of paper work. Reimbursements were competitive. As Medicare evolved into its maturity, so did its complexity, unpredictability and redtape. While in the early stages of the program, reimbursements were adjusted upward to the Medicare Economic Index (MEI), the process gradually succumbed to the government's perennial cost control efforts, and until the recently implemented RVRBS system (discussed earlier), reimbursements compared unfavorably with private income sources. The functioning of professional review organizations (PROs), a payer selected outside body contracted by the provider to audit claim records, has often been viewed as interfering with effective medical practice.

Finally, issues and statistics have already been presented in this chapter regarding physicians' *professional liability*. Practitioner reaction includes what is at times called the practice of "defensive medicine". If such endeavor does exist to the extent depicted, while substantially adding to healthcare cost, it may also be viewed as a possible source of enhanced quality, for, in general, it may be better to overtest than to undertest. The annual cost of "defensive medicine" has at one time been estimated at about $10 billion, or some 13% of the total moneys ($75 billion) spent on physician services[35]. However, the exact delineation of "defensive" in the practice is rarely clear, for if a test is even remotely related to an existing or suspected ailment, it may not be any more "defensive" than necessary. A physician's concern to cover all pertinent contingencies may indeed be as much in the interest of the patient as it may be in his or her potential legal interest, or simply in the interest of practicing prudent medicine. Thus, the concern for "defensive medical practice" may be exaggerated.

References

1   Reinhardt, U. "Manpower Substitution and Productivity in Medical Practices: Review and Research", *Health Services Research*, Vol. 8, No. 3, 1973, fspp.200-227. Also see Reinhardt, U. "Production Function for Physician Services" *Review of Economics and Statistics*, Vol. 54, No. 1, 1972 pp.55-66.

2   AMA, *Medical Groups in the US* 1985, Chicago, IL 1985

3   Kralewski, J.E. Ottensmeyer, D.J. Shapiro, J. "Medical Group Practice Systems: What Can be Learned From the Hospital Sector?", *Journal of the American College of Medicine*, Vol. 9, 1986, pp.1-14

4   Feldstein, M. "The Rising Price of Physician Services", *Review of Economics and Statistics*, Vol. 52, No.2, May 1970

5   Sloan, F. "Physician Fee Inflation: Evidence from the Late 1960s", in Rosett, R. (ed) *The Role of Health Insurance in Health Services Sector*, Watson Academic, New York, 1976

6   Pauly, M. and Redisch, M. "The Not-for-Hospital as Physicians' Cooperative", *American Economic Review*, Vol. 63, No. 1, 1973

7   Holahan, J. et al *Physician Pricing in California*, Urban Institute Working Paper, Report 988-10, 1978. See also Dyckman, Z. *A Study of Physician Fees*, Staff Report, Council of Wage and Price Stability, Executive Office of the President, Washington DC, 1978. Newhouse, J. and Phelps, C. "Price and Income Elasticities for Medical Services", in Perlman, M. (ed) *The Economics of Health and Medical Care*, John Wiley, New York, 1974, pp.139-61.

8   Feldstein, M. "The Rising Price of Physician Services", *Review of Economics and Statistics*, Vol. 52, No. 2, 1970, pp.121-133. See also. Feldstein, M. "Hospital Inflation: A Study in Nonprofit Price Dynamics", *American Economic Review*, Vol. 61, No.5 1971, pp.853-72.

9   Fuchs, V. and Kramer, J. "Determinants of Expenditures for Physicians Services in the United States, 1948-68", *NBER, Paper Series*, 1973. See also Evans, R. "Supplier Induced Demand: Some Empirical Evidence and Implications" in Perlman

10 Newhouse, J. "A Model of Physician Pricing" *Southern Economic Journal*, Vol. 37, No. 2 1970, pp.174-83

11 Newhouse, J. et al "Where Have All the Doctors Gone?", *Journal of American Medical Association*, Vol. 247, No. 17, 1982, pp.2392-96, and Newhouse, J. et al "Does the Geographical Distribution of Physicians Reflect Market Failure?" *Bell Journal of Economics*, Vol. 13, No. 2, 1982, pp.493-505

12 Stano, M. "An Analysis of the Evidence on Competition in the Physician Services Market", *Journal of Health Economics*, Vol. 4, No.3,, 1985, pp. 33-45

13　McCarthy, T. "The Competitive Nature of the Primary Care Physician Services Market", *Journal of Health Economics*, Vol. 4, No. 2, 1985, pp.93-117. See also, Sweeney, G. "The Market for Physician Services: Theoretical Implications and an Empirical Test of the Target Income Hypothesis" *Southern Economic Journal*, Vol. 48, No. 1, 1982

14　Kessel, R. "Price Discrimination in Medicine", *Journal of Law and Economics*, Vol. 1, No.1 1958, pp.20-53. See also Newhouse, J. "A Model of Physician Pricing", *Southern Economic Journal*, Vol. 37, No. 1970, pp. 174-83; and, Havinghurst, C. "Antitrust Enforcement in the Medical Services Industry: What Does it All Mean?", *Milbank Memorial Fund Quarterly*, Vol. 58, No. 1980, pp. 89-124

15　Evans, R. *Price Formation in the Market for Physician Services in Canada, 1957-69*, Queens Printer, Ottawa, 1973. See also, Evans, R. "Supplier Induced Demand: Some Empirical Evidence and Implications" in Perlman, J.(ed) *The Economics of Health and Medical Care*, John Wiley & Son, New York, 1974, pp.162-73; and, studies that rejected this model such as Pauly, M. *Doctors and Their Workshops: Economic Models of Physician Behavior*, University of Chicago Press, Chicago, 1980, and Fuchs, V. *The Health Economy*, Harvard University Press, Cambridge MA. 1986

16　Sloan, F. "Physician Fee Inflation: Evidence from the Late 1960s" in Rosett, R.(ed), *The Role of Health Insurance in the Health Services Sector*, Watson Academic, New York, 1976, pp.321-54. See also Feldstein, 1970

17　Steinwald, B. and Sloan, F. "Determinants of Physician Fees", *Journal of Business*, Vol 43, No. 3, 1974, pp.493-511. See also, Sloan 1976; Holahan, J. et al, 1978; McLean, R. "The Structure of Market for Physician Services", *Health Services Research*, Vol. 15, No. 3, 1960, pp.271-80.

18　Kehrer, B. and Knowles, J. "Economies of Scale and the Pricing of Physician Services", in Yett, D. (ed) *An Original Comparative Analysis of Group Practice and Solo Fee-for-Service Practice*, (DHEW Report), National Technical Information Service, Springfield VA., 1974. See also, Dyckman, Z. *A Study of Physician Fees*, Council of Wage and Price Stability, Staff Report, Executive Office of the President, Washington DC, 1978; and, Feldstein, 1970; Fuchs 1973.

19　Vahovich, S. "Physicians' Supply Decisions by Specialty: TSLS Model" *Industrial Relations*, Vol. 16, No. 1, 1977, pp.51-60; Feldstein, 1970; see also Kehrer, 1974

20　Reinhardt, U. *Physician Productivity and the Demand for Health Manpower*, Ballinger, Cambridge MA. 1975. See also Pauly, 1980; and Ginsburg, P. "Impact of Economic Stabilization Program on Hospitals: An Analysis with Aggregate Data", in Zubkoff et al (eds) *Hospital Cost Containment: Selected Notes for Future Policy*, Prodist Press, New York, 1978, pp.293-323

21　Helbing, C. & Keene, R. "Use and Cost of Physician and Supplier Services Under Medicare", *Health Care Financing Review*, Vol. 10, Spring 1986, pp.109-122

22 *AMA et al. v. Bowen*, US Court of Appeals, 5th Circuit, No. 87-1755, October 14, 1988. 857 F.W. 267 (5th Cir. 1988); *Massachusetts Medical Society et al. v. Dukakis*, US District Court, District of MA., No.85-4312-K, 637 F.Supp 684 (D.Mass 1986); *Whitney v. Heckler* 603 F. Supp 821 (N.D.Ga 1985); and a number of others

23 Hsiao, W.C. and Stason, W.B. "Toward Developing a Relative Value Scale for Medical and Surgical Services" *Health Care Financing Review*, Fall 1979. See also Hsiao, W.C. et al. "The Resource-Based Relative Value Scale. Toward the Development of an ALternative Physician Payment System" *JAMA*, August 1987; Jensen, A.D. "Are Relative Value Scales the Answer?", *Health Affairs*, Spring 1988; Sikora, P.J. RBRVS: A Revolution in Physician Payment" *Group Practice Journal*, Mar-Apr 1988; Hsia, W.C. et al. "Results and Policy Omplications of the Resource-Based Relative-Value Study", *New England Journal of Medicine*, Sept 1988; Hsiao, W.C. "Resource Based Relative Values for Invasive Procedures Performed by Eight Surgical Specialties, JAMA, October 1988; Stevens, C. "How Fast Will Private Insurers Adopt RBRVS?" *Medical Economics*, August 1990]

24 Renoulds, R. *Estimated Changes in Payments to Physicians Under the Medicare Fee Schedule*, American Medical Association Center for Health Policy Research, 1991

25 Relman, A.S. "Dealing With Conflict of Interest" *New England Journal of Medicine*, Vol. 314, 1986, pp. 749-51

26 Gray, B.H (ed) *The New Health Care for Profit*, National Academy Press, Washington DC 1983. Also see, Gray, B.H. *For Profit Enterprise in Health Care*, National Academy Press, Washington, DC 1986

27 Hillman, A. L. "Financial Incentives for Physicians in HMOs. Special Report" *New England Journal of Medicine*, Vol. 317, No. 27, 1987, pp.1743-48

28 AMA, *Socioeconomic Characteristics of Medical Practice*, 1992, pp.17-21

29 Wolfe, L. "A Fatal Error", *New York Magazine*, December 7, 1992, pp. 54-59

30 Danzon, P.M."Medical Malpractice Liability" in Litan, R.E. and Winston, C. (eds) *Liability: Perspectives and Policy*, The Brookings Institution, 1988

31 Kletke, P.R., Marder, W.D. and Silberger, A.B. *The Demographics of Physician Supply: Trends and Projections*. AMA Center for Health Policy Research, Chicago IL, 1987

32 Flood, A.B., Scott, W.R. and Ewy W. "Does Practice Make Perfect?", *Medical Care*, Vol. 22, No. 2., 1984 pp. 98-125

33 Cotter, P.S. "An Analysis of the Changing Pattern in Physician Employment Status", in Gonzales, M.L. and Emmons, D.W., *Socioeconomic Characteristics of Medical Practice*, AMA Center for Health Policy Research, Chicago, 1986

34 Emmons, D.W. *Changing Dimensions of Medical Practice Arrangements*, AMA Center for Health Policy Reserach, Chicago, 1987, pp.20-37

35   Reynold, R.A., Rizzo, J.A. and Gonzales, M.L., "The Cost Medical Professional Liability", *Journal of the American Medical Association*, Vol. 257, No. 20, May 1987, pp.2776-81

Chapter 16
ECONOMIC COORDINATION OF HOSPITAL-PHYSICIAN FUNCTIONS

While there are physician-hospital interactions of a purely professional nature, particularly through physician staff affiliations with hospitals, this chapter concerns itself with coordinated activities motivated almost entirely by economics, profit, tax, and other financial considerations. Hospital-physician function coordination for economic gain is accomplished by way of *joint ventures* whereby the coordinating parties relinquish part of exclusive control, which they would otherwise exercise if undertaken individually, over the project involved in the joint venture. The joint venture creates elements of economic interdependence, profit and risk sharing between the parties. Thus, through joint venture, the participating parties, by their own will, eliminate actual and potential competition between themselves, which competition would have materialized if, barring the joint venture, they entered into the endeavor separately and independently from each other. As a result, the fundamental economic implications, to be discussed in this chapter, are accompanied by significant legal implications by way of antitrust considerations, to be discussed in Part IV of this volume.

Traditional hospital-physician relationships differ from joint ventures in various respects. First of all, while dependent on the organizational form of the venture, control allotment over the venture is a differentiating factor, not normally encountered between institutional and individual providers. Secondly, the joint venture based relationship is separate and independent from any other standard hospital-physician staff relationship, and, as we shall note later in this chapter, may take various forms, such as a partnership, basic contract, or an independent corporate entity.

Finally, the formation of a joint venture entails investments both from the hospitals as well as from the physicians involved, outside the scope of any traditional hospital-staff relationship. In general, joint ventures may be viewed as reflections of a changing economic environment for both the hospitals and physicians, of newly emerging needs for the parties involved, and as a means to an end in terms of strategic, business and financial terms. Thus, hospital-physician joint ventures are a product of emerging needs economic expediencies in modern medical markets.

Emerging Changes and Needs in Medical Markets

The enactment of the PPS in 1983, discussed earlier, placed substantial Medicare reimbursement constraints on hospitals. Prior to 1983, physicians utilized hospital facilities for their patient's care without much interference from outside the scope of their practice. Hospitals, in turn, had a financial incentive to accommodate physician utilization efforts, since they were reimbursed by Medicare based on a costs. The 1983 Prospective Payment System imposed on hospitals significant financial risk per admission, a risk which they now attempt to share with physicians by altering the latter's utilization patterns. In addition, with hospitals investing increasingly in offsite ambulatory therapeutic and diagnostic facilities, functioning as independently profit motivated enterprises, the control of costs becomes paramount, and physician conduct affecting costs has come under increasing scrutiny. Hospital and physician financial interests become closely related. Joint ownership by way of hospital-physician joint ventures renders cost control and profit motive for both parties mutually beneficial.

The growing supply, and surplus in some areas, of physicians increases professional rivalry and competition. We have noted in the previous chapter that patient visits, overall physician real as well as nominal income, has been declining, notwithstanding increases within some subspecialties. On the other hand, the cost of medical education has been consistently increasing, leaving graduating physicians with substantial debt upon graduation. Hospital-physician joint ventures may be viewed as a way to conserve the physician's financial status.

The patient has now also become the customer. All dimensions of care tend to be scrutinized. Group purchasing power, and utilization control procedures, became important elements of cost control. Cost and profit conscious HMOs dominate the provider scene. Technological progress created the opportunities for performing many diagnostic and therapeutic procedures in ambulatory, rather than inpatient, settings. The latter, in turn, created opportunities for the formation of various free-standing clinics, and other independent entrepreneurial healthcare functions, most conducive for hospital-physician joint venture activities.

The Motives for Joint Venturing

Joint ventures serve as a tool for attaining certain financial goals by the participants that they either could not attain by themselves, or could do so only at a much higher cost.

Joint ventures normally provide the capital necessary for providing the desired service, and do so at a much lower market risk to the participants than if they went out and did it alone. For instance, MRI services are often offered by way of joint ventures between hospitals and their radiologists, thus securing adequate demand for the facility. In addition, joint ventures provide physicians with capital which they alone could procure only by risking their personal assets (e.g. by securing bank loans), or by relinquishing control, through obtaining venture capital.

Hospitals have, in the past, constructed buildings for their staff close to the hospital facilities in order to provide convenience for the practitioners, and to facilitate utilization. They used their own capital/debt sources for this purpose. With increasing joint venturing trends, these facilities are constructed with capital obtained through the joint venture, leaving the hospital's apparent financial condition, debt-equity ratio, intact. In the same time, physicians also have a vested interest in maintaining the hospital's financial status at the highest possible level, since a sound hospital operation will attract medical tenants for their building, increasing return on their invested capital.

Joint ventures may bring business and professional talents together. Hospitals may obtain technical expertise by joint venturing with physicians, and the latter may benefit from the hospital's expertise in running an organization. Given the joint profit potential of the project, various types of expertise can be obtained and supplement in the long-run cheaper than by retaining outside consultants.

Traditionally, hospitals relied on physicians for bring in technical talents and their patients for facility utilization. Hospitals, in turn, provided physicians with major capital items of technology, and the environment for practicing for caring for the doctor's inpatients. With the development of diagnostic and therapeutic technology, many inpatient functions are now performed in ambulatory centers owned and operated by third-party providers, generating competitive pressures and pricing constraints. By joint venturing, physicians and hospitals combine their risks and resources to cope with third-party market competition. It also enhances cross-referral opportunities, for the financial benefit of the participants. This is so, notwithstanding certain legal and ethical constraints that some states place on patient referrals by their physicians to facilities owned by the same doctors.

There are other motives of some significance for joint venturing. To the extent that both hospitals and physicians have found some of their patients moving to third-party operated ambulatory healthcare facilities such as home health businesses, outpatient diagnostic services, ambulatory surgery facilities, and HMOs, it became necessary to join forces in order to retain their market share. This trend has been particularly accentuated by the shifting of market dimension emphases on the part of hospital marketing experts, and physicians, from geographical to product line. This is in accordance with the increased degree of function specialization offered by free-standing third-party maintained competing healthcare facilities.

Most Frequent Forms of Joint Venturing

A joint venture may be implemented by way of a variety of legal entities. *Partnership* has often been used to implement a joint venture between hospitals and physicians. The 1914 Uniform Partnership Act defines partnership as an association of two or more persons to carry on a business for profit. Partners in a "general partnership" participate in both the management and control of the property involved, in return for unlimited personal liability for all debts and obligations of the partnership, although the assets of the partnership belong to the organization and not to the partners. In a limited partnership situation, while the general partner's situation is similar to that in a general partnership, the limited partner's liability is limited, not unlike to that of shareholders in a corporation, by the amount of invested capital, associated with no responsibilities or rights to manage the partnership.

Another way healthcare-based joint ventures were implemented is through the general (as distinct from not-for-profit or professional) *corporate* structure, where the corporation, as a separate legal entity in most cases assumes its shareholders' liability. The chartering, functioning and revenue distribution of not-for-profits is restricted in most states. Professional corporations, on the other hand, are usually restricted to the same or similarly licensed professional group in the state, and they do not protect their shareholders from the liabilities of the corporation.

Functionally, physician-hospital joint ventures may occur in a variety of forms, and for a variety of reasons. Thus, physicians may participate with the hospital in the acquisition and development of *magnetic resonance imaging* (MRI), or similar, facilities that could operate on or about the hospital's property for inpatient and ambulatory utilization. Joint venture opportunities have been explored by way of *real estate* development projects, such as hospital parking garage, laundry facilities, or, a physician office building. The latter would contain several physician's suites, hospital operated pharmacy and restaurant, both available to the public, gift shop, and so forth. *Shared service facilities*, such as laundry, credit and collection, data processing, have been the objects of joint venturing between hospitals, physicians, and other, for instance long terms care, institutions.

Preferred provider organizations (PPOs), and Health Maintenance Organizations (HMOs), have been intruding into the hospital primary care markets for some time now. In order to preserve market shares, hospitals have been reacting by forming PPO joint ventures with some of their medical staff. As we indicated earlier, the antitrust ramifications of such joint ventures will be discussed in Part IV of this volume.

The Medicare PPS has put considerable pressure on hospital acute care capacity, and provided inducement to the hospitals to reduce that capacity by *transformation* into other types of facility. Joint ventures can provide the opportunities to achieve this transformation into other types of care facilities. Hospitals may provide physical facilities along with support services, while an expert joint venture partner would provide the staffing, technical and management expertise.

The Prospects for Joint Venturing

Joint ventures among healthcare providers in general have not been very successful. In fact, it has been reported that seven out of ten ventures fail, although for reasons attributable to management problems, rather than to those that may be inherent in healthcare joint venturing.[1] Nonetheless, joint venture activity in healthcare appears to be increasing, particularly since the parties to the venture see it as a way to improve their competitive position and capture larger market shares. Joint venturing also constitutes an access to capital as well as to technical and professional skills. Furthermore, it enhances medical staff loyalty to the hospital.

In addition, the Medicare based prospective pricing system has been increasingly pressuring hospitals to undertake external ambulatory endeavors. The latter is also stimulated by the increasing emergence of independent ambulatory care entrepreneurs to compete with hospitals and physicians. Finally, competition has been intensified by increasing physician-to-population ratios, and persisting excess hospital capacity throughout most parts of the country. Thus, joint venturing is a potentially viable means to cope with these competitive pressures.

In 1987, the AHA conducted a survey of some sixteen hospitals as to their experience and attitudes regarding joint venturing. The hospitals involved ranged from size of over 500 beds (about one-third), to those with less than 200 beds (less than 25%). Over half of the surveyed hospitals reported more than one joint ventures, with the range for the distribution from one to five, and no more than two partners involved for any venture. The forms of joint venture was found mainly in HMO and PPOs (over one-third), followed by MRIs (about one-third), durable medical equipment (25%), physical therapy services (just under 25%), and medical office buildings (16%). Other endeavors involved in joint ventures were diagnostic imaging, linear accelerators, nursing homes, health centers, answering services, reference laboratories, and other endeavors.

Most ventures involved physicians as the partner, with business corporations, other hospitals, and insurance firms playing significant roles as well. The ventures involving physicians or other hospitals were structured mainly as corporations, with partnerships being the second most popular form. The predominant motive for the ventures appeared to have been for-profit, twice as many as those formed with a not-for-profit motive. While physicians participated in more than half of the former motive category, only one-third of the latter involved physicians[2].

References

1   Sandrick, K. "Joint Ventures: Why 7 Out of Ten Fail?", *Hospitals*, December 20, 1986

2   Nathanson, S.N. "Joint Ventures: A Viable Diversification Strategy", *Trustee*, March 1988, pp.10-11. See also Riffer, J. "Ambulatory Care Joint Ventures Rise", *Hospitals*, February 5, 1986. Gilbert, R.N. "Hospital Revenue Diversification: A Case Study in Joint Venture Investing" *Healthcare Financial Management*, April 1986

Chapter 17
COMPETITION AND COST CONTROL IN THE PHARMACEUTICAL INDUSTRY

Drugs clearly perform important functions on the medical scene. While normally prescribed by physicians, they may substitute for some of the physician performed functions, such as surgery in some cases. In addition, drugs function independently as therapeutic agents reducing or eliminating the need for hospitalization, and reducing the explicit and opportunity costs of illness. While drug prices have been consistently increasing over the past few decades, their increases appear to have lagged behind those in expenditures on healthcare service items, with average annual rate of cost increase during 1960 through 1985 of just over 9% compared with over 12% for medical services. Thus, expenditures on drugs, as a percentage of total healthcare expenditures, declined from about 16% in 1950 to about 8% by 1985[1]. In addition, the prescription drug component of the CPI also suggests some relative moderation in the historical costs of drugs. Between 1970 and 1991, the total medical care component of the Consumer Price Index increased some 500% (34 vs. 177 in 1991), while the specific prescription drug component rose by about 420% (47.4 vs.199.7 in 1991), the cost hospital rooms by 813% (23.6 vs. 191.9), and the medical care services component by about 550% (32.3 vs. 177.1)[2].

Structure, Conduct and Performance

Notwithstanding the above, drug manufacturing has long been suspect of various economic malfeasances, such as excessive rates of profit in spite of similarly excessive amounts of promotional expenditures, and various forms of price discrimination by way of selling cheaper to large purchasers than to small ones, and selling brand name drugs at much higher prices than identical generic one. The mainstream of economic thought attributed these maladies to a lack of adequate competition among manufacturers predicated upon high concentration and substantial entry barriers. A *structural* view of the industry.

This view of the industry is based on traditional competitive industrial assessments which, for socially acceptable performance, has consistently sought normal long-run competitive profits, lack of price discrimination, and increased reliance on price competition, instead of noprice competition by way of excessive and competitive promotional expenditures that can only be supported by the existence of significant *monopoly power*. Reducing the duration of patent protection, and third-party reimbursement based on generic drug prices were, among other remedies, urged to cope with the industry's perceived anti-competitive environment.

Recent writers took a more dynamic view of the industry, suggesting that traditional assessments of monopoly power by way of the profit yard-stick overstate profits due to inadequate accounting measures. Furthermore, possible negative effects of an apparently present monopoly power could likely be more than offset by the private and social benefits of competition in terms of R&D expenditures and resulting product innovations. Furthermore, large promotion, particularly of the informational type, expenditures may be viewed simply as a means of communicating with prescribing physicians, and as a tool for overcoming market based entry barriers that may face new entrants into a product market.

The nature, application and significance of concentration ratio as a measure of market/industrial concentration and at least of a multi-firm market power has been discussed earlier in the volume. A relatively recent study estimated the four-firm concentration ratio among drug companies in the aggregate at about 30% (with no single firm having larger than an 8% share), much lower than in the cigarette (80%) and detergents (60%) markets[3].

Looking at individual markets, each with products that are close substitutes for each other, sell in the same price range, and included in the same competitive market according to the traditional market definition criteria, as suggested in the US Department of Merger Guidelines, a different picture emerges. Many classes of drugs within the industry do not compete with other by virtue of their totally different designated functions and targets. Even if one separates therapeutic drugs out of the industry, many non-competing products remain. Thus, one researcher found some 19 different therapeutic drug markets based on consumer substitutability, while another some 70 separately identifiable markets, based on therapeutic effect classification. Yet another study relying on physician prescription patterns yielded 10 markets [3, p. 32-36]. Based on 19 individual therapeutic drug markets, the four-firm concentration was found to range from a high of 95% for anti arthritics to a relatively low of 46% for anzymes-digestants, with an average ratio of 68%[4]. Thus, the four-firm concentration ratio for individual therapeutic drug markets appears to suggest the presence of significant monopoly power, at least in the combined hands of the four largest firms, and in a static sense assuming market stability with minimum or no firm turnover.

If the market in fact demonstrates instability by a a relatively frequent turnover of firms per time period, significant R&D and new product competition may be present among firms. The overall drug industry was found to be the second most unstable, after petroleum, using a traditional Hymer-Pashigian index of instability. The latter measures instability by using two ratios for all firms in a market or industry. One is the ratio of an individual firm's sales during time period "t" to total industry sales during the same time period. The other is the same ratio for the previous time period "t-1". The index is calculated by simply subtracting the "t-1" period ratio from the one for "t"[5]. Firm entry and turnover within the industry were also studied for seventeen therapeutic drug markets over a ten year period 1963 and 1972 inclusive. Fifteen of the markets experienced new entrants with market shares between 10% and 43%, and sixteen of the markets experienced firm exits[6]. Thus, new product developments, as well as entry and exit of firms in many therapeutic pharmacological markets, and the resulting dynamic competition, may overshadow the simple numerical reflection of possible market power conveyed by four- firm concentration ratios.

In terms of *conduct* criteria, three major factors may be examined: R&D and product innovation (may also be viewed as a "performance" criterion), competition in terms of advertising, and the same in terms of price. Patents play an important role in the industry, however, the protection they render to the inventor may be overcome by potential competitors by simply altering dosages, or making minor compound modifications. These apparently minor innovations by way of altering the original product can have substantial social and economic impact.

Thus, for instance, the same drug that was available only as an injection may be modified, for oral applications, by another possibly new firm constituting a major enhancement of social benefit, with significant economic consequences for the incumbent firm[7].

New products normally emerge only pursuant to R&D expenditure. The industry spends some 15% of sales per annum on R&D, third only to information processing and semi-conductors. Over two-thirds of this expenditure is internally financed, with rest covered by universities and the government. It also appeared during the early 1960s that firm size had little to do with the proportion of sales expended on R&D, or the number of inventions generated[8]. Thus, economies of scale in R&D expenditure were not viewed initially as major entry barriers, although subsequent studies appear to have contradicted this view when applied to the late 1960s, and subsequently [3, p.48].

The purpose of expenditures on advertising in drug markets is not entirely clear. One traditional and rather widespread school of thought disapproved of advertising in general, hence in pharmacology, as being wasteful, and consumer manipulative without social benefits. More recent studies appear to hold the opposite view, and attribute to drug advertising expenditures virtues such as being informational for prescribing physicians, and instrumental in facilitating the entry of firms into new markets[9]. In terms of timely informational benefits, it is asserted that physicians operating under time constraints cannot follow up on new drug data from journals or other publications. Thus, drug firm promotional efforts, and visits from drug firm representatives, are attributed in this regard a significant role, and studies appear to confirm that role[10]. However, since the cost of drug advertising is ultimately passed on to the patient, to all patients who use the advertised drug, unfair cross-subsidization and effective income redistribution takes place on the expense of patients of physicians who do not rely on drug advertising as their source for drug information, subsidizing the cost to the patients whose physicians use advertising as their primary source for information on new drugs, modified dosages or compounds.

The benefits, instead of the negative entry barrier effects, of advertising for potential new firms in a market was found to be considerable. Measuring entry as incremental percentage sales in 1972 not present during a prior period, positive relationship was shown between advertising expenditures and new entry of drugs that may not have otherwise been able penetrate a new market [3, pp.44-45].

Price competitive needs to be examined in terms of the drug's relative significance in the market, and in terms of its product life cycle. Significant drugs with substantial therapeutic values will likely be priced initially much above marginal cost in view of the absence of close substitutes. Others, with lesser advantage over their competitors are priced closer to marginal cost. But when viewed in a dynamic context, even initially highly priced drugs will ultimately experience a decline in their price structure as directly or indirectly competing drugs appear on the horizon over time, or substantial quality improvements are implemented in existing drugs, increasing the elasticity of demand for all drugs, and gradually reducing their price[11]. Furthermore, upon patent expiration for an old drug, new drug substitutes are relatively readily approved by the FDA, allowing competitors to enter into specific therapeutic markets, increasing their elasticity of demand, and reducing their price. In addition, it was found that both physicians, and pharmacists filling prescription, may at time act as the patients' agent, leaning toward, or substituting, lower priced drugs for higher ones [11, pp.99-100].

Profitability may be viewed as a *performance* barometer. In that regard, the drug industry appears to have performed very well indeed. During an approximately twenty year period ending in 1975, return on equity in the drug industry was over 60% higher than the same yardstick in the rest of the manufacturing sector[12]. However, the high rate of profit in the industry has come under suspicion as a possible indicator for the presence of monopoly power. The profit (Pa) used as a basis for this argument was calculated by conventional accounting methods: total revenue (TR) minus total cost (TC), divided by stockholders' equity (E), or TR-TC/E=Pa. Pa was, in turn, used as a basis for comparison with the return on capital in other industries, and for the conclusion that the drug industry, for reasons related to the presence of monopoly power, is much more profitable, and unreasonably so, than other manufacturing industries.

The TC variable in the above formula utilized by accounting includes R&D, advertising, and other promotion related expenditures. These are expensed out in the year they are incurred. Yet, it may be argued, while the funds for these items may indeed be expended during a given year, their impact on the operation, performance and profitability of the drug company likely be spread over several years, that is, the time period necessary for them generate results. Consequently, they may better be viewed as time-testable assets, to be depreciated over time, than as a one-time expense. To the extent, therefore, that the TC variable for any time period includes these undepreciated time testable asset elements, the drug companies' profit, and their rate of return on shareholders' equity (in absolute and relative terms), is over estimated. The modified formula would be as follows: economic profit (Pe) is equal to the *ratio* of TR, less TC, less the pertinent asset depreciation (d) *to* E plus the depreciated value of time-testable assets (At-d), or Pe=TR-TC-d/E+(At-d). The addition to shareholders' equity of undepreciated time-testable assets more than offsets, particularly during the earlier years of any increments in these assets) the increase in net income due to the reduced TC element, yielding a lower return on equity, and more in line with those in the rest of the manufacturing sector.

While conventional accounting recognizes the depreciation of fixed assets over time, accordingly reducing corresponding net incomes throughout the manufacturing sector, no such treatment has been accorded to the drug manufacturing sectors time-testable assets. Clearly, the final impact of this amendment upon the drug companies' rate of return depends on the classification and size of expenditures capitalized rather than expensed out every year, the utilized accounting method of depreciation, and the annual rate of increase in capitalized time-testable assets. Thus, the annual rate of return to the drug companies, and the industry, varies inversely with the economic life of time-testable assets. Once applied, the adjusted formula yields a rate of return for the drug industry quite close to, although still somewhat (about 20%) higher than, most other industries in the rest of manufacturing sector, even if similar adjustments are made for time-testable assets in the other industries[13]. The margin of return in favor of the drug industry may be attributed to (a) substantial rightward shifts in the demand function for drugs during the past several decades brought about by the consistent appearance of new therapeutic drugs, facilitated third-party payment mechanisms, and the increased age intensity of the population, and (b) the higher risk factor due to the unpredictability of outcome for R&D expenditures at all, stages of product development, including government approval.

The most recent industry estimate for the total cost of bringing a drug to the market is about $230 million[14].

Drug manufacturing is multinational in scope. Three of recent major merger transactions involved foreign acquirer corporations (Beecham, Roche, and Rhone-Poulenc). Thus, a drug manufacturer must be large enough to survive domestically and abroad. The minimum efficient scale of operation in that regard is estimated to generate about $3 billion in annual sales,[15] yielding enough economies of scale in marketing and research to cope with the costs of failed drugs at various late stages of their development.

Drug Manufacturing and Marketing Under Managed Care

The pharmaceutical industry has been affected essentially by several of the same factors that impacted on the entire healthcare system: the emerging predominance of HMOs and PPOs, purchaser preoccupation with costs and the consequent utilization of purchasing market power through organized purchasing efforts, consolidations within the hospital sector by way of mergers and the emergence of large investor owned and corporate managed hospital chains, and the increasing age intensity of the population. In particular, with almost 60% of physicians belonging to some type of managed care system by 1989[16], and prescribing drugs under specific guidelines instead of pursuant to their own decision often affected by intensive drug industry advertising and sales visits, the pharmaceutical industry needed to reconsider the method of promotion to the individual practitioner. Cought up in the campaign against spiraling healthcare costs, managed care affiliated physicians are often pressured to prescribe certain drugs based on their cost, and particularly generic versions of multi-sourced brand name drugs. HMOs often restrict the choice of drug retailers, limit the daily quantity prescribed, implement drug utilization reviews, and require generic versions of unpatented drugs[17]. In addition, some hospitals began to utilize a preapproved list of drugs, so called "drug formularies", which were subsequently expanded by HMOs into the ambulatory environment[18]. The impact of these constraints on the drug industry becomes particularly significant in view of the fact that by 1989 the cost of almost 50% of retail prescription drug sales were covered by third-party payers[19], many of which emphasized generic drugs, and substitution for lower priced versions of the same drug.

The emergence of drug wholesaling during the 1980s made possible the implementation of a system of discounting and rebates, which were not common place when drugs were distributed directly by the manufacturers to retailers. At the present time, wholesalers are thought to account for about three-quarters of all drug sales [PMA, 1989]. Finally, an increased number of FDA approved over-the-counter (OTC) drugs contributed to the slowing down of the apparent cost inflation of drugs, since most third-party payers do not cover OTC drug purchases, and the latter normally sell for a lower price than prescription drugs. In addition, the proliferation of OTC drugs also increased consumer awareness and education regarding drug utilization. This latter development, along with the reduced autonomy of physicians in prescribing drugs, places drug companies in direct marketing contact with final users, as has long been the case for any other non-medically related consumer item.

The Pharmaceutical Access and Prudent Purchasing Act of 1990 (introduced by Senator David Pryor: S.2605) was designed to allow Medicaid drug price negotiations with drug manufacturers at the state government level, not unlike those that already transpire between drug manufacturers and hospitals, HMOs, mail service retail distributors of drugs, and other large purchasers. The Bill was designed essentially to transform Medicaid from a third-party payer for drugs to a volume purchaser of pharmaceuticals. The Bill also intends to enable states to substitute among drugs within the same therapeutically categories, contrary to industry suggestions to the effect that such substitutions are not in the interest of the patient. Thus, it is becoming evident that market powers on the demand side of the market will continue to exert downward pressure on drug prices, subject to the cost constraints of the manufacturers.

Mail Pharmacy Services (MPS): A Means of Drug Cost Control?

Mail order drug retailing has become a substantial business, and a major competitor for the community based drug store. Traditionally, they serviced remote and rural areas. Now, they are a part of major employer based prescription benefit programs, and service some 100 million prescriptions per year[20]. There are three major consumer groups that rely on and support MPS. First, largest, and the fastest growing, is made up of public sector and corporate employers accounting for almost 50% of the MPS volume, and serviced largely by for-profit sellers (e.g. Medco Containment Services). Secondly, veterans under the VA program, accounting for about one-third of the total volume. Thirdly, members of the American Association of Retired Persons (AARP), consisting of individuals with no drug benefit plans of their own; although no more than about 10% of the potentially huge AARP market utilizes this service, they make up much of the rest of the MPS sector[21].

The total MPS market has grown very fast during the past decade, from under $100 million during the early 1980s to some $1.5 billion by 1989, constituting some six percent of the total US outpatient prescription drug market as of 1989, with its proportion expected to increase to some 15% by the end of 1993[22]. The composition of sales has largely been centering on chronic long-term medications utilized by the elderly segment of the population, typically filling long-term (90-180 days) medication needs[23].

From the employer's point of view, MPS appears offer distinct benefits. Possible plan cost saving, relative to traditional drug plans, of up to 50%. Reduced administrative and transaction costs, particularly for firms with a geographically scattered labor force, due to most MPS' centralized billing and utilization review systems. In addition, a MPS permits the employer to increase health benefits for employees, without significant increases in corresponding costs. From the patients' point of view, MPSs have been found to be private, convenient, reasonably priced, and often educational by way of medication-specific leaflet availability[24].

Questions are often raised regarding the cost differential between MPS and community-based pharmacy plans. In this regard, the cost of prescription drugs may be dissected into two broad components: direct costs, and program costs.

A component of *direct* costs is the cost of the ingredient, that is the drug, itself. The latter, in turn, depends on whether a patented brand name multisource is used or a generic version of the drug is dispensed, the retailer's own cost for the product, and the size of the prescription itself. MPSs generally claim to use generic versions of any drug whenever they can, and apparently do so with some 25% of the dispensed prescriptions. The MPS advantage in this regard is clearly facilitated by a higher long-term maintenance chronic composition of their business compared to the community drug retailer. A larger proportion of these drugs are available in generic form than acute care prescriptions. In addition, given the volume of sales, MPS tend to pay a lower average price to their suppliers than individual retail druggists do, giving the former a further cost advantage.

Another direct cost, dispensing fees, include nondrug product costs such as rent, supplies, payroll, and profit margin. There is a wide range of variations in these fees among community drug store based plans. Medicaid's reimbursement for dispensing fees in 1989 averaged somewhere between $3.50 and $5.50[25]. Lack of reliable data from pharmacies, and from third-party payers in general make it difficult to accurately estimate dispensing fee amounts and proportions. Similar problems prevail for MPSs.

The third direct prescription cost component involves administrative fees, that is, the transaction costs of running the third-party payment plan such as Prudential, or the Blues. While reliable data in this regard is also scarce, these average around 60 cents per prescription in community-based pharmacy plans. Since they are both program administrators as well as dispensers of medication, MPSs normally include these costs with dispensing fees.

Indirect drug program costs include demographic characteristics, such as age and gender distribution, The elderly will consume larger amounts of medication per time unit, and females will continue to do so for a longer time period due to their extended statistical life expectancy. There appear to be no significant difference in this regard between community drug store and MPS plans, although the latter tend to market target the elderly more aggressively due to their need for long-term chronic medication[26].

Another indirect drug program cost is inherent in the characteristics of the drug plan itself. The MPS' larger volume characteristics may yield lower average unit cost per time period. In addition, as an incentive for employees to enroll in MPS based programs, employers may offer plans with lower copayment features than those involved in community-based pharmacy plans, or no copayment at all. This appeared to have at least two impacts: (a) a larger proportion of the plans cost is born by the plan organizer, or the employer, and (b), in situations with copayments, some utilization reductions were noted[27].

A third type of indirect cost falling within the category of transaction system errors may also be significant. These entail costs associated with frauds on the part of users and suppliers, pharmacological malpractice, inventory waste. Once again, a lack of reliable data seems to prevent researchers from drawing cost comparative conclusions between MPS and community-based drug store based plans[28].

The Relative Cost of Pharmaceuticals in the US

The decade of 1980s witnessed sharp increases in drug prices. The PPI and CPI for drugs increased at an average annual rate of 9.6%, compared to the corresponding rate of increase in the general CPI of 4.7%, and the 2.6% increase in the PPI. Although it was argued that drug price index increases may have been overstated by as much as 3% due to sampling biases in favor of higher priced drugs[29]. Much of the increases during the 1980s may be attributed to substantial increases in prescription drug related expenditures which grew at an average annual real rate of almost 5%. Notwithstanding the above, expenditures on prescription drugs and other medical nondurables, as a proportion of total national medical expenditures, decreased from 8.6% to 8.2% during 1990s.

A way to suggest that US drug prices are too high is to view them relative to those charged in the Canadian healthcare system. Thus, a recent Federal Government study sampled some 50 of the top 100 US prescription drugs with Canadian wholesale prices much higher than those in the US[30]. Another US Government study, conducted by the USGAO in late 1992, compared manufacturer's price components for a group of selected drugs in Canada and the US. After screening drugs not sold in the same or comparable dosage in the two countries, or not sold in the same manner (prescription v. otc) in the two countries, or having similar disparities rendering price comparisons meaningless, some 120 drugs were compared. These included 39 of the 50 most commonly prescribed drugs in the US that constitute about a third of all drugs prescribed in this country. In addition to comparing per package factory prices, the costs of common prescription dosages were also compared. Price differences were not weighted by relative sales volume due to a lack of volume information from US markets[31].

The findings indicate that drug manufacturers charge more to US wholesalers in the US than they do to Canadian ones. In general, the drugs included in the study cost about one-third more to US wholesalers than to those in Canada. For individual drugs, the median price differential was found to be above 40%. The range for the entire collection was from -44% (US price being lower) to US price being almost 1000% higher. Specifically, the distribution suggested that about 30% of the drugs were 50-99% more expensive in the US, 27% were found to be 20%-50% higher, and about a quarter of them was 100% to 500%. The tail ends of the distribution indicated 16% for the 0%-19% price difference, and 3% for 500% or more [31, p.12-13]. Some 25% of the drugs cost 100% in the US that in Canada, another quarter of the surveyed drugs had prices 50-99% higher in the US than in Canada, about one-third of the drugs cost 0-50% more in the US, while some 20% of the drugs was less expensive in the US [31, p.14].

The price differentials have not been attributed to differences in production, research and distribution costs. First of all, production and distribution costs constitute only a small portion of total costs. Thus, even if these costs were allocated to each product sold in the two countries, they would not justify major price differences. The cost of R&D is allocated among products consistently, whether sold in the US or in Canada. Finally, the cost of marketing, sales and regulatory compliance, even if allocated to individual drugs, do not differ between the US and Canada. Thus, the reasons for the differences must be sought somewhere else.

The pricing constraints faced by drug companies in Canada, not present in the US, are largely government or regulation related. In 1987, the Canadian Patent Act was revised, and the Patented Medicine Prices Review Board was set up. While the changes created longer market protection for patented drugs by lengthening the prohibited entry time period for generic competitors of patented drugs, the Board also implemented close monitoring of patented drug prices to prevent excessive pricing structures. The Board closely scrutinizes the introductory price levels for drugs patented in Canada after 1987, and subsequent price increases

for drugs that were already in the Canadian market by 1987. Subsequent to public hearings, warranted sanctions in cases of perceived over-pricing include mandating a lower price, or removing the government imposed competitive shield against generic versions of the violating firm's over-priced drug, or against one of its other drugs. The effectiveness of these measures appear to be indicated by higher price differentials for drugs under the Board's control [31, p.15-6].

Another drug price constraint in Canada rests with the purchasing power of the provincial governments, in their capacity as major third-party payers through drug benefit programs. Although nine of the twelve provincial drug benefit programs, including those of Ontario and Quebec, pay for the drug needs of the elderly and the poor only, they do constitute a major restraint on drug price since they cover nearly half of the prescription volume. Ontario, for instance, created a list of reimbursable drugs (a "formulary") along with their maximum price. Drugs are multidimensionally screened prior to being placed on the formulary: effectiveness, price, safety, and availability. Periodic price reviews may subject drugs to removal from the formulary. For instance, in mid-1991, some 10% of the submitted drugs were subjected to negative price revisions, and about 2% was dropped due to persistently excessive pricing. Furthermore, since formularies are published, products and prices, and made available to drug prescribing physicians, they become a prime source of available drug information for the doctors. Provincial drug formularies appear to increase US-Canadian drug-price differentials by as much 500%, with the median price differential for listed drugs being close to 50%, contrasted with only 10% for unlisted drugs [31, p.17-8].

The impact of generic competition on the price of proprietary drugs has been quite interesting. It has been noted that, barring regulatory and purchasing market power imposed pricing constraints, manufacturers tend to increase proprietary drug prices in the face of increased generic competition. The reasons rests with image, perceived quality and reputation. Their ability to raise price in an unregulated and uncontrolled market, thus rests with a lower elasticity of demand emanating from these factors. In Canada, the constraints imposed by the Board, and by the provinces' purchasing market power, place a constraint on drug prices and the ability of manufacturers to react to generic competition in the traditional manner by way of increasing prices [31, p.19-20].

Finally, some conjectures regarding the impact of Canadian drug price controls on industry R&D expenditures, innovations, and product development. One argument has traditionally been that reducing or controlling drugs prices will reduce R&D expenditures, hence reduce the availability of new drugs to fight new and existing diseases. A counter argument postulated that drug price controls would simply reduce drug company profits, instead of the number and quality of forthcoming drugs. In Canada, the patients have it both ways: in the same time that drug companies subjected themselves to drug price controls, they also agreed to increase R&D expenditures in Canada, and they have done so. On the other hand, drug companies might have been able to place themselves in this apparent Canadian cost-profit squeeze, simply due to the minor impact that it will have on their overall financial position: the Canadian drug market represents less than eight percent of the USA's share of the drug companies' international market. Thus, what happens in Canada may have no more than a limited impact on the drug manufacturers' corporate-wide financial condition. What they were willing to accept in Canada, they may not be able to tolerate, or in the long-run survive, in the US. The implementation of Canadian like controls in the US, may indeed yield lower R&D expenditures, or simply just more efficient R&D expenditures with no ultimate impact on the flow of newer and more effective drugs. In fact, if the drug manufacturer's profit margin is squeezed by Canadian type price controls, they may generate a supply elasticity incentive for them to produce more and newer drugs, in order to maintain their statusquo in terms of overall profitability. This response would disregard substantial financial cushions that may already be built into high advertising and other promotional expenditures.

References

1   Waldo, D.R. et al. "National Health Expenditures, 1985", *Health Care Financing Review*, Fall 1986, p.14. Also see Gibson, R. and Waldo, D. "National Healthcare Expenditures", 1980, Health Care Financing Review, September 1981, pp.20-31

2   *Statistical Abstract of the United States*, 1992, p.471

3   Grabowsky, H.G. and Vernon, J.M. "New Studies in Market Concentration" in Chien, I. in *Issues in Pharmaceutical Economics*, Lexington Books, Lexington MA 1979, p.31

4   Vernon, M. "Concentration, Promotion and Makerket Share Stability in Pharmaceutical Industry" *Journal of Industrial Economics*, July 1971, pp. 246-266

5   Cocks, D. "Product Innovation and the Dynamic Elements of Competition in the Ethical Phramaceutical Industry", in Helms, R.B. (ed) *Drug Developments and Marketing*, AEI, Washington, DC 1975

6   Kearney, A.T. *Study of Economics of Entry and Exit in the Pharmaceutical Industry*, Pharmaceutical Manufacteres Assocn, Washington DC., 1974

7   Schwartzman, D. *Innovation in the Pharmaceutical Industry*, Johns Hopkins University Press, Baltimore, MD 1976, p.18

8   Schnee, J.E. Caglarcan, E. "Economic Structure and Performance of the Ethical Pharmaceutical Industry", in Lindsey, C.M. *The Phamaceutical Industry*, John Wiley & Johns, New York, 1978, p.32

9   Leffler, K.B. "Persuasion or Information? The Economics of Prescription Drug Advertising" *Journal of Law and Economics*, April 1981, pp.45-74

10 Avron, J. "Scientific vs. Commercial Sources of Influence on Prescribing Physician Behavior" *American Journal of Medicine*, July 1982, pp.4-8

11 Chien, R.I. *Issues in Pharmaceutical Economics*, Lexington Books, Lexington MA 1979, p.77

12 Campbell, W.J. and Smith, R.F. "Profitability and the Pharmaceutical Industry, in Lindsey, C.M. *The Pharmaceutical Industry*, Wiley, New Yor 1978, p.114

13 Clarkson, K.W. "The Use of Pharmaceutical Profitability Measures for Public Policy Actions", in Chien, 1979, p.117. Also see Comanor, W.S. The Political Economy of the Pharmaceutical Industry", *Journal of Economic Literature*, Vol. 21, September 1986]

14 PMA, Pharmaceutical Manufacturers Association *1987-89 Annual Survey Report*, Washington, DC. 1989. PMA and The Tufts University Center for the Study of Drug Development, April 1990

15 NYT, *The New York Times*, July 29 1989, and the *Wall Street Journal* July 28, 1989

16 Scott-Levin Associates, *Managed Care Survey*, 1989

17 Marion, *Managed Care Digest*, 1989

18 Gold, M. and Hodges, D. "Health Maintenance Organizations in 1988", *Health Affairs*, Winter 1989, p.127

19 Siegelman, S. and Feierman, R. "Annual Pharmacy Business Survey", *American Druggist*, May 1990, p.33

20 Enright, S.M. "Mail Order Pharmaceuticals", *American Journal of Hospital Pharmacy*, Vol. 44, 1987, pp.1870-73

21 Codling, M. *Rapid Growth of Mail-Order Drug Dispensing*, Arthur D. Little, Cambridge MA. 1987. See also Medco Containment Services, *Annual Report*, 1987, Fair Lawn NJ. Find/SVP, *The Market for Mail Order Pharmaceuticals*, New York, 1989

22 Drury, S. "Mail Order Drugs Can Cut the Cost of Prescription Plans, *Business Insurance*, March 1, 1983, p.30. See also Glaser, M. "Lovers and Haters of Mail Rx Service. Debate at Symposium", *Drug Topics*, April 21, 1986, pp.31-32. Navarro, R. "Prescription by Mail", *Medical Interface*, Vol 2, No.10, P.8

23 "Pennsylvania Firm Sees Big Potential For Mail Order" *Drug Topics*, May 14, 1986, pp.20-22

24 Chi, J. "Now Federal Employees Too Are Going With Mail Order Drugs", *Drug Topics*, Nov. 17, 1986, p.26. See also McHugh, J.H. *Mail Order Prescription Service: A Provider Perspective*, Arthur D. Lttle, Cambridge 1987. Jendlin, P.T. "Containing Costs Through Mail Order Generic Cost Plans" *Journal of Compensation and Benefits*, December 1987, pp.162-3. Glaser, M. "Mail Order Rxs: Separating Fact From Fiction" *Drug Topics*, February 56, 1984, pp.42-48, and "Lovers and Haters of Mail Rx Service Debate at Symposium" *Drug Topics*, April 21, pp.31-32

25 NPC, National Pharmaceutical Council, *Employers and Prescription Medicine Benefits*, Reston VA., 1987; and *Pharmaceutical Benefits Under State Medical Assiatance Programs*, Reston VA., 1989.

26 AARP, American Association of Retired Persons, *Prescription Drugs: A Survey of Consumer Use*, Attitudes and Behavior. Washington 1984

27 Soumerai, S.B. et al. "Payment Restrictions for Prescription Drugs Under Medicaid, Effects on Therapy, Cost and Equity", *New England Journal of Medicine*, Vol. 317, 1987, pp.550-57. Also see, Leibowitz, A. et al. "The Demand for Prescription Drugs as a Function of Cost Sharing", *Social Science and Medicine*, Vol. 21, 1985, pp.1063-70

28 Morgenson, G. "What's Not in The Prospectus", *Forbes*, July 1987, pp.61-62. See also, Boston Consulting Group, *Economics of Mail Service Prescription Plans*, New York, 1987, and Christensen, D.B. "Mail Order Prescription Services: Some Reflections", *Medical Interface*, Vol. 2, 1989, pp. 21-23

29 Berndt, E.R "Auditing the Producer Price Index: Micro Evidence from Prescription Pharmaceutical Preparations" *NBER Working Paper*, No. 4009, March 1992

30 HHS, Office of the Inspector General, *Strategies to Reduce Medicaid Drug Expenditures*, 1990

31   GAO/HRD 92-110, *Prescription Drug Charges in US and Canada*, 1992. See also, HCFA, *Manufacturers' Prices and Pharmacists' Charges for Prescription Drugs Used by the Elderly*, June 1990. Frank,R.G. and Salkever, D.S. *Pricing, Patent Loss and the Market for Pharmaceuticals*, A Report to the Office of Technology of Technology Assessment, Dec 1990.

Chapter 18
COST AND COMPETITION
IN DENTISTRY

While the frequency of dental problems is common, the range of dental diseases is relatively narrower than those found in general healthcare. Most of the maladies are limited to dental caries, and periodontal problems. Oral cancer is quite uncommon, and, when it does occur, its treatment is normally conducted outside the confines of a typical dental practice. Other fields of dental practice, such as orthodontics and pedodontics, usually involve preventive rather than disease treating efforts. In addition, cosmetic and corrective dentistry received increasing attention in recent years.

Another element of the major clinical differences between dental care and general health care is that dental problems *per se* are rarely fatal, although treatment complications, even fatalities, often related to anesthesia and by virtue of an occasional malpractice, do occur with some frequency. Furthermore, at the initial stages most dental diseases are asymptomatic, not obviating the need for care. Hence, patient attendance at dental practices are often postponed, or completely bypassed. In general, the frequency of dental care per person par time period appears to vary directly with the patient's education and the level of socio-economic status.

As with the case of general healthcare, dentistry also has at least three major dimensions of economic concern: cost of care, access to service, and the quality of service. In general, the *cost* concerns in dentistry have not been voiced with the same intensity as in other areas of the healthcare sector. One reason may be that dentistry constitutes no more than about 7% of the total expenditure on healthcare[1]. Another expenditure attribute is the historical predominance of privately financed service procurements, instead of the predominance of third-party, particularly government, payers found in the rest of the general healthcare sector. Nevertheless, cost excesses by way of unneeded or improper treatments, and even fraud, particularly under Medicaid, have been alleged, and probably do occur, although formal public reaction has been relatively limited[2]. Dentistry is simply not where healthcare finance is concentrated.

On the demand side, an often cited reason for healthcare costs increases has been the proliferation of third-party payers on the scene, particularly traditional health insurance companies such as the Blues and commercials. Physicians performed examinations, tests, and procedures without a concern for costs, although often with concern for medical malpractice suits, as reimbursements were sure to come. Until recently, dentistry was largely uncovered by insurance carriers. In recent years, dental insurance began to proliferate through work-place based plans, although significant deductibles, copayments, and other cost sharing provisions were often included. Nevertheless, the effective price of dental care for the patient appears to have decreased, prompting an increase in demand[3].

The healthcare literature advanced arguments to the effect that the increased flow of income/expenditure into the healthcare sector financed by insurance and third-party payments made it financially possible, and created the incentive, in medicine to advance research and develop new technology probably for the ultimate benefit of the patient, as well as for that of the provider[4]. In dentistry, it appears that the acceleration of demand for services financed by insurance was at least met, if not surpassed, by an increase in the supply of dentists, both from domestic and foreign sources. If research and development in dental technology advances, it likely happens without any significant impetus from patient revenues[5]. Indeed, while the income of some dentists have recently increased, most dentists have seen their income decline, and, in fact, many perceived a decrease in the size of their overall market. The closure of a number of dental schools in the country, caused mostly by declining enrollments and the accelerating cost of education, further reflects on a market that is apparently shrinking along with a still increasing supply of practicing dentists[6].

The Dental Industry

The profession has traditionally been dominated by solo practitioners working on a fee-for-service basis, normally paid directly by the patient. During recent years, pre-payment plans, group practices, capitation payment systems, and increased regulations, changed somewhat the arena for dental practice. The services provided by the dentist is determined largely by the needs of the patient, although factors such as the patient's ability to pay for the services, the dentist's financial interest in particular payment source, and regulatory constraints may also play a role. In general, the dental provider is motivated by maximizing income per time period, preserving or enhancing the status of his or her practice as well as that of the profession, and by improving the dental health of his patients.

Rational patients intend to maximize their perceived dental well-being subject to the incurred costs, both in terms of time spent at the dentist's office and in terms of the price paid; or conversely, subject to a desired level of dental well-being, minimize the total cost of care, both in terms of time and money. Group purchasers of dental services view the process as a business, and attempt to maximize profits (non-profits, sustain themselves) by lowering expenditures and maintaining the perceived quality of the service.

Recent institutional changes in the profession saw the emergence of offices with two or more dentists where the participants share in the profits as well as in the expenses. Three or more dentist group practices have also evolved, although they by no means dominate the scene. Arrangements whereby one dentist employs the services of other dentists have also evolved, particularly in department store based offices, and in heavily advertised and predominantly business motivated practices. Some hospitals also maintain outpatient dental clinics. Control over employee healthcare costs prompted the emergence of industry or employer owned dental clinics. In addition, nonhospital affiliated publicly owned and operated dental clinics provide dental care to specialized groups such as the US Armed Forces, American Indians, veterans, the medically indigent, and prison inmates.

Statistics offered later in the chapter suggest that group practitioners enjoy an approximate 25% income advantage over solo practitioner, suggesting perhaps that significant production scale economies may exist in medicine. These scale economies could emanate from intra-group specialization generating increased practice proficiency, greater capacity utilization of auxiliary personnel as well as of office space, professional interaction among affiliated practitioners, pooled capital for advanced technological acquisitions and fuller utilization of equipment, and financial economies such as negotiated discounts on equipment pricing and loan arrangements.

A dentist's productivity may be measured in terms of patient visits or gross billing per practice hour. Unfortunately, there do not appear to be convincing data or studies to date that clearly suggesting that a dentist's productivity and efficiency varies directly with firm size. As will be noted later, there does appear to be a trend toward an increase in dental firm size. Such trend may be viewed as a perception on the part of the practitioners that functioning within larger practice units is more profitable, hence may be more efficient. For instance, it appears historically that group practices are inclined to accept more lower paying Medicaid patients, arguably due to a rational decision based on lower production costs and, therefore, higher profits[7].

If one considers an improvement in the quality of service, even at constant cost, an improvement in production efficiency and productivity, then group practices may again score higher than solos. Procedure specialization conducive groups breed increased competence and proficiency at certain procedures. Furthermore, members of the group may function as designed or incidental peer reviewers of each other's work, billing, administrative and complaint handling procedures. Thus, if one assumes away collusive disregard for various aspects of practice malfeasance, groups may possess built-in safeguards for a certain degree of quality and administrative efficiency. The few studies that were conducted on the efficiency of group general and specialized medical practices do suggest that groups offer better care than solo ones. However, the groups considered by the study were mainly those affiliated with major medical centers and universities, rendering the results probably nonrepresentative of the general group practice area[8].

Determinants of Demand for Dental Services

For many years dentistry, like other professions, was void of any significant advertising. Yet, once undertaken, *advertising* turned out to be an important determinant of demand for the service. The American Dental Association (ADA) has traditionally labeled advertising as unethical, a violation of the ADA's "Principles of Ethics". In early 1977, the FTC filed a complaint in order to free up advertising activity in dentistry. A late 1977 Supreme Court decision, involving lawyers, declared organized bans on advertising unconstitutional by way of violating freedom of speech under the First Amendment[9]. At about the same time, the ADA generated a set of criteria for advertising "routine services", where the latter were defined roughly as services performed frequently for a set fee, using standard techniques[10]. By mid-1979, the FTC's case against the ADA was all but settled, with terms including commitment by the ADA not to inhibit in any way truthful advertising of dental services. Subsequently, advertising by dentists has, though gradually, been gaining considerable momentum. By now, some sort of advertising, form of promotion or service marketing may be considered as a prerequisite for a financially successful dental practice. The degree of competition in community based dental services markets rendered "word of mouth" oriented marketing alone all but inadequate for reasonable success.

Based on accepted economic theories of advertising, it may frequently be viewed as having benefits beyond those that accrue to the advertiser of a service of a product[11]. The ultimate motive for an advertiser is probably the enhancement of sales and profitability. However, for the consumer, particularly in the field of services where product or service knowledge is not only limited but are technically and politically constrained, such as in medicine and to a lesser extent dentistry, advertising becomes an essential source of information. In fact, the informational importance of advertising increases directly with the cost of obtaining that information by alternative means. Furthermore, the advertising in otherwise and traditionally relatively unknown and technically not understood, or misunderstood, services such as medicine and dentistry, will likely increase competition in their respective markets because potential and actual consumers become more aware of their alternatives both in terms of price and to an extent quality.

The informational impact of dental services advertising reduces the cost of seeking out the best and lowest priced dentist, and will allow patients to consider pricing and perceived quality alternatives among dentists, prompting them to switch among provider alternatives. Intensified patient switching in dental services will inevitably increase inter-provider competition both in terms of price and quality (broadly defined to include not only the performance of the dentist, but also the location of the dental office, office hours, and the nature of the practice), when dentists attempt to maintain, or increase their patient pools. This phenomenon has become notable in dental markets already. Franchised, retail-based and large-firm practices have proliferated in some parts of the country. In addition, the introduction of advertising in other medical and related markets appeared to have reduced prices, or to reduce the rate of increases in the price structure[12].

In addition to advertising, the emergence of third-party payers, *pre-paid dental plans*, and other measures designed to reduce the out-of-pocket lump-sum dental expenses of the patient also impacted upon the demand for dental services. However, the impact does not seem to reflect an increase in total demand for dental services as much as a change in the composition of existing demand for those services. Increases were found in the frequency of preventive and maintenance care, with the likely outcome of long-term reduction in the dental component of total healthcare costs[13].

On the other hand, two Rand Corporation studies on the impact of pre-paid dental plans on the demand for dental services appear have concluded that on the average, per-capita expenditures, based on the frequency of visits alone, at least doubles, in addition to changes in the demand for service mix. As third-party payer participation increases, the importance of price as a denominator for dental market competition is reduced, shifting the need of cost containment from the consumers to the payers. Finally, by way of reducing the direct cost of care to the patient, prepaid plans reduce the consumer's demand elasticity for dental service, and elevate factors such as perceived service quality, location, provider personality, and other possibly less substantive amenities as prime denominators for service competition among dentists[14].

A determinant of demand for dental services has been attributed to the suppliers of the service themselves. The analysis is conducted within the context of the so called "target income" hypothesis. The essence of the latter is that dentist fees and income tend to increase directly with the provider/population ratio. As provider/population ratio increases, competitive pressures would normally be expected to reduce provider income. To compensate for the income reducing effects of market forces under those circumstances, providers increase their fees to the extent the market permits it, and, additionally, generate (induces) extra demand for their services to maintain some target income level. The inducement of extra demand is perceived to happen by way of the dentist, acting as not only the patient's supplier but also the patient's agent in procuring the service, simply recommending additional treatments. In general, the model postulates that an influx of additional dentists into the community initially reduces net income per practice. Dentists will react by raising prices and generating more service, until their income level is restored either to the previous level, or to a level where the total positive utility of the restored additional income is equal the total negative utility of leisure lost due to working more to accommodate the additional demand generated in the process[15].

While theoretically appealing, and initially prescribed largely to physician behavior, the model may have limited or no applicability to dentistry. In fact, some studies have found a normally expected market standard negative relationship between service supply and fees in dentistry[16]. In addition, the high price elasticity of demand for dental services would support a market controlled resistance to higher dental prices in the face of increased supply. Finally, another study, using Health Insurance Association of America price and utilization data, estimated simultaneously a three-equation model of the supply of, and demand for, dental services, and the dentist/population ratio. Dentist density was used as an explanatory variable in the demand equation in order to test for provider created demand, or target income seeking. Once again, the conclusions do not support the target income hypothesis[17].

There also appears to be a high income elasticity of demand for dental services[18]. As economic conditions improve, and personal income increases, so, it appears, does the demand for dental services. Another study suggested a seventy-five percent increase in the *rate of increase* in dental real income for every one percent increase in the *rate of increase* in real GNP, and vice versa[19]. In addition, significant and similarities have been found between movements in the consumer price index and those in dental fees[20].

Supply Determinants for Dental Services

A number of factors were found to have contribute to the supply of dental services. These include trends toward group and large scale practices, manpower developments and the growth of allied dental services, and regulatory matters. We noted earlier that group practices tend to display higher productivity than solos. Practices with three or more dentists generated about 20% more visits per dentists than solos or two dentist practices[21]. No significant differences were noted between solo and two dentist offices[22].

The market for independent *allied dental services*, such as hygienists, within and outside dentist supervision, appear to have been gaining momentum during the past decade. Their role is particularly important in the preventive segment of dental care. Given a lower investment in human capital, and lower capital equipment requirements for their offices, independent, and quasi-independent (only nominally supervised) allied dental personnel emerges as a significant competitive factor for professional dentists in preventive and restorative markets. This would particularly be the case if the former were marketed under high human traffic circumstances such as department stores, and shopping malls. In addition, the proliferation of allied dental services may be viewed not only as a source of competition for dentists, but also a possible source of expanded markets, if the dispensing of allied services, as it may very well, yield new diagnostic and treatment services for licensed dentists.

Regulatory conditions, particularly at the state level, may have a profound impact on the supply of dentists. and dental services. They have a direct impact on entry conditions. They may also affect the scale and nature of the dental practice itself, the number and composition of assistants used, and the parameters of competition in the dental services market.

While the number of states without reciprocal licensing agreements appears to have declined, the lack of reciprocity among states does contribute considerably to dental service costs. Thus, based on a composite of 12 typical dental service costs, it was suggested that dental service fees in nonreciprocal states were some 15% higher than in states with reciprocity[23]. A lack of reciprocity also restrains the interstate movement of dental professionals, and thus inhibits market adjustments that would take place in response to a shortage of service in one geographical area, and a surplus in another. Hence, the inhibition of interstate migration among dentists may keep fees artificially high in some regions, and unduly low in other regions.

Some states have limited the number of dental offices under single ownership, and inhibited the establishment of so called satellite offices. However, these limitations appear to have vained in recent years, particularly since the restrictions could not as readily be associated with socially motivated healthcare concerns as with attempts to block the growth of chain-operated normally heavily advertising dental practices, such as those that could be frequently found in California.

It is also likely that limits on the number of offices per practice inhibits the attainment of various scale economies. Thus, capital equipment procurement may be done at a lower cost if several units are purchased at the same time. A larger practice, distributing business risks over several patient populated geographical and geo-social areas, may procure financing easier and at a lower cost. These considerations apply to single dentist multi-office situations, as well as to an organized multi-office network operated by several dentists.

Another regulatory issue may pertain to practice ownership, and the use of trade names in dental practices. Historically, licensed dentists had to hold ownership of dental practices, and were normally discouraged from using trade names. Subsequently, the appearance of dental franchises were noted, operating at department store locations, shopping malls, and in large drug stores, and using trade names[24].

In some states, there has also been a limit on the number of hygienists that could be employed by a practice. This resulted in fewer hygienists employed per dentist, expanding range of functions attributed to the hygienists, who worked longer hours. While this regulation may not have had a significant impact on sole practitioners, and two dentist offices, who, at any rate, use a limited number of hygienists, they were bound to have a significant effect on group practices who tended to use a number of hygienists. In essence, the regulation may have had a negative impact on the number of group dental practices.

In general, a number of government policies had decisive effects on the development of dental markets, both supply and demand. For instance, dental schools have been subsidized by the federal government since 1963, causing an over 50% increase in their output capacity during the 60s and most of the 1970s. Furthermore, in addition to subsidizing the institution, the federal government also subsidized the process of education itself. In fact, during the 1970s, until 1981, some three thousand dollars per dental student was handed out by way of additional subsidies. In 1981, the process was halted, and a slim future became predictable. Indeed, both applications and enrollments have dramatically dropped during the past ten years, and several dental schools have seen it necessary to curtail their facilities, or close down altogether[25].

In addition to the cessation of government subsidies, procompetitive public policies became aggressive in general healthcare, as well as dentistry[26]. We have also discussed the FTC's successful action against the ADA because of the latter's historical practice of banning advertising. Those bans have essentially been completely removed from the profession. Finally, support personnel related regulations are now vested with the state governments, and professional as well as financial challenge from this segment of the practice to dentists appears to be growing. Dental hygienists in several states have set up their own business. Technicians have now become "denturists" in some part of the country supplying fitting people with dentures. So called "dental auxiliaries", with no more than two years of training in contrast to a dentist's four, were found in foreign countries to have performed a number of dental procedures when permitted by regulation[27]. The political atmosphere for their utilization in this country could be brought about only by the emergence of a severe shortage of dentists. An unlikely event under the prevailing US dental market conditions.

Statistical Profile of American Dentistry[28]

Dentists are categorized into several groups for the purpose of statistical reporting. An *independent dentist* either owns or shares in the ownership of a dental practice. They may be sole proprietors, partners, in incorporated or unincorporated practices. Owners of incorporated practices, either by solo or with partner, are also viewed as shareholders. *Independent contractors* are practitioners who contractually use the space and equipment owned by other dentists. Their generate income by charging their own patient, or their insurance carriers. A *nonowner dentist* is employed in an another dentist's practice of some form, and is compensated by salary, commission or other prearranged basis. A *solo* dentist owns his or her unincorporated or incorporated (shareholder) practice, and is the only dentist in the office. Thus, solos are a subset of independents. *Non-solos*, therefore, are group practitioners working at least one other dentist in the office. *Total patient visits* include appointments (excluding no-shows), walk-in, and emergency treatments[29].

There do not appear to be significant changes in the *regional distribution* of all dentists between 1985 and 1990. Some migration out of the South Atlantic region appears to have taken place (19.3% in 1985, 16.2% in 1990), but it was largely diffused throughout the country. Nor has there been much change in the *average age* of general practitioners s during the five year period. It appears that the average age of specialists has been lowered somewhat, particularly that of females (44.8 in 1985 to 39.6 in 1990). Some 82% of all dentists still practice as sole proprietors with a ratio of unincorporated/incorporated of approximately 2/1. About 11% practice in partnerships, with slightly more incorporated than unincorporated. A little over 2% function as employee, and some 3% as independent contractors. Over 70% of general practitioners, and 62% of specialists function in practitioner environments. Some 20% of GPs and 24% of specialists work in two-person offices, and a little over 10% of GPs and almost 15% of specialists work in offices with three or more dentists in the office.

There has not been much change in most aspects of *practice intensity* between 1985 and 1990, and not much difference between GPs and specialists in this respect. Specifically, dentists spend around 48 weeks per year in their offices. However, the number of hours per week appears to have gone down from about 42 to a little over 37 between 1985 and 1990, possibly due to the allied dental service activity, although almost all of the hours spent in the office is devoted to treating patients in some form or another. As in 1990, much of the treatments performed by GPs is in the operative area (34%), followed by prosthodontic (19.4), preventive (13.3), and diagnostic (11.7) work, in that order. For specialists, the emphases seem to have been orthodontics (36.3%), followed by oral/maxillo-facial surgery, periodontic, and endodontic work (all between about 13% and 18%).

The 1991 ADA data has broader coverage. Thus, the number of *dental offices* per practice became more pertinent in the latest set of data. No more than about 5% of GPs have more than one private office, compared with over 34% of specialists in this respect. Most of those with multiple offices in the GP category have two office practices (83.3%), some 11% with three offices and just over 5% with four offices. The distribution for specialists is similar (67.5% two offices, 24% three offices, and about 8% for four office).

Most dental practices utilize a complete set of needed *equipment*. However, roughly three times as many specialists operate their own dental labs as GPs (20.5% v. 7.2%). For GPs, the most frequently utilized equipment items include composite light curing units (97.8% of GPs), ultrasonic or sonic scaling units (87.9%), high speed air handpiece with fiber optics (71.4%), automatic x-ray film processor (70.6%), sterilizable (autoclavable) handpiece (68.3), and nitorus oxide analgesic equipment (58.3%). It appears that a smaller proportion of specialists utilize most of these equipment.

It is interesting to note the proliferation of computer utilization among dental practitioners. Published 1986 statistics do not even speak to that issue, possibly due to lack of collected data, or to a much lower frequency of computer use in the profession. At any rate, by 1990, 44%

of GPs and over 55% of specialists used computers in their practice. Among those GPs that did use computers, over 92% had their in-house computer facilities, and they used them mostly for patient accounting, processing insurance forms, word processing, maintaining treatment records, patient scheduling, and similar functions for both GPs and specialists.

In terms of *patient composition*, there do not appear to be any dramatic changes between 1985 and 1990. While the bulk of the patient population fall within the age range 15-64, the proportion of those predictably increased somewhat from 1985 (16.61%) to 1990 (21%). Similar increase was registered for specialist in that age category. Additionally, no significant changes occurred during the five year period in terms of the proportion of those patients who were covered by private insurance program (63% for GPs in 1991), covered by public assistance program (5.4%), and completely uninsured (31,8%). The proportions for specialists are quite similar. A typical patient visited GPs 3.3 times per year, and 7.1 times went to specialists. The number of weekly office visits, including those to hygienists, in 1990 was 78 for GPs (94% scheduled), and about 104 for specialists (96% scheduled). On these visit, 75% of the patients went to see their dental GP, and 90% their dental specialists.

The *net income* (personal income minus practice expenses, before income taxes) of dentists from the general independent private practice of dentistry considerably improved between 1985 and 1990. In 1985 the mean net income was $65,810 (median:$60,000). In 1990, it was $89,900 (median: $80,000). Top earnings were at about $120,000. Specialists fared considerably better. In 1985, the mean income of dentists in specialized practice was $108,390 (median:$98,500). By 1990, mean net income increased to $148,520 (median:$130,000). Earnings capacity, both in terms of mean and median, appears to peak out during the relatively broad age range 45-54 for GPs. Earnings data for specialists shows a distinct peak during age 45-49, leveling off considerably thereafter. The number of years it takes to generate peak earnings after graduation is between 20 and 24 for GPs, and 15-19 for specialists.

There are no major differences in earnings among geographical regions, suggesting a relatively free-flow of dental service resources among state lines. For GPs in 1990, the mean range was from $83,840 (East South Central Region) to $101,240 (Pacific Region). Comparable data for specialists indicates a low of $124,480 (New England) and a high of $165,500 (South Atlantic - with very close levels for the Pacific region as well). The likely mobility of dental resources through various regions of the country is also suggested by a notable similarity in the average age of independent practitioners in each region. The 1990 mean age range for GPs was from a low of 44.5 years (Mountain) to a high of 48.8 years (Pacific), and 44.4 years (East South Central) to 48.8 years (New England), for specialists.

Nonowners and independent contractors have earned substantially less than their owner colleagues. For comparable number of hours worked per year (around 1,600-1,700), nonowner GPs earned about half (mean:$48,780) of their owner colleagues in 1990 ($38,670 in 1985). Independently contracting GPs earned even less, at a mean of $50,370 ($48,210 in 1985), indicating not only a much lower earning capacity than their owner colleagues, but also a much less significant increase since 1985. Corresponding earnings by specialists in these categories is only slightly higher.

Most dentists employed at least one staff member on a full-time or part-time basis. Almost all dentists employed a chairside assistant. Between 60% and 70% of practitioners employed dental hygienists on a full-time or part-time basis.

Prognoses

The dental profession is, and has been for some years, under transformation. There has been a dramatic increase in the number of professional and allied practitioners. Overhead costs have dramatically increased. The imposition of new OSHA rules regarding intensified sterilization of dental instruments, prompted by the AIDS predicament, further increased the cost of practice to the practitioner, and to the patient. Multi-sources of payments, and related elaborate bureaucracies necessitating voluminous and increasing paperwork, compounded the administrative costs involved in practicing dentistry. Third-party payers, motivated by savings, closely scrutinize the procedures applied.

In addition to these changes, the ownership foundation of a large proportion of dental practice has also undergone transformation. The number of professional dental corporations has significantly declined, as the frequency of sole proprietorships increased. This follows an increase in dental professional corporations between 1975 and 1987. Thus, the dramatic decline of professional corporations in dentistry appears to concentrate on the post 1987 period[30]. The reasons seem to rest with pertinent changes in the tax laws, implemented by the 1986 Tax Reform Act, and the shift from a professional corporation status to that of an "S corporation", yielding a lower tax rate for individual as well as corporate entities involved.

The current relatively high dentist-to-population ratio is seen as headed for reversal. While the number of dental professionals is expected to peak during the late 1990s at about 143,000, the following two decades is expected to witness an approximately 10% decline in their numbers[31]. In addition, the Bureau of Census, anticipates the US population to increase to some 383 million by around 2050[32]. Some argue, therefore, that planners of dental professional service capacity, and projected dental school contractions, closures, or expansion, as the case may be, should be implemented while keeping these long-term projections in mind.

References

1   The latter part of the chapter will examine in detail the major statistical dimensions of the industry.
2   Kudrle, R.T. "Dental Care", in Feder, J., Holahan, J., and Marmor, T. (eds) *National Health Insurance: Conflicting Goals and Policy Choices*, The Urban Institute, Washington, 1980, pp.579-605; see also Bailit, H.L. Raskin, M. Reisine, S. and Chriboga, D. "Controlling the Cost of Dental Care" *American Journal of Public Health*, Vol. 69, No.7, 1979, pp.699-703
3   Manning, W. G.Phelps, C.E. *Dental Care Demand: Point Estimates and Implications for National Health Insurance* The Rand Corporation, Santa Monica, 1978.
4   Harris, J.E. "Commentary" in Pauly, M.V. (ed) *National Health Insurance: What Now, What Later, What Never?* American Enterprise Institute, Washington DC 1980, pp, 260-69
5   Evans, R.G., Williamson, M.F. *Extending Canadian Health Insurance: Options for Pharmacare and Denticare* University of Toronto Press, Toronto, Ont. 1978, p.125
6   The followimg dentals school have closed their doors in recent years: Oral Roberts University was the first one (1986); Emery University (1988); Georgetown University (1989); Farleigh Dickinson University (1991); Washington University in St. Louis, MO. (1991); and, Loyola University of Chicago Dental School has just graduated its last class (1993).
7   Kushman, J.E. "Participation of Private Practice Dentists in Medicaid", *Inquiry*, Vol. XV, 1978, pp. 225-33. See also Bailey, R.M. "Economies of Scale in Medical Practice" in Klarman, H.E. (ed) *Empirical Studies in Health Economics*, Johns Hopkins Press, Baltimore MD. 1970, pp. 255-73; Ross, N. "Impact of the Organization of of Practice on the Quality of Care and Physician Productivity", *Medical Care*, Vol. 18, No. 4, pp.347-59; Luft, H.S. "Trends in Medical Care Costs: Do HMOs Achieve Their Savings? Rhetoric Evidence" *New England Journal of Medicine*, Vol. 298, No. 24, 1978, pp. 1336-43.
8   Schoen, M.H. "Dental Care and the HMO Concept" *Milbank Memorial Fund Quarterly*, Vol. 53, No. 21975, pp 173-93; see also Perkoff, G.T. Kahn, L., and Haas, P. "The Effects of Experimental Prepaid Group Practice on Medical Care Utilization and Costs", *Medical Care*, Vol. 14, 1976, pp.432-39;
9   Bates v. State Bar of Arizona 93 US 2691 (1977)
10 ADA, *Guides for State Boards of Dental Examiners on the Definition of Routine Dental Services for Purposes of Dentits' Advertisement*, Chicago 1977.
11 Stigler, G.S. "Economics of Information", *Journal of Political Economy* Vol. 49, No.3, June 1961, pp.213-25

12   Feldman, R. Begun, J. "Effects of Adevrtising: Lessons from Optometry" *Journal of Human Resources*, Vol. 13 (Supplement), 1978, pp.247-62; Cady, J. *Restricted Advertising and Competition: The Case of Retail Drugs*, American Enterprise Institute, Washington DC 1976

13   Bailit, H.L. and Raskin, M. "Assessing Quality of Care and Dental Insurance" *Inquiry* Vol. 15, No. 4, December 1978, pp.358-70.

14   Manning, W.G. and Phelps, C.E. *Dental Care Demand: Point Estimates and Implications for National Health Insurance,* Rand Corporation, Santa Monica CA 1978; see also Clasquin, L.A. *Mental Health, Dental Services, and Other Coverage in the Health Insurance Study* Rand Corporation, Santa Monica CA 1978.

15   Sloan, F.A. Feldman, R. "Competition Among Physicians" in Greenber, W. (ed) *Competition in the Healthcare Sector: Past, Present, and Future,* Federal Trade Commission, Washington DC 1978, pp.57-131

16   Shepard, L. "Licensing Restrictions and the Cost of Dental Care" *Journal of Law and Economics*, Vol. 21, April 1978, 187-201

17   Musgrave, G.L. "A Market Model of the Distribution of Dentists" *The Target Income Hypothesis and Related Issues in Health Manpower Policy*, DHEW Publication No. HRA80-27, 1980, Department of Health Education and Welfare, Washington DC., pp.60-82

18   See Manning, Dental Care Demand...

19   House D.R. "Dentists' Incomes, Fees, Practice Costs, and the Economic Stabilization Act: 1952-76" *Journal of the American Dental Association*, Vol. 99, November 1979, pp. 857-61.

20   Bureau of Economic Reserach and Statistics, "Dental Fees and Inflation" *Journal of the American Dental Association*, Vol. 93, July 1976, pp. 129-133

21   Kushman, J. Scheffler, R. Miners, L. Mueller, C. "Non-Solo Dental Practice: Incentives and Return to Size" *Journal of Economics and Business*, Fall 1978, pp. 36-38.

22   Douglass, C.W. and Day, J.M. "Cost and Payment of Dental Services in the United States" *Journal of Dental Education*, Vol. 43, No. 7, 1979, pp. 330-48.

23   Shepard, L. "Licensing Restrictions ....", pp.187-201

24   *The Advertising Dentist*, Vol. 1, No. 6 June 1980, pp.22-24; also see "Drug Store Dentist" *Medical Care Review* October 1979, 945

25   See fn.#6 above. In addition, much of this information is based on a conversation with H.B. Waldman, DDS, of the State University of New York at Stony Brook, NY.

26   Note earlier references to the 1975 case of Goldfarb v. Virginia Bar Association, and similar decisions involving the professions

27   McBride, O. "Restrictive Licensing of Dental Paraprofessionals" *The Yale Law Journal*, Vol. 83, 1974, pp.802-26; See also Kudrle, R.T "The Implications of Foreign Dental Coverage for US National Health Insurance" *Journal of Health Politics, Policy and Law* Winter 1981.

28 The following are based on American Dental Association, *Survey of Dental Practice*, 1986, 1991

29 On a regional basis, the ADA reports its data as follows: New England (CT,ME,NH,RI,VT,MA); Middle Atlantic (NJ,NY,PA); East North Central (IL,IN,MI,OH,WI); West North Central (IA,KS,MN,MO,ND,NE,SD); South Atlantic (DE,MD,DC,FL,GA,NC,SC,VA,WV); East South Central (AL,KY,MS,TN); West South Central (AR,LA,OK,TX); Mountain (AZ,CO,ID,MT,NV,MN,UT,WY); Pacific (AK,CA,HI,OR,WA).

30 Much of this discussion is based on Department of Treasury, IRS. *Source Book: Corporate Income Tax Returns, Sole Proprietorship Returns,* and *Partnership Returns,* GPO, Washington DC. for the years 1957-1991. Also cited by Waldman.

31 AADS Manpower Committee. *Manpower Project Report No.2,* American Association of Dental Schools, Washington DC, 1989. Cited in Waldman H.B., "Marked Increase in the General Population and Decreasing Numbers of Dentists in the 21st Century", unpublished paper.

32 Pear, R. "New Look at the US in 2050: Bigger, Older and Less White", *New York Times* December 4, 1992, p.A1. Also, Chief of Population Projections, Bureau of Census. Cited in Waldman.

PART FOUR

COMPETITION AND ITS ENFORCEMENT IN HEALTHCARE

Chapter 19
HEALTHCARE AND ANTITRUST:
AN OVERVIEW

E arlier in the volume, we have examined systematically the
fundamental issues addressed by the antitrust laws. The statutes
were reviewed, and some of the landmark cases analyzed. The next
several chapters will take a closer look at the application of the antitrust
statutes to healthcare markets. Specifically, we will study some major
competitive restraints that were found to have occurred in healthcare
markets, and were dealt with by way of antitrust enforcement. In the
course of this review, the basic elements of healthcare competition will
repeatedly surface, and their social importance highlighted. Furthermore,
frequent references will be made to explicit and implied consequences
for prevailing cost conditions, in relation to the anticompetitive situation
under scrutiny.

The Propriety of Competition
Enforcement in Healthcare

The application of antitrust principles to healthcare issues has not
had universal support. Indeed, significant debates took place over the
years whether the healthcare field is one where the enforcement of
competitive standards is appropriate, needed, or may even be harmful[1].It
was less than two decades ago that the Supreme Court held that the
"learned professions" are subject to the antitrust laws[2]. Prior to Golfarb,
the learned professions were explicitly excluded from the realm of "trade
and commerce", the expressed focus of competition enforcement[3].

The competitive restraint issue in Golfarb centered on the propriety of a minimum legal fee schedule published by a county bar association, and even enforced by the Virginia State Bar. The defense's contention was that bar members belonged to one of the learned professions, and that competitive environment was not conducive for the practice of those professions. However, the Supreme Court saw it differently: "In the modern world it cannot be denied that the activities of lawyers play an important part in commercial intercourse, and that anticompetitive activities by lawyers may exert a restraint on commerce" [2, p.788]. It was also noted that the Virginia State Bar's 1962 Minimum Fee Schedule Report had expressed concern to the effect that lawyers have slowly been committing economic suicide as profession. Thus, Golfarb henceforth substantively included all learned professions, including the medical profession, into the arenas of commercial competition as far as the antitrust laws were concerned.

A subsequent Supreme Court decision essentially reaffirmed the Goldfarb doctrine, suggesting that, while the professions may be different from other commercial endeavors for antitrust purposes, the focus of antitrust concern should remain the same for the professions as it is for other commercial activities. Reasonableness must be evaluated in terms of competitive impact, and not policy considerations that the competitive constraint are designed to augment[4]. In this case, the Society adopted an ethical standard attempting to preclude competitive bidding among its members based on the rationale that "competition among professional engineers was contrary to the public interest... [and] ... the practice of awarding engineering contracts to the lowest bidder, regardless of quality, would be dangerous to the public health, safety and welfare" [4, pp.684-85]. In rejecting the argument, the Supreme Court indicated that the "Sherman Act reflects a legislative judgment that ultimately competition will produce not only lower prices, but also better goods and services" [4, p.695].

These two cases then laid down the foundation for subsequent competition policy to the effect that the application of antitrust rules to the professions will likely lower cost without compromising the quality of service, and attempted or actual competitive restraints cannot be justified by arguments vested in "public interest".

Competition, Cost Containment and Antitrust in Healthcare

A prime policy issue in healthcare today is cost containment. While on its face the issue seems simple enough, namely to reduce the level of, or the rate of increase in, healthcare expenditures, its application is often contradictory to antitrust principles. For instance, health planning is inherently contradictory with free entry and independent market action. This problem has been magnified in the past by the nonconventional nature of demand and supply in healthcare markets, and the traditional lack of incentive to reduce prices due to undiscriminating third-party reimbursements. Throughout much of healthcare policy development history, the patient has seen healthcare as essentially a "free" good. In fact, these demand-supply distortions in healthcare were the basis of the argument in a relatively recent healthcare related antitrust case to distinguish the healthcare sector from other professions, such as engineering and law[5]. The counterargument to the effect that antitrust laws should firmly be enforced in healthcare may be based on the traditional lack of price competition in the sector.

As an alternative to antitrust enforcement, healthcare professionals have at times advocated private self-imposed regulation. For instance, the 1977 Voluntary Effort was organized under the sponsorship of various hospital, physician, supplier and insurer organizations. In a request for a business review by the US Department of Justice, the American Hospital Association, The American Medical Association, and the American Federation of Hospitals, proposed that (a) national steering committee be established to reduce hospital expenditure growth rates, to coordinate a limitation on the supply of hospital beds, and constrain hospital capital expenditures; and, (b) state cost containment committees be set up to monitor hospital costs. The Department of Justice declined to approve the proposals, noting that their implementation would be in violation of various antitrust provisions.

A major conflict between cost containment efforts and the principles of antitrust enforcement rests in the antitrust proscription of virtually *any type* of interference with the market's pricing system, including those that may specifically be designed to set maximum prices, and not only minimum prices. The concern is that maximum prices may ultimately turn out not to be price ceiling, but price floors instead[6].

A Concise Review of
General Antitrust Principles

The function of the antitrust laws is to attempt to combat competition inhibiting conduct under structurally conducive environments in the market place. While this appears to be a loaded statement, a review of the earlier parts of this volume should easily shed light on its essence. Some conduct, although appearing to be anticompetitive, may not be of social concern because of the absence of structural prerequisites, such as a minimum level of market shares, and entry barriers. Other conduct, while innocuous in nature, may at the least be suspect because the prerequisite market structural conditions are present. In general:

> The Sherman Act was designed to be a comprehensive charter of economic liberty aimed at preserving free and unfettered competition as the rule of trade. It rests on the premise that the unrestrained interaction of competitive forces will yield the best allocation of our economic resources, the lowest prices, the highest quality and the greatest material progress, while at the same time providing an environment conducive to the preservation of our democratic political and social institutions. But even were that promise open to question, the policy unequivocally laid down by the Act is competition[7].

Thus, ultimately, the antitrust statutes were designed to protect social interest rather than private ones, for its is social welfare that competition would theoretically be expected to enhance. In healthcare, social interests are generally seen to be represented by the patient and the ultimate, sometime private and often third-party, payer.

The major antitrust statutes are the *Sherman Act*, with its two substantive sections, 1 and 2, prohibiting contracts, combinations and conspiracies in restraint of trade; and, prohibiting monopolization, attempted monopolization and conspiracies to monopolize, respectively. The *Clayton Act*, along with the Robinson-Patman Amendment to its Section 2. The latter proscribes competition restraining price discrimination among different purchasers. Section 3 deals with exclusive dealing, total requirements, and tying, contracts resulting in a substantial lessening of competition. Section 7 is concerned with mergers and joint ventures in restraint of trade, and with a tendency to create monopoly in any geographic or product line dimension. Finally, the Federal Trade Commission Act, Section 5 proscribes "unfair methods of competition", also covered under the Sherman and Clayton Acts; the FTC is also concerned with unfair deceptive trading practices, such as false advertising, and commercial misrepresentations to the public. Most of past competition restraining acts were covered under more than just one specific statute.

The two federal agencies responsible for the enforcement of antitrust statutes are the United States Department of Justice, equipped with both criminal and civil weapons, and the Federal Trade Commission (FTC) that may bring civil actions only. Additionally, private persons may sue for treble damages empowered by Section 4 of the Clayton Act. These private litigants may include physicians and other individual healthcare providers, and institutional providers as well as third-party payers. In addition, a state as a "person", or as a representative of its citizens ("parens patriae"), may bring antitrust actions to recover damages incurred pursuant to Sherman and Clayton Act violations. Some violations of the Sherman and Robinson Patman Acts, mostly price fixing efforts, may also be felonies, generating a three year prison sentence, and fines double the gain or loss or $250,000, whichever is greater - for individuals, and one million dollars for corporations.

The Sherman Act's proscription of contracts, combinations or conspiracies assumes at least two independent entities acting in combination with the intent or effect of unreasonably restraining interstate trade. In the absence of a formal agreement, the presence of a conscious awareness of the scheme is sufficient[8]. The latter is often a matter for juries to decide.

Some restraints of trade are analyzed by the courts in terms of their reasonableness, their purpose and commercial impact. The *"rule of reason"* is applied to appraise their ultimate impact for competition and society. Thus, exclusive physician-hospital contracts, or staff privilege restrictions, are not likely to be found violative unless their competitive impact is substantial[9]. More generally:

> Every agreement concerning trade, every regulation of trade, restrains. To bind, to restrain, is of their very essence. The true test of legality is whether the restraint imposed is such as merely regulates and perhaps thereby promotes competition or whether it is such as may suppress or even destroy competition. To determine that question the court must ordinarily consider the facts peculiar to the business to which the restraint is applied; its condition before and after the restraint was imposed; the nature of the restraint and its effect, actual or probable. The history of the restraint, the evil believed to exist, the reason for adopting the particular remedy, the purpose or end sought to be attained, are all relevant facts[10].

Thus, an unreasonable restraint of trade must entail a substantial foreclosure of competition in a product or service within a geographical area, with, particularly in the case of medicine, a negative impact on the quality of care, or on the price and availability of service[11].

Other practices may have such a pernicious effect on competition that are presumed to be *de facto* unreasonable, and unlawful *per se*, without the need to engage in any further inquiry as to precise harm, or business justification[7]. In general, these practices include price-fixing whether directly or indirectly interfering with the market's pricing mechanism[5]; horizontal division of business based on product or geography between two or more actual or potential competitors[12]; unjustified horizontal group boycotts aimed at excluding a business from a market[13]; and, tying agreements, where the seller of one product with substantial monopoly power forces the buyer to purchase another one of his products in the market of which it has no monopoly power 11].

Most antitrust dramas, particularly in monopolization and merger cases, play out in the "relevant market", with product and geographical dimensions. The product dimension of a relevant market includes all substitutes with a significant positive cross-elasticity of demand coefficient. Thus, it may include a cluster of services in an inpatient general acute care hospital environment, or a group of medical specialties or subspecialties, e.g. cardiac surgery[14] The geographical dimension of the relevant market is the area of effective competition encountered by the seller within which customers readily migrate in response to a relatively small price change. In healthcare service markets, this area usually entails a county, or some adjoining counties within which patients are willing to travel in order to receive the best perceived service value[14].

In Sherman section 2 cases, issues of monopoly power, monopolization, and attempted monopolization often dominate. The presence of monopoly power, measured in terms of the relevant market share, is indicated by the ability to exclude competitors and control price. In general, but not in all cases, an above 60% market share already indicates adequate monopoly power, and a 90% market share, particularly in view of the alleged conduct, is normally found convincing[15]. Monopolization proscribed by section 2 of the Sherman act involves the willful (instead of through natural growth and development) acquisition and/or possession of monopoly power, and the abuse of such monopoly power by way of exclusionary, predatory and anticompetitive techniques.

Attempted monopolization may exist even with a 30% market share if the intent to monopolize is shown, along with a dangerous probability that it will succeed. Some or all of other factors that may also play an important analytical role include the state of technology, the relative size of competitors, entry barriers or a lack thereof, product differentiation, firm life cycles and turnover, and market share trends.

Anticompetitive mergers, acquisitions and joint ventures are the concern of section 7 of the Clayton Act. In order to assist the business and legal communities, the US Department of Justice has issued a number of Merger Guidelines over the years, starting with 1968 through 1992. Market share decisions are now made based on the Herfindhal-Hirschman Index (HHI) that takes into account the market shares of all firms in the market, as well as market concentration. Earlier in the volume, we have extensively analyzed the various versions of the Guidelines, including the most recent one.

The Robinson Patman Act amendment of section 2 of the Clayton Act proscribes price discrimination, or conduct that amounts to price discrimination, among competitors in restraint of trade. In fact, the discriminated buyer may be viewed as much of a culprit as the discriminating seller if the former solicits or knowingly receives the discriminatory treatment. Viable defenses that may be invoked include corresponding cost differences, good faith meeting of competition in the discriminated market, and a non-profit buyer, such as a hospital.

There are a number of defenses and exemptions to antitrust enforcement. The most fundamental issue that needs to be dealt with in the federal (not state) courts is the presence of harm to *interstate commerce*, either by the alleged anticompetitive activity being in interstate commerce, or that the conduct complained of significantly impacts interstate commerce. *State actions* are also exempted from the federal antitrust laws. Immunity is granted even to private activities undertaken pursuant to explicit state declared intent to restrict competition, or under a state's active control, supervision or involvement in the challenged activity. Some healthcare related cases applied state action exemptions to peer reviews of medical staff privileges[16]. The Local Government Antitrust Act of 1984[17] limits damage recovery to injunctive relief under the antitrust statutes from any local government, government officials or employees acting in an official capacity[18]. The exemption may also apply to publicly owned hospitals, although there does not appear to be any firm confirmation to that effect.

The *"business of insurance"*, regulated by state law, is also exempted from the antitrust laws by the McCarran-Ferguson Act, although the exemption does not cover traditional *per se* violations. In this context, the "business of insurance" entails only taking and spreading risk, but not efforts to reduce costs. Thus, peer review committees charged with assessing the reasonableness of chiropractic charges, or an agreement between an insurance company and drug stores to reduce the cost of drugs to policy holders was not considered part of the "business of insurance" by way of allocating risk; they were simply cost reducing efforts[19]. The antitrust laws do not apply to efforts, under the First Amendment to the Constitution, aimed at *petitioning the government* either, even if such effort is designed or results in competitive restraints, provided that the efforts themselves are not *a priori* aimed at restraining competition and to injure competitors[20].

The *professional review process* is exempted from antitrust provisions by the Health Care Quality Improvement Act of 1986, provided the process follows the Act's guidelines. The Act essentially defines "professional review" as a deliberation focusing on physician competence or professional conduct, aimed primarily at furthering the quality of care, and undertaken pursuant to facts. The results are typically reported to the Board of Medical Examiners. Finally, the FTC may not have access to antitrust weapons against *nonprofit organizations;* its jurisdiction includes entities that function for their own profit, or for the profit of their members. It was the latter provision that was used by the FTC when taking action against the AMA in 1980[21].

United States Department of Justice Activities

In addition to private enforcement under Section 4 of the Clayton Act, there are three levels of government enforcement in antitrust. The *United States Department of Justice* [USDJ] has been active in healthcare markets for a number of years. The latter share enforcement authority over the federal statutes with the *Federal Trade Commission*. Thirdly, state attorney general's offices have also played an important role.

The USDJ's activities have been quite intense, particularly in recent years[22]. In 1992, several criminal proceedings by way of grand jury investigations, under way or concluded, were conducted. In Baltimore, two generic drug manufacturers and their top executives were charged with conspiracy to fix the price of Dyazide, a generic anti-hypertension drug, involving some $75 million dollars worth of trade in the product. The executives involved have either pled guilty, serving a 21 month sentence, or will soon be tried[23].

In 1990, three Tucson dentists and two of their professional corporations were convicted in federal district court for price fixing. One of the dentists and his professional corporation got a new trial, the other two were acquitted. The Court of Appeals affirmed a new trial for one of the dentists, and reversed the lower court's decision to acquit the other two, indicating its concern for competition in the healthcare sector[24]. In early 1993, the main figure in the Tucson dental price fixing conspiracy entered a plea of *nolo contendere* to the felony indictment, and was ordered to perform 250 hours of community service, valued at about $35,000.

Two major civil actions in 1992 by the USDJ may be mentioned. A Sherman 1 case against the Hospital Association of Greater Des Moines, involved a conspiracy among its five member hospitals coordinating limitations on their advertising budget, and precluding image promotion or quality comparisons among them. Consumers, potential patients, of competing institutional healthcare providers were denied essential price, quality and service information. The case was concluded with a consent decree and an imposed antitrust compliance program.[25].

In a second matter, the USDJ brought action against the Greater Bridgeport IPA, alleging conspiracy among its 670 members that precluded (essentially boycotted) individual practitioners from contracting with an HMO when contract negotiations between the collective IPA and the HMO broke down over fee related issues. The consent decree settling the case included proscriptions of (a) collective agreements among IPA members precluding individual IPA members from independently dealing with third-party payers one way or another, (b) an IPA functioning as the exclusive negotiating agent for its members. Once again, an antitrust compliance program was imposed[26].

Hospital *mergers* have been a major part of USDJ enforcement efforts. Geographic market delineation issues played their usual important role. As suggested in the 1992 Horizontal Merger Guidelines, discussed extensively earlier in this volume, a relevant geographic market for two merged hospitals would include a region within which there is a ready migration of patients as a result of a "small but significant and nontransitory" price change on the part of the merged hospitals. Specifically, if a price increase by the two merged hospitals diverts enough patients, either on their own or by the decision of third-party payers, to hospitals in other areas to render the price increase unprofitable, then those areas, with the hospital therein, should be included in the relevant market. The diversion will depend not only on the newly emerged price differences between the two regions, but also on institution factors such as the ability or willingness of physicians to get staff privileges at other hospitals, the willingness of patients to switch doctors, and noninstitutional barriers such hospital images, and patient loyalties.

Patient origin data has often been utilized to delineate geographic markets, and they can be useful. However, in large urban areas substantial patient traffic may be found between the merging hospitals and outlying areas, and between the merging hospitals' own region and other areas with other nonmerging hospitals, in either direction. Nevertheless, if *third-party payers* with the discretionary decision to switch do not consider the other hospitals as reasonable substitutes for the merging hospitals, they may not be included in the relevant geographic market. In that event, sole reliance on patient origin data would over-size the relevant geographical market, to the likely detriment of the plaintiff.

Once the relevant market is delineated, and the market power of the merging, and merged, firm is determined, potential impact on competition, and on the consumers, may be assessed. Utilizing concentration measurements, including the HHI (discussed earlier in the volume), may not provide a persuasive picture due to the involvement of clearly qualitative, instead of the more objective quantitative, issues. Thus, a merged hospital with market may indeed be able raise prices above more competitive levels. In addition, however, if the two merging institutions have enjoyed an identity and stature in the region better and more favored than the rest of the hospitals, in other words were uniquely good substitutes for each other in contrast to other hospitals in the region, then the merger may take on added negative significance due to the inability of the other institutions to reposition themselves into a more competitive posture with the merged organization possibly because they may be too small, have no reputation, are unfavorably located, or have a limited range of services[27].

In view of the number mergers in the hospital sector, the USDJ's antitrust enforcement efforts appear to be relatively controlled. In fact, it appears that less than 10% of the hospital mergers that occurred between 1987 and 1991 were actually investigated by the USDJ, and only about 20% even of those investigated brought actual antitrust challenges. In addition, it also appears that the USDJ recognized that in small community or rural environments there is simply no market for even two competing hospitals: a type of healthcare naturally monopoly exists. The records indicate that between 1987 and 1991, the USDJ did not challenge any of the mergers that occurred between hospitals with 100 or less beds, or any hospital merger in communities with a population under 200,000. This may also reflect a recognition by the USDJ of important efficiency considerations that may be present when hospitals with substantial excess capacity, often the case in small-town environments, merge[28].

In addition to outright mergers, *joint ventures* have played an important role on the general scene of antitrust enforcement by the USDJ. The issues generally fell into two broad categories: (a) current price information exchange among competing providers, and (b) physician-hospital joint ventures target marketing their services at managed care plans and other third-party payers. The exchange of price data may be both competitively beneficial, or detrimental, depending on the purpose and the extent of the exchange practice, and on how widely, if at all, the data is disseminated among consumer groups and third party-payers. A limited and exclusively restricted price data exchange program will most likely benefit only the providers in a collusive environment, and not the uninformed consumers, competition or efficiency.

Physician-hospital joint ventures often take the form of provider controlled PPOs and IPAs, ones that are *not* third party-payers or managed care plans themselves. In fact, they are formed for the specific purpose of jointly target marketing their services to managed care plans and third-party payers. Thus, the risk of competitive restraint emanates from the joint exercise of market selling power by otherwise potentially competing providers who, barring the joint venture, would sell their services to third-party payers or to managed care plans.

Once again, the delineation of relevant product and geographical market dimensions becomes important, and the response to a significant price increase by third-party payers, managed care plans, healthcare insurers, employers, and government reimbursement programs, becomes the yardstick of measurements. In particular selective contracting practices enable managed care plans to be more responsive to "small but significant" price changes than most other types of third-party payers. Thus, their conduct is often the center of attention. In general, relevant healthcare *product* markets appear to center on specific medical specialties, while the *geographical* dimension, substantially depending on the involved product market itself, is likely to be locally based, such as a county. The likelihood of competitive restraints in a delineated product and geographic market further depends on the ease of potential entry into that market.

Finally, the USDJ's efforts to maintain a competitive environment in healthcare markets involves *business reviews* that present competitive issues. The Department may be solicited to review a specific proposed business conduct with respect to that conduct's legality under the antitrust laws based on the Department's interpretation of the facts as they were submitted and when they were submitted to the Department. The product is a Business Review Letter (BRL)[29]. Thus, favorable BRLs were issued in a case involving an accounting firm collecting and publishing current list prices for hospital services in Georgia, and in another one where an accounting firm collected and evaluated average PPO affiliated provider charges for kidney and liver transplants as cost inputs for future price determination. A favorable BRL was issued even in a case where a single agent negotiated fees and other contract terms with third party payers on behalf of some 20 separate and non-competing physician groups affiliated with a Cleveland hospital[22].

Federal Trade Commission Activities

Antitrust concerns in the healthcare field gained considerable recognition with a 1943 decision where the AMA and a local medical society was found to have engaged in a conspiracy to boycott a prepaid healthcare plan in Washington, D.C. The fact that the AMA wanted to protect the "economic status of the medical profession", or the allegation on the part of the AMA that the plans were "illegal" did not mitigate the courts' concern for the preservation of competition in the interest of society[30].

Notwithstanding the 1943 AMA decision, antitrust enforcement in healthcare did not gain momentum for over thirty years mainly because of the effective utilization of such defenses as state action, interstate commerce, and McCarran-Ferguson, as well as perceptions to the effect that the "professions" may be beyond the reach of antitrust law enforcement. The 1975 Goldfarb decision changed all that[31]. A county bar's minimum fee schedule constituted price fixing under Sherman 1, the "learned professions" and "state action" defenses could no longer be invoked, and meeting the interstate commerce requirements were made easier. Three years later, the Professional Engineers case[32] striking down an ethical rule against competitive bidding, and seven years later the Maricopa case[33] deciding against a schedule of maximum fees charged by medical society members to insurance companies, confirmed the cessation of the professions' immunity from antitrust enforcement.

The Federal Trade Commission's "flagship case" in the healthcare field may be the one against the AMA, with the latter having been found to have illegally suppressed truthful *advertising* by physicians[34]. This case also challenged the AMA's "contract practice" that essentially forbade physicians to underbid other practitioners or community standard fees in contracted transactions with hospitals and HMOs[34].

Boycotting HMOs was the issue in two cases which ended in consent decrees[35], and by way of another consent decree, the American Society of Anesthesiologists agreed to cease prohibiting salaried practice by its members[36].

Perhaps the most common issue in recent years, however, centered on access, or denial of access, to *hospital staff privileges*. The dispute in a substantial number of cases focused on whether by denying healthcare providers, physicians and allied healthcare professionals, access to hospital facilities by formal contracting restrains competition in the relevant product and geographic markets with incumbents in those situations, that is, with those who are already on contracts, often exclusive contracts, with the hospitals involved[37]. In addition to, and along with, competitive considerations, however, the issue of care quality is also relevant. Thus, a hospital granting staff privileges only to highly qualified practitioners invokes issues of both competition and quality of care, in fact, the former in terms of the latter. On the other hand, the system of privilege granting may be abused to the detriment of competition, for instance where a group of practitioners control hospital practices in this regard[38].

Indeed, it may be argued that the practice of privilege granting can be used by the hospital as an anticompetitive leverage, a tool of monopolization, in one or more product markets. The point may be illustrated by the following "power play" scenario. Medical Center A is the only tertiary care institution in the county, or even in an adjacent tri-county area. A multispecialty group practice (MGP) forms a couple of miles down the road. Most of the physicians in the MGP, at its formation, hold staff privileges at Medical Center A. In some major product lines, such as cardiac surgery, the MGP receives patients from the county, but its members perform the cardiac procedure at another hospital, two or three counties away. Similar situations may develop in other product lines. The MGP diverts patients away from the Medical Center, and the latter finds itself with a major source of competition a couple of miles away. It reacts by threatening MGP affiliated staff members with a revocation of their staff privileges. In response, several major players leave the group practice, and the latter folds. In situations like this, the product line delineation is usually not the issue. However, whether a medical center in a situation such as this may be held accountable for monopolization, or attempted monopolization, under Sherman 2, will likely depend on the size of the relevant geographical market, and the medical center's market share. In rural areas, a tertiary care medical center, probably the only one in the region, would clearly have considerable exposure in this scenario. In urban and metropolitan areas, with the presence of a number of other similar tertiary care centers, the likelihood of the medical center's conduct to be found in violation of Sherman 2, particularly in major product lines such as cardiac surgery where inter-regional patient migration normally significant, is much smaller because of diluted market shares.

Another issue that the FTC dealt with was *physician control* of medical payment (e.g. Blue Shield). An anticompetitive consequence of such control would be by way of eliminating or inhibiting price competition among participating physicians, foreclosing potential competition from alternative third-party payment plans, or excluding competing providers from the coverage[39]. Physician controlled medical malpractice insurance companies came under scrutiny for indirectly inhibiting competition from allied health professionals. Thus, the FTC challenged a mutual insurance company providing medical malpractice coverage to a large proportion of Tennessee's physicians for refusing to cover doctors who supervise independent nurse-midwives, but insured those who supervise the same type of nurses in their employment[39].

Physician interfere with *cost containment* efforts was also scrutinized by the FTC. State medical and dental societies have been challenged for attempted or outright boycotts of third-party payers in order to secure adherence to society established or supported fee schedules. In Michigan, Medicaid and the Blues were boycotted in order to compel them to adopt physician and medical society established fee schedules[40]. An association of dentists in Indiana was fund to have boycotted insurance companies that attempted to review patient diagnostic X-rays in order ascertain the applicability and propriety of charges[41]. The FTC has also been active in connection with hospital mergers.

The FTC's law enforcement activities are augmented by the issuance of Advisory Opinions. These included, among many other items, commenting on ethical codes governing professional association members' advertising, and a hospital's exclusive contract with a group of radiologists[42].

In addition to the Federal enforcement agencies, State attorney generals have been playing an important role in antitrust enforcement. In fact, it has been noted that the decentralized system of the American healthcare delivery renders federal antitrust enforcement alone, without state level participation, rather difficult[43]. Antitrust enforcement in healthcare took on momentum during the mid-1970s, at the time when states attorney generals began to take a look at their healthcare scene. Between 1975 and 1983, ten states filed twenty antitrust complaints in healthcare. The State of Ohio alone filed seven of these actions, and apparently it was Ohio that filed the first antitrust action of any type in healthcare in the US[44]. Indeed, Ohio was acknowledged as the leading State in the field of State Attorney General conducted antitrust enforcement[45]. An early antitrust healthcare case dealt with a boycott of welfare recipients by members of the alliance of dental society[46]. Another case attempted to resolve the issue of a conspiracy between a county medical society and its members to exclude HMOs from a community[47]. A third case was filed against the Joint Commission on Accreditation of Hospitals (JCAH) alleging an unlawful combination and conspiracy to restrain competition between psychologists and psychiatrists in JCAH accredited facilities[48].

The substantial number of actions in the healthcare field brought by antitrust enforcement agencies may be grouped into a number of somewhat discretionary, but nevertheless meaningful, categories: (a) Physicians and Allied Health Personnel; (b) Provider Pricing; (c) Horizontal Conduct Restraints; (d) Hospital Exclusions.

Physicians and Allied Health Personnel

In this category, *staff privilege denials* took up the largest proportion of enforcement time. The precluded physician normally complains of restraint of competition by way of group boycotts either involving the medical staff on board and the hospitals, or the medical staff among themselves, or individual staff members and the hospital, or the hospital and an outside group of physicians by way of an exclusive contract. In general, a corporation and its officers are viewed as a single entity, one that cannot conspire with itself[49]. However, if some members of the organization is found to have personal economic interest going beyond the interest of his institution, then those members may be viewed as separate legal entities capable of conspiring among themselves or with the institution. The economic motives of the individuals involved are an essential ingredient of the issue. Thus, individual or several medical staff members may act in their own personal economic interest, have an "independent personal stake", when excluding a physician from staff privileges, and could be found to have boycotted the excluded physician in restraint of competition[50]. Otherwise, if no such personal vested interest can be found on the part of alleged conspirators, then the conspiracy itself in restraint of trade may not exist[51]. In addition, hospitals have normally been given considerable freedom of choice if that choice was shown to be a result of genuine concern for the quality of care[52]. In general, when applying the rule of reason to staff privilege denial or revocation cases, the following factors appear to have played an important role in the courts' decision: (a) the reasons involved, (b) the standards applied, (c) the consistency of the standards with hospital objectives, (d) the relevant product and geographic markets affected, (e) the extent to which (1) the action reduced the patients' choice of physicians, or (2) the plaintiff is excluded from the relevant market, or (3) other competitive injures occur[53].

In addition to a conspiracy action under Sherman 1, staff privilege denials or revocations may also involve Sherman 2 by way of monopolization, or attempted monopolization allegations. In general, these cases have not been very rewarding for plaintiffs due to the presence of other competing hospitals in the relevant market, yielding a smaller market share for the defendant than would be necessary to find monopoly power, hence the possibility of monopolization. If the hospital can show valid reasons for its actions, the attempted monopolization allegation may not survive either[54].

Physicians may find themselves with reduced or revoked staff privileges pursuant to a decision of a committee of their peers, aimed at evaluating utilization or credentials. *Peer reviews* of utilization appraises the need and propriety of a particular service, while that of credentials looks at education, experience, and the potential for the quality of care, in view of the hospital's standards. Antitrust and competitive concerns in this context become relevant if the peer review process is abused for the private economic gains of otherwise competing participants in the review process.

Finally, in some fields of specialty, such as anesthesiology, radiology, and pathology, the practitioners' affiliation with a hospital is often formulated by way of *exclusive contracts*, precluding other providers from gainfully performing the services covered by those contracts. In fact, these contracts may provide for the contracted doctors to administer the involved clinical department. The courts have viewed these contracts under the rule of reason, and sought to establish a valid rationale for the hospital's action by way of entering into these contracts[55]. Arguments in favor of these contracts included greater control and standardization of procedures, more predictable scheduling of facility utilization by support staff, easier monitoring of standards, improved physician competence due to higher frequency of procedure performance, full-time availability of services. On the other hand, anticompetitive effects in this context were ascribed to the extent to which alternative providers were precluded in the relevant market, seller dominance, foreclosed entry, high concentration of potential employer hospitals in the market, and the duration of the exclusive contract. In particular, an exclusive contract in healthcare would be viewed as unreasonably anticompetitive if the contract foreclosed a significant proportion of providers in the market, or a substantial proportion of patients were denied their choice of doctors in the particular specialty[56].

Another possibly anticompetitive dimension of hospital-physician exclusive contracts is a tying arrangement. In Jefferson Parish, it was indicated that in order to have a substantially anticompetitive tying arrangement, the exclusive contract granting hospital must be selling two separate products, specifically in that case acute care hospital in-patient services (tying product) and anesthesiological services (tied product), and, secondly, the hospital must have the market power in the tying product to impose the tied product on its patients. Anesthesiological services were found to be a relevant product market, however, no evidence was found of the hospital having a monopoly power in the tying product in the relevant geographical market: only 30% of the patients residing in the market entered into the defendant hospital, with at least twenty other hospitals present in the same geographic market. Patients had a clear choice among a number of anesthesiological service providers, in addition to those offered by the defendant hospital. The hospital did not have the monopoly power to either impact on the practice of noncontracted anesthesiologists, or to force patients to use its own contracted providers. Thus, either by way of an exclusive dealing arrangement, or of a tying arrangement, the defendant hospital's market share will most likely be an important determinant of the degree of anticompetitiveness involved in the contract. The necessary substantial restraint on competition is more likely to be present in rural areas where physicians and patients have the facilities of only one hospital available to them, in contrast to urban or metropolitan areas where there is usually a multitude of hospital facilities available[57].

Provider Pricing

A major issue in this category may involve *price fixing* among *physicians*, hospitals or their professional associations. We may recall that price fixing is normally viewed as any interaction among competitors with the purpose or effect of interfering with the market's pricing mechanism, regardless of the ultimate results, that is, whether the price is raised, lowered, stabilized, or whatever[58]. In general, price fixing is viewed as a *per se* violation by the courts. The scenario typically involves agreements among doctors, hospitals or other healthcare providers, or their associations, either as to prices paid for inputs, or charges for services. Thus, a fee schedule promoted by a medical foundation as an alternative to prevailing health insurance plans in order to contain medical costs was found *per se* unlawful, in spite of counter arguments to the effect that the plan was reasonable, non-mandatory, and that participants could also relate to other plans. The participating physicians were viewed as independent and competing contractors[59].

Reported pricing fixing cases involving *hospitals* were relatively rare. However, institutional provider association involvement in litigations of this type were more frequent. Thus, action was brought against nursing home associations for alleged conspiracies to raise the price of services provided under the state Medicaid program[60], or against a state hospital association and its member hospitals for fixing the price of services and products supplied through the Indian Health Service[61].

Third-party payers, such as insurance companies, HMOs, PPOs now normally solicit advice from physicians (professional peers) regarding the medical necessity of proposed treatments or procedures, or regarding fees as to whether they are usual, customary, or reasonable ("UCR"). The committee of peers that conducts this *peer review of fees* normally contains competing physicians, thus making the process conducive for possible price fixing, exchange of price information, or the avoidance of price competition in other ways[62].

Outside professional organizations, consultants, and accounting firms often conduct *hospital price surveys*, for general publication and marketing. Significant restraints on price competition may emanate from these surveys. The elements of such restraint would normally include current and future pricing on specific services, and references to specific competing hospital names. Less competitive risk in this regard would be involved with surveys of historical and aggregate data, and without identifying specific institutions[63]. Carrying it one step further, procompetitive benefits may also be generated by these independently conducted surveys that contain provider specific price and quality information. For instance, they can facilitate informed healthcare purchases by third-party payers such employers and insurance companies[64].

Vertical price fixing may also exist between a hospital and its contracted physicians. It is possible that, by policy, a hospital may seek to approve, or dictate to their contracted doctors, what to charge for services such as radiology, pathology, or anesthesiology. Since the contracted providers are not employees of the hospital, in fact, they are independent contractors, this may amount to vertical price restraints. So far, not many cases took issue with this type of conduct, and when the problem arose, the rule of reason, instead of the *per se* approach, was applied by the courts[65].

Finally, another provider pricing issue that poses anti-competitive concerns involves *price discrimination* by way of selling, or knowingly buying, commodities at discriminating prices. Thus, a healthcare provider, hospital or physician, may sell supplies or drugs to competing commercial entities at different prices; or, be knowingly charged a price different from those charged to competing providers in the process of purchasing supplies. Many of these transactions, while anticompetitive, may, in fact, be socially acceptable due to the various defenses included in the Robinson-Patman Act, as discussed earlier in the volume. In addition, non-profit providers, when purchasing for their own internal use, are exempt from antitrust scrutiny[66].

Horizontal Conduct Restraints

There appear to be five major areas of horizontal conduct restraint which have, or could have, received antitrust attention: (i) combined procurements, (ii) combined services, (iii) joint ventures, (iv) alternative delivery systems, and, (v) structural transformations (mergers and acquisitions). A number of cases, as well as Antitrust Division Business Review Letters, seem to have advanced some basic principles of competitive restraints and social concerns in this context.

Combined procurements take mostly the form of group purchases of supplies. Initially, these efforts have been designed to reduce costs by way of a proper exercise of purchasing power, and avoid a duplication of efforts and supplies. On the other hand, they may turn out to be of competitive concern if they are viewed, for instance, as a group boycott against competing, but excluded suppliers. They may also be interpreted as competition restraining exclusive dealings contracts, or an attempt to monopolize. In addition, purchasing providers not included in the combined procurement effort may perceive a restraint of competition by way of them being group boycotted, or simply being a victim of price discrimination by virtue of not benefiting from the reduced supply price that the group might extract from suppliers[67].

The factors that appeared to have determined whether these efforts were in fact considered anticompetitive included (1) the market share of the contracted transactions, thereby the volume of excluded purchaser (provider) and supplier business; (2) the obligation of provider members to procure exclusively through the group effort; (3) the number of options or alternatives available to not included purchasers or suppliers; (4) the length of the contracted time period, thereby the time during which competition is foreclosed; and, (5) the presence or absence of open bidding in the process of selecting suppliers.

The Justice Department has remained relatively passive in relation to group purchase efforts by hospitals. So long as there is free access to the group by all hospitals in the area, member hospitals may purchase from not contracted hospitals, and the contracts are executed individually between the hospitals and the suppliers, no significant danger to competition is perceived.

Joint actions by providers may involve the procurement or sharing on certain services. Thus, some hospitals may jointly operate certain departments, MRI or other radiological facilities. The result may be reduced average cost of service production. Arragements of this type could also create at least the impression of group boycotts, horizontal market allocation, monopolization or exclusive dealings. The number of other provider alternatives in the area, impact on competition, and the assessment of individual provider's ability to offer the same service independently, all impact upon a conclusion as to whether or not significant competitive restraints are involved in such situations.

We noted earlier that *joint ventures* constitute an important element in provider interaction. These involve the operation of some facilities or providing certain services. Thus, hospitals may agree to form a joint venture for the purpose of operating ambulatory facilities, HMOs, long-term care facilities, diagnostic or therapeutic radiological centers, and the like. The ultimate restraint on competition in joint venture situations are normally assessed in terms of the following factors: (a) the likelihood of the parties entering into the market barring the joint venture, i.e the likelihood of eliminating potential competitors; (b) the presence of other potential entrants into the market; (c) the market power of the parties to the joint venture; and (d) the prevailing level of concentration in the market.

Provider formation of *alternative delivery systems (ADS)*, such as HMOs and PPOs, may meet competitive scrutiny. The issues normally involve price fixing, boycotts, exclusive contracts, and monopolization or attempted monopolization[68]. The underlying considerations include the manner of provider fee setting by the ADS, and, the extent, if any, of provider exclusion from the ADS. In the case PPOs, no significant competitive restraint is perceived by the enforcement authorities if the participating providers constitute less than 20% of the relevant market, or if the PPO is organized by nonprovider third-parties such as insurance carriers, and the latter negotiates fees separately with each provider[69].

Finally, the important area of *mergers and acquisitions* that substantially lessen competition under Clayton 7, as well as Sherman 1 and 2. The anticompetitive impact of a merger between two hospitals is normally assessed within the context of a relevant market, and the merging parties' share in that market. The anticompetitive impact generated by the merger is perceived to vary inversely with the size of the delineated relevant market, and directly with the merging parties' share in that market [70]. Premerger notification ("Hart-Scott-Rodino filing") of the Federal Trade Commission and the Department of Justice under Section 7a of the Clayton Act is required when (a) one of the merging parties has over $100 million in total assets or sales, and the other over $10 million, and (b) the acquisition price of the assets involved is over $15 million [71]. Lastly, hospital mergers are not exempted from antitrust scrutiny under the state action doctrine, or under federal health planning laws [72].

The following chapters will take a closer look at competitive issues in the healthcare industry, and the impact of competition enforcement there.

References

1 Borsody, P. "The Antitrust Laws and Healthcare Providers", *Akron Law Review*, Vol 12, p.417 (1979); Bovbjerg, K. "Competition v. Regulation in Medical Care: An Overdrawn Dychotomy", *Vanderbil Law Review*, Vol. 34, p. 965 (1981). See also Rosoff, L. Antitrust Law and the Healthcare Industry, St.Louis University Law Journal, Vol. 23, p.446, (1979); and, Symposium on the Antitrust Laws and the Health Services Industry" *Duke Law Journal*, 1978, pp.303-697.

2 Golfarb v. Virginia State Bar 421 US 773 (1975)

3 FTC v. Raladam Co. 283 US 643, (1931), "the medical profession is not a trade", p.653.

4 National Society of Professional Engineers v. US 435 US 679 (1978)

5 Arizona v. Maricopa County Medical Society, 457 US 332 (1982

6 Albrecht v. Herald Co. 390 US 345 (1968). Also see, US v. Socony-Vacuum Oil Co 310 US 150 (1940).

7 Northern Pacific Railway v. US, 356 US 1,4-5

8 Monsanto v. Spray-Rite Service Corp., 465 U.S. 752 (1984)

9 Tampa Electric Co. v. Nashville Coal Co. 365 v. 320 (1961)

10 Chicago Board of Trade v. US, 246 US 231, (1918) p.238

11 Jefferson Parish Hospital District No2.v.Hyde 466 US 2 (1984), p.31

12 Timken Roller Bearing Co. v. US 341 US 593 (1951)

13 FTC v. Indiana Federation of Dentists 106 S.Ct. 2009 (1986)

14 Robinson v. Magovern 521 F.Supp. 842 (W.D.Pa.,1981), one county. See also Jefferson, 1984 for radiology in the City of New Orleans; Mays v. Hospital Authority of Henry County 596 F.Supp. 120 (N.D. Ga.1984) for radiology in a county; and, Gonzales v. Insignares 1985-2 Trade Cas (CCH) P.66,701 (N.D. Ga.,1985), also a single county.

15 Weiss v. York Hospital, 745 F.2d 786 (3d Cir.1984) - market share over 80%; see also Hayden Publishing Co. v. Cox Broadcasting Corp 730 F.2d 64, (2d Cir. 1984) p. 69, note 7 - "a party may have monopoly power in a particular market, even though its market share is less than 50%"; and, US. v. Aluminum Company of America 148 F.2d 416, 424 (2d Cir. 1945)

16 Patrick v. Burget 800 F.2d1498 (9th Cir. 1986); see, however, Posner v. Lankenau Hospital 645 F.Supp. 1102 (E.D. Pa. 1986); and, Quinn v. Kent General Hospital Inc. 617 F.Supp. 1226 (D.Del. 1986)

17 Pub. L. No. 98-544, 15 USC 34-36

18 Palm Springs Medical Clinic Inc v. Desert Hospital 628 F.Supp 454 (C.D. Cal. 1986 - state action exemption was applied to a hospital district created pursuant to state law

19 Union Labor Life Insurance Co. v. Perino, 458 US 119 (1982); see also Group Life and Health Insurance Co. v. Royal Drug Company, 440 US 205 (1979)

20   United Mine Workers v. Pennington 381 US 657 (1965); Eastern Railroad Presidents Conference v. Noerr Motor Freight Inc 365 US 127 (1961); see alsoCalifornia Motor Transport Co. vTrucking Unlimited 404 US 508 (1972), and Hospital Building Co. v. Trustees of Rex Hospital 691 F.2d 678 (4th Cir. 1982)

21   American Medical Association v FTC 638 F.2d 443 (2d Cir.1980)

22   The following is based on a speech by Robert E. Bloch, Chief, Professions and Intellectual Property Section, Antitrust Division, USDJ, February 19,1993.

23   US v. Robert Shulman Crim. No. HAR-92-0446 (D.Md. 12/9/92), and US v. Bolar Pharmaceutical Co. Inc.et al. Crim No. 92-0454 (D.Md 12/17/ 1992).

24   US v. A. Lanoy Alston, DMD, PC et al. 974 F.2d 1206 ((thCir. 1991).

25   US v. Hospital Association of Greater Des Moines, Inc. et al. Civil No. 4-92-70648 (S.D. Iowa 12/22/92)

26   US v. Greater Bridgeport Individual Practice Association Inc. Civil No. 595 CV00575 (D.Conn. 9/30/92)

27   US Department of Justice and Federal Trade Commission, *Merger Guidelines*, April 2, 1992.

28   Testimony of Charles A. James, Acting Assistant Attorney General, Antitrust Division, before the Joint Economic Committee Regarding Healthcare Mergers in the 21st Century (June 24, 1992). See also Burda, D. "Mergers Thrive Despite Wailing About Diversity", *Modern Healthcare*, October 12, 1992, pp. 26-32; and *Report of the Secretary's Task Force on Hospital Mergers*, Department of Health and Human Services, January 1993; cited in Mr. Bloch' s speech.

29   28 C.F.R. Section 50.6

30   American Medical Association v. US. 317 US 519 (1943)

31   Goldfarb v. Virginia State Bar 421 US 773 (1975)

32   National Society of Professional Engineers v. United States 435 US 679 (1978)

33   Arizona v. Maricopa County Medical Society 457 US 332 (1982)

34   FTC v. American Medical Association 94 FTC 701 (1979). See also American Medical Association v. United States 317 519 (1943)

35   FTC v. Forbes Health Systems Medical Staff 94 FTC 1042 (1979)

36   FTC v. American Society of Anesthesiologists 93 FTC 101 (1979)

37   Hyde v. Jefferson Parish Hosp Ditrict 513 F.Supp. 532 (E.D. LA 1981); Robinson v. Magovern 521 F.Supp 842 (W.D. Pa. 1981); Smith v. Norther Michigan Hospitals Inc. 518 F.Supp 644 (W.D. Michigan);

38   FTC v. Forbes Health Systems Medical Staff 94 FTC 1042 (1979)

39   Virginia Academy of Clinical Psychologists v. Blue Shield of Virginia 624 F.2d 476 (4thCir.1980); FTC v. Medical Service Corp of Spokane County 88 FTC 906 (1976); FTC v. State Volunteer Mutual Insurance Co. 102 FTC 1232 (1983).

40   FTC. v. Michigan State Medical Society 101 FTC 191 (1983)

41 FTC v. Indiana Federation of Dentists 101 FTC 57 (1983); FTC v. Texas Dental Association 100 FTC 536 (1982); FTC v. Indiana Dental Association 93 FTC 392 (1979).

42 FTC v. American Academy of Ophthalmology 101 FTC 1018 (1983); FTC v. Burnham Hospital 101 FTC 991 (1983)

43 Marmor, T.R., Boyer, R. and Greenberg, J. "Medical Care and Procompetitive Reorm" Vanderbil Law Review, Vol. 34, May 1981 pp.1025.

44 Weller, C. D. "On 'FTC Sings the Blues' and Its Respondents", *Journal of Health Politics, Policy and Law*, Volume 7, Summer 1982, pp.547-58.

45 Salmans, S. "Critics Say Lack of Incentives Hurt Insurers Efforts To Curb Medical costs" *New York Times* March 31, 1982, p.12. See also Commentary, "Enforcement of State Antitrust Laws Gains Momentum: Ohio Sets Pace in Suites", *Federation of American Hospitals Review*, Vol. 14, June 1981, pp.23-26.

46 Antitrust Complaint, Ohio Ex. Rel. Brown v. Alliance Dental Society Civ. No. 76-96 (Ohio Court of Common Pleas, 1/27/76)

47 Antitrust Complaint, Ohio Ex. Rel. Brown v. Mahoning County Medical Society, Civ. No. 76-168Y (N.D. Ohio, August 24, 1976).

48 Antitrust Complaint, Ohio Ex. Rel. Brown v. Joint Commission on Accreditation of Hospitals, Civ. No. 2-79-1158 (S.D. Ohio 12/14/79)

49 Harvey v. Fearless Farris Wholesale Inc. 589 F.2d 451, 455 (9th cir. 1979)

50 Weiss v. New York Hospital 745 F. 2d 786, 813 (3d Cir 1984); Williams v. Kleaveland 534 F. Supp. 912, 920 (W.D. Mich, 1981); Robinson v Magovern 521 F.Supp. 842, 907 (W.D. Pa 1981)

51 Feldman v. Jackson Memorial Hospital 571 F.Supp. 1000 (S.D. Fla. 1983); Smith v. Northern Michigan Hospitals 703 F.2d 942, 950 (6th Cir 1983); McMorris v. Williamsport Hospital 597 F.Supp.899, 914 (M.D.Pa. 1984); Pontius v. Children's Hospital 552 F.Supp. 1352, 1374 (W.D.Pa. 1982).

52 Kaczanowski v. Medical Center Hospital of Vermont 612 F.Supp.912 (W.D. Mich. 1981)

53 Pontius v. Children's Hospital, at 1372; McElhinney v. Medical Protective Co. 549 F.Supp. 121 (E.D.Ky 1982); Robinson v Magovern, at 915-25.

54 Potters Medical Center v. City Hospital Association 800 F.2d 568 (6th Cir 1968).

55 Tampa Electric v. Nashville Coal 365 US 320 (1961); Smith v. Northern Michigan Hospital, at 950; Dos Santos v. Columbus-Cuneo-Cabrini Medical Center 684 F2d 1346 (7th Cir. 1982); Belmar v. Cipolla 475 A.2d 533 (N.J. Supt Court, 1984).

56 Jefferson Parish Hospital District No.2 v. Hyde 466 US 2, 3-4 (1984)(in concurring opinion).

57 Kuck v. Bensen 649 F.Supp 68 D.Me. 1986); Gonzales v. Insignales and Rockdale County Hospital Authority, 1985-2 Trade Cas. (CCH)P.66,701 (N.D.Ga. 1985); Mays v. Hospital Authority of Henry County 596 F.Supp. 120 (No.D.Ga, 1984).

58 US v. Socony-Vacuum Oil Co. 310 US 150, 221 (1939)

59 Arizona v Maricopa County Medical Society 457 US 332 (1982)
60 US v. Montata Nursing Home Association, 1982-2 Trade Cas. (CCH) P.64852 (D.Mont.1982); US v. South Carolina Health Care Assoc'n, 1980-2 Trade Cas. (CCH) P. 63316 (D.S.C. 1980).
61 US v. North Dakota Hospital Association 640 F.Supp. 1028 (D.N.D. 1986); Ohio v. Greater Cleveland Hospital Association, 1983-2 Trade Cas. (CCH) P.65,685 (N.D. Ohio, 1983)
62 Ratino v Medical Service of District of Columbia (Blue Shield) 718 F.2d 1260, 1270 (4th Cir. 1983).
63 Antitrust Division BusinessReview Letters to: Maryland Health Care coalition (2/10/82), Southwest Michigan Health Systems Agency Inc (3/2/82), Stark County Health Care Coalition of Canton, Ohio (8/30/85). FTC Staff Advisory Opinions in: American Dental Association (8/26/85), Utah Society of Oral or Maxillofacial Surgeons (2/8/85), North Texas Chapter of American College of Surgeons (12/12/85).
64 Antitrust Division Business Review Letter to Sydney N. Herman, representing Lexecon Health Service, Inc (6/20/86)
65 Konik v. Champlain Valley Physicians Hospital Medical Center 733 F.2d 1007, 1019 (2d Cir, 1984); Rockland Physician Associates v. Grodin 616 F.Supp. 945 (S.D.N.Y. 1985)
66 Abbott Laboratories v. Portland Retail Druggists Association Inc. 425 US 1 (1976); De Modena v. Kaiser Foundation Health Plan Inc. 743 F.2d 1388 (9th Cir 1984)
67 Northwest Wholesale Stationers Inc v. Pacific Stationery & Printing Co. 472 US 284, 295 (1985); White & White Inc v. American Hospital Supply Corporation 723 F.2d 495, 508 (6th Cir. 1983); Antitrust Advisory Letter to Ohio Hospital Association (6/9/82), FTC Staff Advisory Opinion to Louisiana Health Care Association (4/23/82)
68 Arizona v. Maricopa County; also see Pennsylvania Dental Association v. Medical Service Association 574 F.Supp. 457 (M.D. Pa. 1983); Ball Memorial Hospital Inc. v. Mutual Hospital Insurance Inc. 784 F.2d 1016 (1985).
69 Antitrust Division Business Review Letter to Health Care Management Associates and Medical Services Association, Inc (9/21/83); FTC Staff Advisory Opinion to Private Healthcare Systems (9/24/85); FTC Staff Advisory Opinion to Association for Quality Health Care Inc (8/28/86)
70 FTC v. Hospital Corporation of America 106 FTC 455 (1985)
71 15 U.S.C. Sect. 18a.
72 State of North Carolina v. P.I.A. Asheville Inc 740 F.2d 274 (4th Cir. 1984); see also FTC v. American Medical International Inc 104 FTC 1 (1984)

Chapter 20
MARKET DELINEATIONS AND COMPETITIVE IMPACT IN HEALTHCARE

It has often been noted in this volume that market definitions normally play a crucial role in antitrust decisions. They have proven to be particularly essential in monopolization and merger cases. Having defined the relevant market, the expert would normally calculate market shares, with often decisive contribution to the outcome. It should now be also noted that the standards and techniques used in connection market power measurements in non-healthcare cases also apply to cases from the healthcare industry, although interpreted within healthcare specific fact contexts.

Although market definition issues have remained essential, non-market share factors have also gained considerable acceptance in nonhealthcare cases[1]; to a lesser extent in healthcare, due to the presence of third-party payers, and the predominance of economic regulation[2]. We will also note that in some cases market definition issues carry relatively little significance. The courts simply infer markets from the conduct at issue, or an implied cost-benefit assessment of a detailed market definition study does not warrant the expenses and time involved.

Basic Premises of
Market Delineation - A Review

A major theme of antitrust enforcement centers on coping with anticompetitive efforts aimed attaining or exercising power to control price, or to preclude competitors and competition from a market. Market power may be abused by a single firm, or by a group of firms, and the definition of the market, along with market power measurement, is essential in either situation. Yet, some authorities argue that the need for market definition is conditional upon the availability, or nonavailability, of other pertinent factors. Thus, a recognized legal scholar of antitrust suggest that

> Market definition becomes crucial only when there no other discoverable facts establishing the existence and degree of market power more directly and with tolerable accuracy. One would never need to define the market if he could accurately establish the firm's demand and cost curves - the quantities that could be sold at various prices, and the costs of producing those quantities. That information would directly establish both the presence of market power and the magnitude of potential monopoly profits. The firm's demand curve would reflect the availability of any substitutes, without need for identifying them or their closeness[3].

Another well-known scholar in the field suggested that

> Market definition.... is merely and aid for determining whether power exists. To define a market in product and geographical terms is to say that if prices were appreciably raised or volume appreciably curtailed for the product within a given area, while demand held constant, supply from other sources could not be expected to enter promptly enough in large enough amounts to restore the old price or volume.... A 'relevant market' then is the narrowest market which is wide enough so that the products from adjacent areas or from other producers in the same area cannot compete on substantial parity with those included in the market[4].

Since market power could not in general be measured directly, the process has traditionally entailed two steps: (a) delineation of the relevant market, and (b) application of certain yardsticks such as market shares, to infer market power. This is so, notwithstanding the fact that relatively recently econometric techniques have been developed to directly estimate market power[5].

The need to know the extent of market power pervades, although does not dominate, antitrust enforcement, particularly when such power cannot be established by assumption. Thus, in merger cases under Clayton 7, market definitions and market power measurements are generally needed. In Clayton 7 merger cases, market definition is generally a prerequisite for the conclusion of the case. The statute proscribes "substantial" lessening of competition in "any line of commerce... in any section of the country". It was clearly stated by the Supreme Court:

> .. determination of the relevant market is a necessary predicate to a finding of a violation of the Clayton Act because .. substantiality can be determined only in terms of the market affected[6].

Under most circumstances, market definition is essential in Sherman 2 cases. Thus, a case involving monopolization or attempted monopolization related issues can hardly be decided without market delineation and market power measurement. In an early decision, the Supreme Court interpreted Sherman 2 as having

> both a geographical and distributive significance; that is, it includes any portion of the United States and any one of the classes of things forming part of interstate or foreign commerce[7].

Even in more recent decisions, the Court emphasized the need for market related measurements in Sherman 2 cases:

> To establish monopolization or attempt to monopolize a part of trade or commerce, under Sect. 2 of the Sherman Act, it would then be necessary to appraise the exclusionary power ... in terms of the relevant market for the product involved. Without a definition of that market there is no way to measure ability to lessen or destroy competition[8].

It appears that the need for market related measurements is reduced when we are dealing with conspiracy or combination to monopolize, "because proof of the agreement to commit an illegal act and proof of an overt act establishes the violation"[9]. On the other hand, "a minimal showing must nonetheless be made as to the product and geographic context of the alleged conspiracy"[10].

In Sherman 1 cases, market power may be presumed as a matter of law, or may be determined by appropriate measurements. The issue is related to whether the method of analysis is to follow the *per se* doctrine, or that of *rule of reason*.

> In the first category are agreements whose nature an necessary effect are so plainly anticompetitive that no elaborate study of the industry is needed to establish their illegality - the are 'illegal per se'". In the second category are agreements whose competitive effect can only be evaluated by analyzing the facts peculiar to the business, the history of the restraint, and the reasons why it was imposed[11].

Historically, under the *rule of reason* method, market analyses have normally been performed. With the application of the *per se* rule, market power has normally been presumed, reducing or eliminating the need for market related studies. Yet, recent cases appeared to have ignored a clear line of demarcation between the two approached within the context of the need for market analyses. Thus, "there is often no bright line separating per se from rule of reason analysis .... [the] essential inquiry is ... whether or not the challenged restraint enhances competition"[12]. The assessment of competitive restraint may be based on actual market studies, or, warranted by the nature of the practice and surrounding circumstances, on presumptions.

Where market studies were performed, a number of different standards were applied by way of *product market* measurements. (a) *Reasonable interchangeability* and the cross-elasticity of demand were considered as appropriate tests in some cases.

> A market is composed of products that have reasonable interchangeability for the purposes for which they are produced - price, use and qualities considered". Or, "...cross elasticity of demand between products is the responsiveness of the sales of one product to price changes of the other. If a slight decrease in the price of cellophane causes a considerable number of customers of other flexible wrappings to switch to cellophane, it would be an indication that a high cross-elasticity of demand exists between them; the products compete in the same market.[13].

(b) *Peculiar characteristics and uses* standard was applied in another case[14]. (c) *Production interchangeability* test was applied in other cases, along with the possible relevance of a closely related cross-elasticity of supply.

> ... the market is viewed from the production rather than consumption standpoint; the degree of substitutability in production is measured by the cross-elasticity of supply. .....[it] refers to the ability of firms in a given line of commerce to turn their production facilities towards the production of commodities in another line because of similarities in technology between them. Where the degree of substitutability in production is high, cross-elasticities of production will also be high, and again the two commodities in question should be treated as part of the same market[15].

(d) The notion of *submarkets* dominated the analyses in an often quoted case involving shoe manufacturing and retailing.

"Submarkets" are subsets of a broader identified market entity.

within [a] broad market, well defined submarkets may exist which, in themselves constitute product markets for antitrust purposes. The boundaries of such a submarket may be determined by examining such practical indicia as industry or public recognition of the submarket as a separate economic entity, the product's peculiar characteristics and uses, unique production facilities, distinct customers, distinct prices, sensitivity to price changes, and specialized vendors[16].

(e) A *cluster of products or services* has also been used as standards for market definition. Thus, in a case involving commercial banking the Court suggested that "... the cluster of products ... and services ... denoted by the term 'commercial banking' composes a distinct line of commerce"[17]. (f) Earlier in the volume, we have extensively examined the standards for market delineation advanced by the 1982, 1984, and most recently the 1992 US Department of Justice and Federal Trade Commission Merger Guidelines. Finally, (g) The National Association of Attorney Generals (NAAG) provided some standards for market power measurements:

Each product produced in common by the merging parties will constitute a provisional product market. The provisional product market will be expanded to include suitable substitutes for the product which are comparably priced. A comparably priced substitute will be deemed suitable and thereby expand the product market definition if, and only if, considered suitable by customers who account for 75% of purchases[18].

In delineating the geographical dimension of the relevant market, the US Department of Justice Merger Guidelines have been widely applied in the cases. The relevant market constitutes and area

..such that a hypothetical firm that was the only present or future producer or seller of the relevant product in that area could profitably impose a 'small but significant and nontransitory' increase in price[19].

Finally, the NAAG defined the relevant geographic market

... where the customers of the merging parties readily turn for the supply of the relevant product.... To this group of suppliers and locations will be added suppliers of buyers closely proximate to the customers of the merging parties ... Utilizing the locations from which supplies of the relevant product are obtained by members of the protected interest group, the geographic market will be defined as the area encompassing the production locations from which this group purchases 75% of their supplies of the relevant product[20].

In summary, there is a set of elements that appear to have dominated market definition efforts in major cases. For *product markets* these were (1) reasonable interchangeability[21], (2) cross elasticity of demand[22], (3) significant price and quality differences[23], (4) different customer classes[24], (5) peculiar characteristics and uses[25], (6) production flexibility[26], (7) specialized vendors and unique facilities[27], and (8) industry and public recognition[28]. For geographical market, the most prominently applied elements included (1) customer locations[29], (2) supplier locations[30], (3) alternative locations available to customers[31], (4) transportation costs and related barriers[32], (5) pricing patterns[33], and (6) industry recognition[34].

Physician and Physician-Substitute Market Issues

There does not appear to be a wealth of case history establishing relevant markets for individual healthcare providers. Many courts rendered opinions without resorting market definitions, and when market definitions were generated, they were quite limited in scope. Cases involving horizontal conduct restrains (e.g. price fixing), essentially dispensed with market definitions as not essential for the conclusion[35]. In one case the it was noted that ".. [in a case] where [a] policy takes the form of a horizontal agreement among the participating dentists to withhold from their customers a particular service that they desire ... no elaborate industry analysis is required to demonstrate the anticompetitive character of the ... [conduct]". In response to an argument that market definition was called for as a matter of law, the court noted that the purpose of market studies is to examine potential adverse affects on competition. With the "proof of actual detrimental effects, such as a reduction of output" can mitigate or eliminate the need for market studies[36]. This conclusion was reinforced by the logical assertion that the relevant product was dental services, and that those services tended to be dispensed locally on a community basis.

Other decisions similarly inferred the presence of a relevant market, favorable or unfavorable to a claimant, from the presented facts[37]. Decisions which did rely on market definitions utilized relatively narrow product markets with considerably broader geographical dimensions[38]. Finally, issues which involve competition between physicians and physician-substitutes were normally resolved by relying on service categories alleged to be the arena of competition, rather than extensively defined markets[39].

In general, it has been concluded that some categories of individual provider services do compete with others, and that some physician activities may be substituted by physician substitutes' services[40].

In addition, HMOs and PPOs were thought to compete in many areas with individual providers. Thus, if viewed as group practices, alternative delivery systems might be included in a relevant market with primary care, or even specialized, private practitioners[41].

On the other hand, alternative delivery systems may also be thought of as offering a product quite different from that of private practitioners, and that the former may only compete among themselves, while the latter belong in their own separate market[42]. In addition, alternative delivery systems have also been viewed as a form of insurance, thus belonging to a market with health insurance companies[43]. It may be noted that government agencies have tended to view alternative delivery systems in the same relevant market as individual providers. Thus, according to the FTC,

> the actions of a medical society or other organizations comprised of competing physicians, and the actions of a plan controlled by a group of competing physicians, are treated as the concerted activity of the physician group[44].

Or, "the proposed PPO will be an organization composed of competing providers and hospitals, and as such could present antitrust concerns.."[45].

In terms of their geographical dimensions, physicians' markets are normally examined by looking at factors such as referral patterns, the locale of hospital staff privileges, office locations, and, to some extent, the geographic region of the relevant "patient origin".

Institutional Provider Markets

There is an issue whether or not the nature of the relevant market for a hospital or nursing home depends on the type of the alleged violation, i.e. whether Sherman 1 or 2, or Clayton 7. Some writers support the notion that the same market definition standards govern in all relevant substantive provisions of the antitrust laws[46]. On the other hand, a 1958 case suggested that "Equating the language of Section 7 to the concept of market does not, however, mean that the Section 7 market is the same as the market for the purposes of other sections of the antitrust laws"[47].

Clayton 7 hospital cases usually defined the product market in terms of the cluster of services offered by a hospital, and not in terms of a specific service. Patient origin data, and physician affiliation statistics, are normally used to delineate geographical market dimensions. Thus, a 1977 decision delineated the product market as simply ".. the delivery of short-term care community hospital services to doctors and patients.."[48]. More recently, an opinion suggested "the cluster of general acute care hospital services" as the relevant market's definition. The market of a service cluster was rendered relevant due to the uniqueness of service clusters in acute care hospitals emanating, for instance, from their availability around the clock; and, from the complementarity of the various services available within one institutional and physical setting, such as an acute care hospital. In addition, due to legal barriers to entry, the cross elasticity of supply for hospital services is low; furthermore, acute care hospitals have been recognized by pertinent regulatory statutes and other healthcare providers as separate and distinct from other care centers, and outpatient facilities. In spite of the possible availability of each service within the cluster elsewhere, "the benefit that accrues to the patient and physician is derived from their complementarity"[49].

The outpatient service components of the hospital's total service cluster do add some complexity to the issues in that non-hospital affiliated outpatient clinics compete with the hospitals in terms of many of those services. A resolution of this dilemma, in the face of a recognized separate hospital cluster service market, appears to rest with the assumption that outpatient care may in fact be a separate product market; however, only those outpatient services not offered by freestanding outpatient case facilities. Hence, the relevant hospital product market may be defined as a cluster of inpatient hospital services, plus those outpatient services no offered by independent clinics[50]. In cases involving specialized services, psychiatric hospitals, product markets were typically defined in terms of those specialized services[51].

The *geographical* dimensions of hospital markets may be viewed in static or dynamic terms. A static approach would likely utilize patient origin, or patient flow, statistics, along with data on physician privilege locations. The dynamic approach would examine the geographical breadth and scope of responses to hypothetical price increases and/or quality reductions. Given the recognition of patient and physician preferences for geographical proximity to home, the two studies likely yield similar results[52]. In addition, some cases took into consideration regulatory regions, such as Health Service Areas (HSAs) as a basis for geographical markets, with the rationale that major hospital capital expenditures, such as construction, are normally regulated. The acceptance of this approach is by no means consistent. In some cases the court accepted this approach[53], in others the FTC rejected it[54].

Under *Sherman 1*, the issues most often litigated were tying arrangements, and exclusive contracts or group boycotts. The relevant product markets were typically hospital services, or a particular hospital service, while the geographical market was found to be quite local and narrow[55] Some courts did not seek a market definition at all since the defendant was presumed to have had market power[56], while others sought detailed market studies to support claimed market power on the part of the defendant[57]. Finally, even when no product market definition was advanced, the court found a measurement of the geographical dimensions of the market sufficient.

> The geographic dimension of the market is arguably the most important consideration since the geographic dimension establishes the boundaries within which a particular product is presently available ... even without [product market] information, however, the relevant market in this case can be sufficiently defined by identifying the geographical dimension of the relevant market[58].

The relevant market was found to be a region of within thirty miles or thirty minutes from the hospital, and patient flow data, along with licensed beds and patient days statistics did not support the presence of market power.

In *Sherman 2* cases, the service cluster approach to product market definition has not consistently prevailed. The aggregate of inpatient hospital care was found to be the relevant product market in a 1984 Pennsylvania case, and not individual hospital services. "Where several goods or services are generally offered by the same provider ... the market for antitrust purposes includes all of those goods and services. ... The patient may require several different types of services during his stay at a hospital depending on the course of his treatment. ... a consumer of hospital services makes one 'purchase decision' - where to be hospitalized - ... further decisions concerning his treatment are relatively insulated from any competitive effects"[59].

Other cases viewed specific hospital services, instead of their cluster, as the pivotal point for market power measurement. In fact, narrow product markets have often yielded relatively large geographical markets. It was observed that geographic markets often expand as the scope of the product market narrows. The hospital's...

> ...coverage reaches its geographic maximum in the delivery of *tertiary* [emphasis added] care because most community hospitals could not economically and safely provide such care. Thus, each type of medical service has particular geographic market[60].

Third-Party Payer Markets

Market measurements in antitrust cases relating to third-party payers concentrated on health insurance as a line of commerce, or viewed insurers as purchasers of healthcare services in provider related markets. Thus, a 1986 case found "healthcare financing for consumers" as the relevant product market, and noted that the cross-elasticity of demand among various types of healthcare financing was quite high, and found no submarkets[61]. In another case, a claim was declined because no market power measurements were offered in the medical insurance market in California[62].

Blue Shield was found to be a major purchaser of medical services for the account of others in Massachusetts, although was not found to have unreasonably monopolized that relevant product market[63]. Blue Shield was viewed as a combination of physicians, instead of policy holders in another case. While to an extent an insurer, it was viewed mostly as a quantity purchaser of health care services[64]. A related issue, whether alternative delivery systems, HMOs and PPOs, should be considered as being a part of the same product market as health insurance companies, appears to command split decision. Finally, the accepted geographic dimension of the medical insurance product market appears to be broad. On the other hand, the relevant geographical market for HMO and PPO operations may be viewed as local, since they contract with providers and solicit subscribers from the same locality.

In the chapters following, we will take a closer look at the cases and the issues pertaining to antitrust in healthcare delivery.

References

1   US v. General Dynamics Corporation 415 US 486 (1974), and US v. Waste Management Inc 743 F.2d 976 (1984)
2   FTC v Hospital Corporation of America 106 FTC 361, 489-96 (1985). See also Rosenblatt, J. "Health Care, Markets and Democratic Values" *Vanderbilt Law Review*, Vol. 34, p.1067 (1981).
3   Areeda, P. and Turner, D. *Antitrust Law*, Little Brown, Boston, MA. 1978, pp. 330-31.
4   Sullivan, L. *Handbook of the Law of Antitrust*, West Publishing Co., Mineapolis, MN 1977, p.41
5   Baker, J.B. Bresnahan, T.F. ""The Gains from Merger or Collusion in Product-Differentiated Industries" *Journal of Industrial Economics*, Vol. 33, 1985, p.427. Also see by the same athours "Empirical Methods of Identifying and Measuring Market Power" *Antitrust Law Journal*, Vol. 61, Issue 1, Summer 1992, pp. 3-16.
6   Brown Shoe v. United States 370 US 294, 324 (1962)
7   Standard Oil Co. v United States 221 US 1 (1911)
8   See e.g. Walker Process Equipment Inc v. Food Machinery & Chemical Corp 382 US 172 (1965)
9   American Tobacco Co. v. United States 328 US 781, 789 (1946); Salco Corp v. General Motors Corp 517 F.2d 567, 576 (10th Cir. 1975); US v. Consolidated Laundries Corp 291 F.2d 563, 573 (2d Cir.1961).
10 Alexander v. National Farmers Organization Inc. 687 F.2d 1173, 1193 (8th Cir. 1982)
11 National Society of Professional Engineers v. US, 435 US 678 (1978); see also Northwest Wholesale Stationers Inc. v. Pacifi Stationery and Printing Co. 472 US 284, 289 (1985); Arizona v. Maricopa County Medical Society 457 US 332, 343 (1982); and, Continental TV., Inc v. GTE Sylvania Inc 433 US 36, 9, (1977)
12 National Collegiate Athletic Association v. Board of Regents of the University of Oklahoma 468 US 85, 104 (1984)
13 See e.g. US v. E.I. duPont de Nemours & Co 351 US 377,400,404 (195)
14 US v. E.I. duPont de Nemours & Co. 353 US 586, 593-4 (1957).
15 US v. Columbia Steel Corp 334 US 495 (1948); Twin City Sportservice, Inc. v. Cahrles O. Finley & Co. 512 F.2d 1262, 1271 (9th Cir. 1975)
16 Brown Shoe v. United Sates 370 US 294, 325 (1962); also see US v. Grinnel Corp. 384 US 563, 572 (1966)
17 US v. Philadelphia National Bank 374 US 321, 356-7 (1963), also see US v. Grinnel Corp.; FTC v. British Oxygen Co. 86 FTC 1241, 1345 (1975); American Medicorp v. Humana Inc 445 F.Supp 589 (E.D. Pa, 1977); FTC v American Medical International Inc 104 FTC 1 (1984); FTC v. Hospital Co. of America 106 FTC 361 (1985)

18 *Horizontal Merger Guidelines of the National Association of Attorneys General*, Sect 3; reprinted in Antitrust and Trade Regulation Reporter (BNA) S-5 (Mar 12, 1987).

19 US Department of Justice and Federal Trade Commission, 1984 *Merger Guidelines*, Sect. 2.31.

20 NAAG, *Guidelines*, Par 3.2

21 US v. Continental Can 378 US 441, 455-58 (1964); Pennsylvania Dental Association v. Medical Services Association 745 F.2d 248, 260 (3d.Cir 1984); White & White Inc. v. American Hospital Supply Cor. 723 F.2d 495, 502 (6th Cir.1983); SmithKline Corp v. Eli Lilly & Co. 575 F.2d 1056, 1064 (3d Cir.1978); Robinson v. Magovern 521 F.Supp. 842, 878 (W.D. Pa. 1981).

22 Pennsylvania Dental Association; US v Aluminum Co. of America (Rome Cable) 377 UD 271, 276-77 (1964); Borden Inc v. FTC 674 F.2d 498, 507-510 (6th Cir.1981); SmithKline.

23 FTC v Warner Communications, Inc. 742 F.2d 1156, 1163 (9th Cir.1984); US v Black and Decker Manufacturing Co. 430 F.Supp.729, 738-40 (D.Md.1976); FTC v Liggett & Meyers Co. 87 FTC 1074 (1976).

24 Avnet Inc. v FTC 511 F.2d 70 (7th Cir.); Robinson v Magovern; US v Waste Management Inc., 743 F.2d 976, 979-80 (2d Cir.1984); Harnischfeger Corp v Paccar, Inc. 474 F.Supp. 1151, 1156-7; US. v Manufacturers Hanover Trust Co. 240 F.Supp.867 (SDNY, 1965).

25 SmithKline v Eli Lilly, p.1064; Robinson v Magovern p.878; Abex Corp v. FTC 420 F.2d 928, 931-32 (6th Cir. 1970).

26 Spectrofuge Corp v. Beckman Instruments, Inc. 575 F.2d 256, 280 (5th Cir 1978); Calnetics Corp v. Volkswagen of America, Inc. 532 F.2d 674, 691 (9th Cir, 1976); In re Municipal Bond Reporting Antitrust Litigation, 672 F.2d 436 (5th Cir., 1982); Twin City Sportservice, Inc. v. Charles O. Finley & Co. 512 F.2d 1262, 1271 (9th Cir.,1975); Whitten v. Paddock Pool builders Inc. 508 F.2d 547, 552-53 (1st Cir, 1974); J.H. Westerbeke Corp v. Onan Corp., 580 F.Supp 1173, 1186 (D.Mass. 1984); US v. ATT 524 F.Supp 1336, 1375-76 (D.D.C. 1981); Science Products Co. v. Chevron Chemical Co., 384 F.Supp.793, 797-98 (N.D. Ill. 1974); JBL Enterprises, Inc. v. Jhirmack Enerprises, Inc. 509 F.Supp 357 (N.D.Cal 1981).

27 American Medical International Inc. v. FTC 104 FTC 617 (1984); US v. Tidwater Marine Services, Inc. 284 F.Supp.729, 738-40 (D.Md.1976); Weeks Dredging and Contracting, Inc. v. American Dredging Co. 451 F.Supp. 468, 487-89 (E.D. Pa.1978); Monfort of Colorado, Inc. v. Cargill, Inc. 591 F.Supp 683, 698 (D.Colo.1983); Crown Zellerbach Corp. v. FTC 296 F.2d 800 (9th Cir, 1961).

28 Avnet, Inc. v FTC 511 F.2d 70 (7th Cir 1975); FTC v. Beatrice Foods Co. 86 FTC 1 (1976); FTC v American Medical International 104 FTC 617 (1984); White & White v. American Hospital Supply Corp.; American Medicorp Inc., v. Humana Inc. 445 F.Supp 589, 601-03 (E.D. Pa. 1977); Elco Corp. v. Microdot Inc 360 F.Supp.741 (D.Del.1973); US v. Pennzoil Co. 252 F.Supp. 962 (W.D. Pa. 1965).

29   US. v. Philadelphia National Bank 374 US 321, 357 (1963); US v. Mrs
     Smith's Pie Co 440 F.Supp. 220, 230 (E.D. Pa. 1976); American Key Corp.
     v. Cole National Corp. 762 F.2d 1569, 1580 (11th Cir. 1985); Jim Walter
     Corp v. FTC 625 F.2d 676, 681-83 (5th Cir 1980).
30   Lorain Journal Co. v. US 342 US 143, 146 (1951); Gearhart Industries,
     Inc. v. Smith International Inc. 592 F.Supp 203, 212 (N.D. Tex 1984);
     Gonzales v. Insignares, 1985-2 Trade Cas. (CCH) P.66,701, 63,335 (N.D.
     Ga 1985); US v. Grinnell Corp, 575; Marathon Oil Co. v. Mobil Corp 669
     F.2d 378, 381 (6th Cir. 1981).
31   US v. Dairymen, Inc 660 F.2d 192, 195 (6th. Cir 1981); Case-Swayne Co.
     v. Sunkist Growers, Inc 369 F.2d 449, 458 (9th Cir. 1966).
32   US v. General Dynamics Corp 415 US 486, 490-91 (1974); Case-Swayne
     Co. v. Sunkist, 449; Cackling Acres, Inc. v. Olsen Farms, Inc 541 F.2d 242
     (10th Cir 1976); Hecht v. Pro-Footbal Inc. 570 F.2d 982, 988-89 (D.C. Cir
     1977); US v. Empire Gas Co 537 F.2d 296, 304-5 (8th Cir 1976); Robinson
     v. Magovern, 882; US v. Hammermill Paper Co. 429 F.Supp 1271, 12 78
     (W.D. Pa. 1977); also see FTC. v. Procter & Bamgle Co. 386 US 568, 571
     (1967).
33   Jim Walter Corp v FTC, 682; Monfort of Colorado Inc. v. Cargill Inc, 700;
     US v. Grinnell Corp 575; US. v. Hammermill Paper Cio., 1278.
34   F&M Schaefer Corp. v. C. Schmidt & Sons, 597 F.2d 814, 817 (2d Cir.
     1979); US v. Kimberly Clark Corp 264 F.Supp. 439, 458 (N.D. Cal 1967);
     US v Philadelphia National Bank, 361.
35   Arizona v. Maricopa County Medical Scicty 457 US 332, 339-52 (1982).
     See also Pennsylvania Dental Association v. Medical Service Association
     815 F.2d 270, 275 (3d Cir. 1987); Feminist Women's Health Center Inc. v
     Mohammad 586 F.2d 530,535 (5th Cir. 1978); FTC v Michigan State
     Medical Society 101 FTC 191, 263-64 (1983).
36   FTC v. Indiana Federation of Dentists 476 US 447, 460-61 (1986)
37   Konik v. Champlain Valley Hospital Medical Center 733 F.2d1007 (2d.Cir);
     Gonzales v. Insignares; Litman v. A. Barton Hepburn Memorial Hospital
     679 F.Supp.196 (N.D.N.Y.,1988);
38   Collins v. Associated Pathologists Ltd. 844 F.2 473 (7th Cir, 1988); Robinson
     v. Magovern; Pontius v. Children's Hospital 552 F.Supp. 1352 (W.D. Pa.
     1982).
39   Wilk v. American Medical Association 719 F.2d 207 (7th Cir., 1983),
     remanded 671 F.Supp 1465 (N.D. Ill. 1987); Bhan v. NME Hospital Inc.
     772 F.2d 1467 (9th Cir 1985), remanded 669 F.Supp. 998 (E.D. Cal. 1987);
     Nurse Midwifery Associates v. Hibbett 549 F.Supp 1185 (M.D. Tenn. 1982);
     Virginia Academy of Clinical Psychologists v. Blue Shield of Va. 624 F.2d
     476, 485 (4th Cir 1980); Blue Shield of Virginia v. McCready 457 US 465,
     483 (1982); Weiss v. York Hospital 745 F.2d 786 (3d Cir.1984).
40   Kissam W.L., et al "Antitrust and Hospital Privileges: Testing the
     Conventional Wisdom" *California Law Review*, Vol. 40, 1982, pp.641-62.
41   Havinghurst, C.C. "Competition in Health Services: Overview, Issues and
     Answers" *Vanderbilt Law Review*, Vol. 34 (1982), pp.1117-29

42 Colton, D.J. Rubin, C.L. "Traditional Antitrust Analysis and Alternative Health Care Delivery Systems: Can Old Tools Harvest New Answers" *Journal of Reprints for Antitrust Law and Economics*, Vol. 27, No.1, pp.217-318;

43 Note, "Prepaid Prescription Drug Plans Under Antitrust Scrutiny: A Stern Challenge to Health Care Cost Containment" Northwestern University Law Review, Vol, 75, pp.506-528.

44 FTC *Statement of Enforcement Policy Regarding Physician Agreements to Control Medical Payment Plans*, 46 Fed. Reg. 48982, 48983 ()ct. 5, 1981).

45 *Business Review Letter* from William F. Baxter to Hospital Corporation of America (Sept 21, 1983);

46 Areeda, P. *Antitrust Analysis*, Little Brown & Co., Boston, MA. #rd Ed. (1981), par 621 at p.886; Comment, "Relevant Geographic Market Delineation: The Interchangeability of Standards in Cases Arising Under Section 2 of the Sherman Act and Section 7 of the Clayton Act", *Duke University Law Journal*, 1979, p.1152.

47 US. v. Bethlehem Steel Corp 168 F.Supp. 576, 588 (S.D.N.Y. 1958); see also Posner, R. *Antitrust Law: An Economic Perspective*, (1976), pp. 128-29; Baxter, W.F. "Responding to the Reaction: The Draftsman's View California Law Review, Vol. 71 (1983), pp.623-25; Werden G. "A Closer Analysis of Antitrust Markets" 62 *Washington University Law Quarterly* 647-53 (1985).

48 American Medicorp Inc v. Humana 445 F.Supp.589 (E.D. Pa., 1977)

49 FTC v. American Medical Internation Inc 104 FTC 1 (1984)

50 Hospital Corporation of America v. FTC 106 FTC 361, 465-66 (1985)

51 US. Hospital Affiliates International Inc 1980-81 Trade Cas (CCH) par 63,721 (E.D.La.1980); US v. Beverly Enterprises, Inc. 1984-1 Trade Cas (CCH) Par. 66,052 (M.D. Ga.June 1984)

52 Hospital Corp. of America v. FTC, at 468-72

53 American Medicorp Inc. v. Humana, at 5899-604

54 US. v. Hospital Affiliates International Inc, at par. 77,852

55 Jefferson Parish Hospital District v. Hyde, 466 US 2, 21 (1984); Goss v. Memorial Hospital System 789 F.2d353,355 (5th Cir.1986); Ball Memorial Hospital Inc. v. Mutual Hospital Insurance Inc. 603 F.Supp. 1077, 1084 (S.D. Ind. 1985); Konik v. Champlain Valley Hys. Hospital Medical Center 733 F.2d 1006, 1017 (2d Cir. 1984). See also Bhan v. NME Hospitals Inc 669 F.Supp 998 (E.D. Cal 1987)

56 Oltz v. St Peter's Community Hospital

57 Gonzales v.Insignares 1985-2 Trade Cas.(CCH) par 66,701 (N.D.Ga 1985)

58 Bhan v. NME Hospitals Inc. at 1019-20

59 Weiss v. New York Hospital 745 F.2d 768, 826 (3d Cir.1984)

60 Robinson v. Magovern 521 F.Supp. 842, 878-83 (W.D. Pa. 1981)

61 Ball Memorial Hospital Inc. v. Mutual Hospital Insurance, Inc 603 F. Supp 1077-81 (S.D. Ind. 1985); Metropolitan Life Ins. Co. v. Adler 1988-1 Trade Cas (CCH), par.67,907 (S.D.N.Y. 1988)

62   Barry v. Blue Cross of California 805 F.2d 866 ((th Cir 1986)
63   Kartell v. Blue Shield of Massachusetts Inc 749 F.2d 922-28 (1st Cir 1984)
64   Virginia Academy of Clinical Psychologists v. Blue Shield of Virginia 624
     F.2d 476-82 (4th Cir. 1980)

Chapter 21
COMPETITION ENFORCEMENT AND HEALTHCARE INTERMEDIATION

During the 1970s and even the early 1980s, the price of healthcare attracted little or no social and political attention. Competition on the healthcare scene, to the extent that it existed, was seen in terms of quality instead of price. The consumers of healthcare were not "rational" in the context of traditional neoclassical micro-standards, as they had no profit maximizing motive. Nor were the providers concerned with costs. They charged what the market would accept, and the market would normally and without much scrutiny pay whatever was charged. In essence, insurance protected both the consumer and the provider from financial responsibility. While markets for "standard" goods and services rely on the direct interaction between the buyers and sellers, no such interaction would prevail in healthcare markets. In fact, healthcare intermediators, having always been ready to compensate for medical services consumed by the patient, often pursuant not even to the decision of the consuming patient but to that of the supplying physician, and having been able to recoup and increase their financial worth by simply raising premiums, insulated the normal buyers-seller control on market price. Patients had the incentive to increase demand, providers presumably further stimulated that demand, and the intermediators simply covered the tab.

As healthcare costs spiraled, however, the sector began to gain social and political attention. Initially at least, however, instead of implementing market structure related remedies, various politically funded regulatory measures were chosen, and imposed on the existing structure. When the various regulatory measures have not brought about their desired effects, attention was spread to the possible benefits of traditional economic competition in healthcare markets. The potential benefits of the bulk purchasing power possessed by alternative delivery systems (ADS), initially mostly HMOs, came into focus. In the case of staff HMOs, the institution itself became the traditional providers' direct competitor. Furthermore, non-HMO affiliated providers, both individuals and institutions, also faced competition from IPAs due to latter's generally lower price and cost structure. Thus, the traditionally lucrative medical market pie had to be shared. Competition among providers, aimed at maintaining the traditional economic statusquo became a major dimension of medical practice. Intra-provider rivalries, within physician groups, among hospitals, and among various physician institutional practice settings (e.g. ambulatory and surgical clinics) and hospitals intensified. In addition, the 1975 Golfarb decision opened the antitrust door to the healthcare sector as well.

Nevertheless, coping with competitive restraints in healthcare by way of antitrust has, particularly during the initial periods of enforcement, remained a difficult task. The often indispensable market study in antitrust cases could not effectively be conducted in healthcare markets where the players, particularly the consumers, are not assigned traditional roles. Assessing the impact of a conduct on competition by way of market definitions and market power measurements was difficult where there has not been competition in the first place, and the consumers are uninformed about product price, product quality, and make product choices not by relying on these conventional variables but on the suggestions, often mandates, of the provider of the very products and services they ultimately receive.

Nevertheless, the courts appeared to have resisted these difficulties, even by way of applying the *per se* rule, with the latter calling for conclusions regarding the competitive impact of a conduct relatively early in the litigation process[1]. Furthermore, the intensified entry of HMOs and PPOs onto the scene created to an extent a somewhat traditional market-like environment where purchasers with market power interact directly with sellers, likely with comparable market power, and transact with prices, quality and profits in mind. A large segment of the sector is still dominated by traditional healthcare delivery. Providers still think and compare in terms of traditional practice patterns. They may try to resist ADSs at one time, or complain if they are excluded from one at another time. The rest of this chapter will review some of the major antitrust issues pertaining to healthcare intermediators.

HMOs and Competitive Restraints

A number of competitive restraint varieties may occur in connection HMO activities. The major types include restraints such as price fixing, tying arrangements, exclusive dealing, boycotts, and monopolization.

The standards for *price fixing* was decisively set back in 1940 in connection with the collective activities of several oil companies attempting to prevent the bottom from falling out from under gasoline prices[2]. Any interference, in any form, with any result, with the market's price making mechanism is viewed as price fixing, and a *per se* violation of Sherman 1. An HMO enters into two sets of price agreements. It contracts with its providers, and essentially it also contracts with its subscribers. When dealing with subscribers, the HMO functions as an insurance company, it is in the "business of insurance", hence likely enjoys antitrust immunity under the McCarran Act, or the state action doctrine, discussed earlier in the volume. However, there are potentials for competitive restraints on the other front, that is when contracting with providers, particularly for an IPA based HMO where the providers contract with the HMO as to fees, among other participation factors, instead of having the otherwise independent individual providers to competitively bid for HMO contracts.

Relevant fact situations were present in the *Maricopa case*[3]. Two nonprofit medical foundations had at least 70% of the area's physicians as their members. Member providers collectively established maximum fees for their services to subscribers of certain insurance plans. The foundations' other functions, such as peer utilization review and administrative functions performed as a PPO, were not at issue in the case. Furthermore, member providers had no financial interest, no investments, in the foundations. The foundations were not economically integrated practices. The two federal lowers courts viewed the agreements in contention as *rule of reason* issues. The Supreme Court, on the other hand, applied a *per se* analysis, concluding that the maximum fees agreed upon by members through their foundations were in effect joint price fixing efforts on the part of providers who would have otherwise independently competed with each other. The Court disregarded its, and the lower courts', lack of experience at that time in the healthcare sector as a possible factor for mitigating and otherwise *per se* issue. The Court's concern for competitive restraints did not rest with price agreements between providers and insurers, for that was viewed as both essential for conducting the health insurance business, and socially acceptable.

The socially unacceptable, illegal, anticompetitive restraint was found in the conduct of the providers themselves when they, each independent provider being part of a coordinated group, set fees, including maximum fees, for services which they offered and rendered individually. Essentially, otherwise competing physicians chose not to compete but colluded, through their foundations. Thus, the foundations became a vehicle for a price fixing conspiracy, given the fact that a foundation by its very nature is not the same as a partnership of joint venture:

> The foundations are not analogous to partnerships or other joint arrangements in which persons who would otherwise be competitors pool their capital and share the risks of loss as well as the opportunities for profit. In such joint ventures, the partnership is regarded as a single firm competing with other sellers in the market[4].

If the providers had a financial interest in the foundations, or their interaction with respect price would have been implemented through pre-paid health plans, then the rule of reason, instead of the *per se* approach would have likely been applied in the adjudication of the conduct.

During the Maricopa proceedings, the defendants referred to an earlier case where an organization of music copy right holders collectively agreed on the terms, including the license fee, for licensing their proprietary composition. The issue in that case was price-fixing, since organization members did not compete among themselves in terms of the license fees charged to secondary players of their music. They simply used the collectively determined blanket rate[5]. Yet, instead of viewing it as price fixing, the Supreme Court considered the newly created practice of blanket licensing as a "new product", and the collectively determined license fee as the price for that new product. The manner whereby the flat fee was set, that is collectively, was seen by the Court as an indispensable prerequisite for the creation of the new product. The argument in Maricopa that the defendants were also creating a new product, a new healthcare delivery system, was rejected. The practice of organized providers agreeing on a maximum fee to be accepted from holders of certain insurance contracts did not, in view of the Court, constitute the creation of a new healthcare delivery system. Instead, it was viewed as a way of collectively setting fees for certain transactions by those independent providers who would have otherwise competed with each other.

On the other hand, an HMO may be considered as a new product by way of a novel healthcare delivery system, in contrast to older systems. Providers contract with the HMO entity instead of among themselves. In essence, the horizontal aspects of provider interaction is replaced by the vertical dimension of dealing with the HMO. In fact, this relatively favorable consideration of the HMO makes it, as we will see later on in this chapter, a less risky undertaking than would a PPO be in terms of collective pricing practices.

Incidentally, in Maricopa, the Supreme Court's decision was followed by a permanent injunction in the US District Court (Arizona) against the associations and foundations getting involved in any activity that resulted in reduced competition in price, or in terms of other variables, among competing providers.

Completely merged plans were differentiated from partially merged ones in the past by the FTC[6]. In a completely merged plan, such as group or staff model HMOs, participating providers have fully integrated their practices, with no part of their practice left to compete with each other. Other hand, a partially integrated plan leaves participating providers to compete with each other in some service areas. In the former case, no significant anticompetitive issues are perceived if the plan involves no more than about 30% of the practitioners in the area. In the latter situation, the group's share in the relevant product market would be an important factor analyzed by way of the rule of reason approach.

Another area of inquiry may address the HMO's ability to offer a large collection of healthcare services. This could give rise to a claim of *tying contracts* to the detriment of competing providers. The allegation of tying contracts involves the seller using its market power in the "tying product", the product of prime interest to the consumer, and making its acquisition by the buyer conditioned upon the purchasing the "tied product", in which the seller normally has no particularly large market power, with the buyer having marginal interest. The resolution of the dispute normally proceeds by way of an examination of the seller's market power in the tying product market. If the latter inquiry points to no significant market power, no *per se* competitive restraints are perceived under the Sherman Act. Thus, if an HMO does not possess a power in an appropriate geographical market so as to make alternative medical service choices for potential patients difficult, the HMO's usual package of services would not be viewed as a tying arrangement contrary to society's interest, and substantially anticompetitive under the antitrust rules.

A case in point in the healthcare field was decided in 1984[7]. A contract between a group of anesthesiologists and a hospital was alleged to be an illegal tying contract, excluding other anesthesiologists from working at that hospital, and foreclosing inpatients at that hospital from choosing a specialist in that field from outside the contracted group. The tying product was hospital inpatient services, while the tied product was the service of anesthesiologists. The prerequisite in this case, as in any case involving illegal tying contract allegations, was a proof to the effect that the hospital had monopoly power in the market for inpatient hospital services, leaving potential hospital inpatients who wanted to use other anesthesiologists with no significant choice by way of alternative hospital services. The court found no such proof in this case. In addition, although not as deciding factors, certain economies and medical advantages were noted in the involved arrangements.

Under Sherman 1, *boycotts* have received *per se* attention, and they may be pertinent to HMO conduct. The conduct typically involves an agreement among a group of providers not to deal with another provider or organization, notwithstanding the legitimacy of an individual provider deciding independently not to deal with another organization. An early healthcare case involved the AMA's practice and code of ethics at the time[8]. According to the latter, member physicians were sanctioned, even excluded from local societies, or blocked from getting local hospital privileges, if they participated in pre-paid plans. The Court found this practice in *per se* violation of Sherman 1.

In recent years, most of the boycott cases focused on the manner whereby hospital privilege denials and other conduct on the part of fellow physician competitors precluded some physicians from practicing medicine in an environment, including hospitals, to which they felt entitled. Thus, so called "physician cartels" (physicians groups already possessing hospital staff privileges) with their own economic interests overriding that of the hospital and the community, often exercised through medical societies (e.g. AMA) were attacked as boycotts under the *per se* rules. Similar, although not per se, situations exit when a physician is denied staff privileges by a hospital, and issues of care quality and efficiency arise. Upon applying the rule of reason, the courts will seek relevant market power measurements in order to determine if the complainant has adequate number of alternative and comparable practice opportunities available. These situations can, and mostly have, come about without the direct involvement of an HMO. In fact, when HMOs were involved in boycott situations, they were more likely the victims, instead of the perpetrators. Thus, HMOs may be boycotted by individual providers through the latters' denial of professional services to the HMO. If the denial is pursuant to a proven concerted action, then a *per se* boycott may be at hand. The proof of conspiracy may be complicated if the HMO entity competes with otherwise fee-for-service physicians by way of substantially lower prices. The withholding of service by providers from the HMO may thus be the result of independently made and purely economically motivated decisions[9].

An area of HMO vulnerability in antitrust may be found in connection Sherman 2 issues, in particular *monopolization* and attempts to monopolize. We have examined these issues extensively earlier in the volume. The issues may be reiterated by reminding the reader that monopolization and related issued under Sherman 2 center on the existence of monopoly power (the ability to control price and exclude competition), its willful acquisition and abuse (in contrast to market power acquired through exceptional business skills, products or services). The magnitude of monopoly power is presented within a relevant market, both in its product and geographical dimensions, and evaluated along with evidence of conduct and performance, prevailing intensity of market competition, and ease of entry by potential competitors. Once a certain level of monopoly power is shown to exist, the manner whereby that power is used needs to be examined in terms of whether is inhibits competition through various methods such as excessive mergers, controlling supply contracts, using purchasing leverage, predatory pricing, precluding new entry, and the like.

These issues may readily bear upon HMOs. HMOs are actual and potential competitors to most types of other healthcare intermediaries, such as Blue Cross and Blue Shield Plans, commercial health insurance companies, and other HMOs. So called defensive HMOs, established by existing fee-for-service physicians, may be set up to deal with other incoming new HMO competition. Existing insurance concerns may discriminate against new HMOs by denying services such as reinsurance, billing, marketing, or sell these services at discriminatory prices. IPA type HMO physicians may find themselves denied by existing insurance concerns the opportunity to join other provider groups. Finally, established healthcare intermediaries may engage in temporary price predation to prevent the emergence of a new HMO on the scene, or to prevent its initial expansion necessary for the first stages of economies and possibly survival. If a refusal to deal is involved, the question, one again, is whether it is a product of a concerted action on the part of several incumbents (a Sherman 1 issue), or a unilateral action on the part of one firm; in the latter case, the next resolves around the firm's market power and how it uses that power.

PPOs and Competitive Restraints

The PPO is a compromise of a sort between the fee-for-service arrangement and the HMO. It aims at reducing costs with less infringement on the patients' and practitioners' autonomy. In essence, a PPO is a contract between providers and patients, a third-party payer being the middle-person. The contract normally covers provider fee discounts and some utilization review, along with securing a volume of patient flow to the providers. Providers find PPOs attractive because they continue to be paid on a retrospective fee-for-service basis, assume minimum or no financial risk, no major disruption occurs to practice patters as in group practice HMOs because their non-PPO associated practice remains intact. Patients, on the other hand, may still choose their own doctor, even outside the PPO. If they choose a PPO provider, instead one outside the PPO, however, their personal out-of-pocket expenses are less, and their co-payment lower. Thus, providers contract to give fee-reduction and allow some oversight of their service utilization patterns in return for more business, and a pre-arranged faster reimbursement. PPO chooses providers, most likely acceptable to patients, based on their track record in terms of quality of service, and service utilization. Major procedures and excessive specialist use are avoided by second opinion programs.

The *social benefits* of PPOs are generated largely by way of attempting to overcome traditional medical market imperfections. Historically, price competition in medicine has been averted by organized and politically aggressive medical societies. Patients, third-party payers, and employers bowed to the notion of physician "sovereignty", by staying away from practice and utilization reviews, fee negotiations, and quality scrutiny. The physician was willfully protected on his or her own turf by the "ignorance" of those outside the medical world, which ignorance tended to be capitalized upon by the practitioners. Medical markets, in turn, were rendered void of the normal social benefits that could be found in non-medical markets. A consumer who did not know the product, who was willfully prevented from learning about the product, who could not assess and compare the quality of the product, hence the product was often chosen for him or her by the provider (supplier), did not know the true price of that product and nor did he or she care because of third-party payer buffers, could not have possibly made rational purchasing decisions, so fundamental for the functioning of a socially beneficial market, even if he or she desired to do so. This was compounded by the fact that traditional third-party payers rarely scrutinized charges submitted by physicians. Competition among providers was largely absent.

PPOs may succeed at remedying some of these traditional medical market maladies in a number of ways. Information about price is distributed. Quality of care becomes an important provider choice criterion. Dealing with multiple providers at the same time, economies of scale may be attained in information gathering both as to price and quality, and disseminated to consumers. The latter are given the incentive to deal with chosen providers and utilize the information by financial incentives, such as lower co-payments.

Given the antitrust theme of the chapter, we must now look at the possible market and competition related problems generated by PPOs. Risks of PPO related competitive restraints emanate from a variety of sources. These include (a) provider inclusion into, or exclusion from, a PPO; (b) the manner whereby provider fee schedules are set; (c) the market share of the PPO and the resulting impact of PPO action on the market.

Prior to dealing with these issues, let us briefly review the various PPO organizational forms, that is who may sponsor a PPO. These alternatives have a direct bearing on the likelihood, and severity under the antitrust rules, of competitive restraints. In general, PPOs may be grouped into three categories. A PPO may be set up entirely by independent *entrepreneurs*; the entrepreneur, essentially a healthcare services broker, may be a private individual or business outside the healthcare field who undertakes a group of providers to provide the service at a contracted rate, under a set of circumstances. A *purchaser* based PPO is organized by a third-party payer; it recruits providers, one or more hospitals and normally a substantial number of doctors, to participate in the plan. A *provider based* PPO is organized by a hospital or a group of physicians; they create a network of services and market it to those who pay for them, normally third-party payers. Once set up, the PPO is marketed to large purchasers of healthcare services, such as health insurance companies, and self-insured employers. The PPO reimbursement discount to physicians ranges from around 10% to 20%. The first PPO was established by Blue Shield in 1983, a purchaser based program. By 1985, the Blues had 11 PPO plans operating in nine states. Preferred providers were contracted at a predetermined fee, which could not be exceeded by excess billing directly to the patient. Any copayment by patients would be deducted from the fee to the contracted providers. Providers not participating in the PPO may continue to treat the Blue's patients, if those patients choose them. However, in the latter case the fees are likely to be higher; in contract to the 100% PPO coverage, only 50% of the fees may be covered; patients treated by nonparticipating doctors pay directly and then seek reimbursement for a part of their costs, in contrast to the payment procedure involved with participating providers where the patient is removed from the payment process.

The anticompetitive implications of a PPO, in terms of who is *excluded or included,* depends in large part on the plan's sponsor. Thus, in *payer-sponsored PPOs,* the sponsor has the right to unilaterally exclude a provider based on fees, utilization, geography, or other considerations. This discretion to decide is even higher in nonprovider or third-party payer but entrepreneur/broker based PPOs. A third-party payer may be concerned with competitive restraints if two or more of them horizontally concert not to deal with a provider, or if one payer agrees with two or more physicians to exclude another provider (both scenarios constitute Sherman 1 *per se* group boycotts). However, even purely unilateral third-party payer actions may be of social concern if the payer is so large in the relevant market that substantial monopsony power may be attributed it (Sherman 2 monopolization issues may be relevant).

In *provider sponsored* PPOs, the competitive consequences of exclusion may be more significant, although by no means definitive. First of all, the exclusion is likely to be the product of an agreement among the competitors of the excluded provider, which may amount to a *per se* group boycott under Sherman 1. If so, the outcome is relatively simple, for no proof of competitive restraint or of damages for that matter is required beyond proof of the actual boycott. If, on the other hand, the rule of reason is applied by the court, the competitive impact of the boycott needs to be analyzed. However, competitive impact needs to be proven not only by way of the injury sustained by the excluded provider, for the occurrence of that injury may very well be the case, but also in terms of injury to *competition* in the relevant product and geographical markets. If the excluded provider/competitor is relatively small, the latter proof may turn out to be an unmet challenge. Thus, much depends on the doctrine accepted by the court, and that may also be difficult to predict. In a 1985 case, the Supreme Court indicated that

A plaintiff seeking application of the *per se* rule must present a threshold case that the challenged activity falls into a category likely to have predominantly anticompetitive effects. The mere allegation of a concerted refusal to deal does not suffice because not all concerted refusals to deal are predominantly anticompetitive[11].

Furthermore, the relevant product market itself may complicate matters. A PPO is a multiproduct joint venture like organization whose functions include utilization review, risk sharing, collective facilities shared by participating providers, rather than a simple cartel among competing providers. An individual provider is not in these service categories, hence not a competitor. If viewed as a joint venture, a PPO is free to chose its participants just as any other joint venture by way of, for instance, a partnership might.

Provider fee schedules within a PPO context received considerable attention. Price fixing *among competitors* is a *per se* violation of Sherman 1. However, uniform pricing applied by an organization within which the providers are under common ownership, hence do not compete with each others in terms of price, or if the providers do not compete with each other because they are in different product or geographical, or both, both markets, price fixing will not likely be an issue of concern. Since participating providers in most PPOs otherwise independently compete, price-fixing concerns in these situations can be real.

In this regard, we have already seen from the Maricopa decision that any price related agreement among otherwise competing providers by way of an organization where there is no "risk sharing" or "integrative efficiencies" is a *per se* competitive restraint. However, the difference between the competitive impact of horizontal and vertical price agreements needs to be emphasized. A horizontal price agreement takes place among competitors, who would otherwise compete in terms of price, and other variables. A vertical price agreement is bilaterally implemented between the buyer and a seller, a "natural" contractual process with little or no social concern for competitive restraint. In payer-sponsored PPOs, if the organization negotiates with each provider, without the providers themselves interfering with each other's negotiation or agree among themselves to somehow impact on those negotiations, no significant competitive restraint are likely. Thus, in situations like that, the key is in the independence with which each provider negotiates bilaterally with the PPO, rather than by collective agreement among the providers or through a third party coordinating effort.

The third dimension of a PPO's competitive concern involves the organization's *size*. This is particularly important when the PPO is provider sponsored. The size in this context is viewed in terms of the proportion of all providers in the region involved with the PPO, and the consequent possible of foreclosure of other PPOs in the same geographic market from having access to and use of these providers. If the PPO ties up a significant proportion of providers in the market, plus it requires exclusivity thereby foreclosing other PPOs, serious competitive concerns may arise. Thus, significant proportion and exclusivity are both necessary for noting a likely restraint on competition. A small PPO, even with exclusivity, will likely generate competition by way of other providers setting up their own PPO. A large PPO, without exclusivity, will likely end up sharing many its providers with other PPOs, due particularly to the providers' financial incentives involved.

Some relatively recent opinions illustrate the point. In the Ball Memorial case, which appears to be the first major participation by a court in a PPO case, the plaintiffs were 80 acute care hospitals in Indiana. They had attempted through the courts to stop Blue Cross from implementing a PPO, alleging price fixing and monopolization[12]. The court denied the motion, declaring the PPOs as part of the insurance market, including other insurance companies, HMOs, third-party payers, other PPOs, and even government programs such as Medicare. The court considered the PPOs as an additional competitive option available to the healthcare insurance consumers.

A PPO with exclusivity provisions and a large market share received the attention of the Department of Justice not too long ago. The Stanislaus Preferred Provider Organization (SPPO) was found, by USDJ investigation, to operate for the purpose of foreclosing other PPOs from being formed, thus restraining competition in the relevant healthcare delivery market. SPPO included exclusivity in its contracts, and the contracted providers represented between 50% and 90% of the total number of providers in the relevant California geographical markets[13].

Blue Cross - Blue Shield
and Competitive Restraints

The first Blue Plans were established around the mid-1930s, sponsored largely by physician and hospital associations in order to improve access to hospital and medical care for those covered, and to facilitate the collection of fees. The initial provider control of the Plans has been largely replaced by state regulation. Nevertheless, provider control of the plans is major concern for competition enforcement, cost control, and the providers themselves. Presently, the Plans are largely state legislated, tax-exempt, and contract with subscribers on the one hand, and with providers (physicians, hospitals and pharmacies) on the other.

In view of the "input-output" nature of their functions, the Plans maintain two sets of contracts: participating provider contracts to secure input at an agreed rate, and subscriber contract with patients to secure the nature and price of output. The provider get direct, and relatively prompt, reimbursement for his charges at a rate considered to be "usual, customary and reasonable" (UCR). Along with the no balance billing to patients provision, UCR may be viewed as cost containment oriented, hence socially desirable. Nevertheless, many providers have rebelled against this system of reimbursement by the Blues by filing antitrust complaints, alleging constraints on free market price formation and undue market power on the part of the Plans.

In a 1981 action, pharmacists objected, unsuccessfully, to the Plans' ability to set prices at levels they considered too low[14]. The district court, refusing to find *per se* illegality, looked upon Blue Shield as a purchaser, hence the transactions were merely between buyers and sellers, not conducive for *per se* horizontal price fixing activity. Furthermore, the constraint on reimbursed prices was part of a contract consummated voluntarily between the buyer and seller, without any indicating of a vertical price fixing. Similar issues arose in another case involving pharmacies a year later. Reimbursement rate ceilings incorporated in provider contracts with the pharmacies were alleged to have been *per se* price fixing under Sherman 1. Once again, it was noted that Blue Shield was not in the same product market as the pharmacies, that is drug retailing, and nor was it in competition with drug manufacturers. Thus, horizontal price fixing was out of the question. No vertical price fixing was perceived either because the reimbursement ceiling had no impact on drug retail prices charged to non-Blue Shield customers or on the price charged by pharmacies not participating in Blue Shield plans. "Failure to make more money was not the kind of problem" that concerned Congress when passing the antitrust laws[15].

Two years later, an often discussed case centered on the issue of prohibiting balance billing by physicians, a provision included in participating provider agreements. A group of Blue Shield participating physicians in Massachusetts alleged that the prohibition of balance billing, along with the price constraints involved the UCR level reimbursements, constituted Sherman 1 and Sherman 2 violations. The lower court agreed with the doctors, and found the balance billing prohibition a restraint on competition in the market for physician services. As to Sherman 2 issues, the court also found that restrictive provisions in provider contracts, the UCR payment system, and the proscription of balance billing, were a manifestation of purchasing monopoly (monopsony) power possessed by Blue Shield in Massachusetts, resulting in unreasonably low fees for providers[16]. The district court did not accept Blue Shield's argument that the practice yielded lower healthcare prices hence contributed to cost containment, citing the often argued antitrust principle to the effect that lower prices do not vindicate competitive restrains. Accepting the physicians' argument against the contractual prohibition of balance billing, the district court cited Maricopa where the uniform healthcare price resulting from the collective action there was seen as discouraging innovating healthcare delivery both in terms of basic practice and procedures and equipment applications. Thus, the proscription of balance billing was seen by the court as an impediment to innovative and progressive medical practice[16].

The Court of Appeals reversed the lower court's decision, advising that the relationship between Blue Shield and the contracted providers should be seen as a buyer-seller interaction where both parties come together and contract willingly and independently on negotiated price and quality of service terms. Finding competitive restraints by virtue of that contract would void the buyer's ability to enforce its terms. It was further pointed out that the negotiated fees were not low so as to consider them predatory in the healthcare market; they were simply low enough to allow patients to benefit from Blue Shield's purchasing power which the patients themselves individually could not have. The fact that the prices were biased lower was seen as a welcome contribution to cost containment efforts, a notion which, if the practice was in any way seen as part of a horizontal price-fixing effort, would have no merit.

It is clear that the introduction of competition into medical markets as a means of cost containment paved the way for antitrust actions to promote and preserve that competition. Reimbursement restrictions, particularly those contracted with the Blue Plans, have been challenged as being anticompetitive, simply as a defensive measure by providers aimed at preserving or promoting a financial status quo. The lower courts in the federal system have typically found reimbursement restrictions socially acceptable and in the interest of the consumer, and the Supreme Court has not yet had an occasion to rule on the issue.

References

1   See the 1982 Maricopa decision, to be discussed at length later.
2   US v. Socony-Vacuum Oil Co 310 US 150 (1940)
3   Arizona v. Maricopa County Medical Sosciey 457 US 332 (1982)
4   Maricopa at p. 356
5   Broadcast Music Inc. v. CBS 441 US 1 (1979)
6   FTC, *Physician Agreements to Control Prepayment Plans*, 46 Fed. Reg 48,982 (1081)
7   Jefferson Parish Hospital District No.2 v. Hyde 466 US 2 (1984)
8   AMA v. US 317 US 519 (1943); see also Kissam J. et al. "Antitrust and Hospital Privileges: Testing the Conventional Wisdom" California Law Review, Vol. 70, 1982, p.595.
9   Feminist Women's Health Center Inc v. Mohammad 586 F.2d 530 (5th Cir. 1978), cert den 444 US 924 (1979)
10 FTC Advisory Opinion to Health Care Management Associates, June 7, 1982
11 Northwest Wholesale Stationers Inc. v. Pacific Stationers & Printing Co. 105 S.Ct. 2613 (1985)
12 Ball Memorial Hospital Inc. et. al. v. Mutual Hospital Insurance Inc. 603 F.Supp. 1077 (S.D. Ind. 1985)
13 Pursuant to a threat by the US Department of Justice to file an antitrust suit, SPPO was disolved
14 Sausalito Pharmacy v. Blue Shield 544 F.Supp. 230 (N.D.Cal 1981), aff'd 677 F.2d 47 (9th Cir.1982)
15 Medical Arts Pharmacy Inc v. Blue Cross and Blue Shield Inc 518 F.Supp.1100 (D.Conn 1981), aff'd 675 F.2d 502 (2d Cir.1982)
16 Kartell v. Blue Shield Inc. 582 F.Supp.734 (D.Mass 1984), rev'd 749 F.2d 922 (1st Cir.1984). See also, 592 F.2d 1191 (1st Cir.1979); 542 F.Supp.782 (D.Mass.1982); and 384 Mass. 409 N.E.2d 313 (1981)
17 Kartell v. Blue Shield Inc. 749 F.2d 922 (1st Cir.1984)

Chapter 22
COMPETITION IN THE
PHYSICIAN SECTOR

Physicians have traditionally not considered themselves as competitors of each other. They may have viewed themselves as a select, even exclusive, group of professionals living within their own world of relative, often absolute, prosperity, shielded by carefully guarded possession of knowledge, information and perceptions, and by the ignorance, even awe, of medicine on the part of many outsiders. For many years, the antitrust courts have accommodated this environment by considering professional activity as essentially too mature to be regulated from the outside, not possessing the necessary commercial content thought to be appropriate for the originally conceived antitrust statutes. Thus, medical practitioners did not have to compete because their conduct enjoyed antitrust immunity. At least until 1975. In 1975, the Golfarb decision, discussed earlier in the book, changed all that. The scope of antitrust enforcement has been extended to the business of professions, including, initially in a somewhat uncertain way, medicine. Since 1975, a number of antitrust actions were brought against practitioners and groups of medical practitioners because of conduct yielding perceived or actual competitive restraints in the relevant markets.

Questions have been raised whether the judicial enforcement of competition in medicine is appropriate, is in the interest of the patients, and consistent with medical ethics. A medical writer summed up the problem as follows:

> In the final analysis, where does the public interest lie - in strengthening the profession's fiduciary commitments to patients or in encouraging entrepreneurialism and commercial competition among physicians?

It is clear that we cannot have it both ways: the kind of free-wheeling business competition envisioned by antitrust law is simply not compatible with the ethical obligations of doctors to their patients.[1]

On the one hand, the solution to the problem appears to be very complex. On the other, if one views antitrust laws simply as a means of implementing or preserving fair competition in the market place, in any market place, as a Congressional mandate, the solution becomes less complex, and more concentrated upon the issue of whether medicine is "commerce" in a "market" or is it something beyond and above that where, in society's interests, this Congressional mandate cannot and should not apply. The courts, in many cases since 1975, appeared to have provided the answer. Indeed, we will note that a number of cases involved not the regulator against the regulated, that is, the US Justice Department or the FTC against medical practitioners, but one practitioner, or practitioner group, against the other, protecting their own interests, and purely economic interests at that, instead of protecting ethical principles. While the cases at times divulge information regarding the non-economic dimensions of an arrangement, such as increased quality of care as a result of some collective practice, economic considerations such as efficiency, competitive foreclosure, price pressure on incomes, outright income diminution, and so forth, are often not far behind. Thus, there is no question that, at least in the view of the judiciary, and of those directly involved in the marketing and distribution of medical services for their own livelihood and income, including most of the providers themselves, medicine is commerce carried out in markets for income, and often for a profit motive.

Credentialing and Group Boycotts

It occurs relatively frequently that physicians apply but are denied *staff privileges* at certain hospitals. The denial often involves the presence of other physicians, or physician groups, at the hospital already performing the functions which the petitioning provider is seeking to perform. The denial of staff privileges, at least on the surface, redistributes income generated in the hospital environment to those already in place there from those who seek the privileges. Largely because of that, although with other lesser motives as well that accompany the financial ones, physicians file antitrust law suites in considerable numbers. In addition to reinstatement, or instatement, a major part of the filed claims is the alleged financial damages which the excluded physician incurs, presumably as a result of the exclusion. Economics and income play a major role in these dramas. In fact, in most instances, if there is no economic loss, there is essentially no case, for an element of such a cause of action is the presence of some loss, in particular financial loss. Furthermore, according to some recent data, some 35% of the filed claims during the mid-1980s, when the precedents in these areas were evolving, involved exclusive contracts between hospitals and physicians, or physician groups, and the denial of physician privileges at hospitals[2].

While staff privilege related decisions at a hospital, normally promulgated by existing medical staff, may ultimately be motivated by self-serving financial and competitive considerations, other reasons are also often invoked. Indeed the involved litigation can be extremely complex, messy, personality bound, and can reveal some of the finest intricacies of intra-hospital personnel politics, pure and not so pure, politics which the patient may never see or learn of, but politics that may very well impact on the quality of care. Thus, physicians have lost staff privileges because they were alleged to have an "uncooperative attitude" or a "disruptive personality", when in fact, the staff privilege revocation may have simply been motivated by peer jealousy of the victim's successful practice outside the hospital, or by the victim's aggressiveness in otherwise competing with his peers[3]. Foreign medical graduates, or new residents, were excluded due to lacking board certification, or for not having medical malpractice insurance coverage[4].

Practitioners denied staff privileges normally claim a restraint of competition under Sherman 1 and 2. The relevant language, rather vague and open to interpretation, is as follows:

> Every contract, combination in the form of trust or otherwise, or conspiracy, in restraint of trade or commerce among the several states, or with foreign nations, is declared to be illegal [Sherman 1]. And, ... Every person who shall monopolize, or attempt to monopolize, or combine or conspire with any other person or persons, to monopolize any part of the trade or commerce among the several States, or with foreign nations, shall be deemed guilty of a felony ... The words 'person' or 'persons' wherever used in this Act .. shall be deemed to include corporations and associations existing under or authorized by the laws of either the United States ...[territories and foreign countries][5].

In fact, the medical staff of a hospital has been viewed as a combination of individual providers, and actions taken by them meeting the requirements of "contract", combination, or conspiracy" under Sherman 1[6]. Furthermore, the Congressional mandates of the Acts have consistently been interpreted not as the protection of individual competitors against the "unfair" conduct of others, but rather as the protection of competition in the interest of society. While the combination or conspiracy of providers aimed at using their collective power to gain competitive advantage is significant, it is viewed more to be in society's interest to ascertain that all qualified providers have access to the market place, and that patients have complete freedom of choice[7].

A problem often needing resolution in actions brought by individual providers against groups was meeting the interstate commerce requirements of the Act. In particular, the question may be raised as to how much impact on interstate commerce, if any, does an individual provider's exclusion from a specific hospital have? If there is an impact, to what extent? How much impact is needed to meet the Act's requirements? Thus, in a North Carolina case, alleging conspiracy by the defendants in preventing the claimant from expanding and relocating his hospital in Raleigh, the Federal Circuit Court of Appeals found no sufficient impact on interstate commerce to meet Sherman Act requirements, with the decision having been subsequently reversed by the Supreme Court. The Court considered factors such as the impact on interstate purchases of medical supplies, out-of-state management fee payments, and interstate financing procurements, amounting to thousands of dollars, to be substantial in terms of their affect on interstate commerce. In other words, allowing the plaintiff to expand and relocate his hospital, substantially increased interstate commerce in terms of interstate financing and purchased merchandise movements attributable to the claimant's expansion and relocation[8]. In general, a partial list of factors considered by the courts when assessing impact on interstate commerce may include the following: patient migration; medication, supplies and equipment procurement; geographical character of the defendant's activities; any connection between interstate commerce and the alleged activities[9].

Conspiracy under Sherman 1 must involve at least two entities with independent economic interests. Thus, intra-entity interaction (such as between a corporation and its officers, and other agents acting on behalf of the corporation with a common economic interest) will not suffice[10]. However, when an entity and its officers or employees have independent economic interests, such as actually or potentially competing medical staff contributing to a hospital's decision on granting or revoking staff privileges, the plausibility of conspiracy under Sherman 1 was accepted[11]. Yet, even under situations of this type, courts hesitated to conclude conspiracy in view of the fact that hospitals must inherently rely in large measure on competing physicians to make admitting decisions; and, conspiracies were even less likely found in cases where the consulted internal physicians were not competitors, and, additionally, their contribution was only a relatively small part of an elaborate administrative decision to admit or to revoke and insider[12].

With respect to *group boycotts*, physicians do not enjoy a trade union's immunity when group members make collective decisions relating to offering their services. Anticompetitive intent and consequence can be read into a group of staff members pressuring an administration into denying privileges to an applicant. Yet, the conduct, inherently horizontal, involves more than one entity, although its target may or may not be in the same product market. A hospital's decision is by its nature a unilateral one in relation to a staff privilege applicant, even though it uses existing staff input into its decision. On the other hand a collective decision by a group of physicians not to deal with another entity, such as a hospital by diverting patients to another, is clearly a horizontal group boycott in restraint of trade under Sherman 1.

An institutional scenario was played out in a 1984 case involving chiropractors against the AMA, JCAH, other medical associations and private physicians[13]. The applied standards for concluding that a group boycott was present required the complete absence of a possibility for an independent action on the part of the defendants, and the presence of a specific design to achieve the boycott. The presence of an opportunity to conspire was not seen as a restrain on competition. In this case, the AMA was found to have organized the boycott based on a resolution that viewed chiropractors as members of an unscientific cult and propagating a view that it was unethical for physicians to associate in any way with chiropractors[14]. Two other associations (The American College of Physicians, and the American Association of Orthpedic Surgeons) were found to have knowingly joined the boycott.

Another case, at about the same, time involved a hospital based professional boycott. An osteopath sued a hospital and its medical staff for failing to grant him admitting privileges[15]. In general, the court felt that a hospital's medical staff may engage in professional self-regulation by excluding a provider for inadequate competence and poor professional conduct, motivated by public service and ethical norms. However, those standards were not found to have been met in this case. In general, these and a number of other cases also centered on the relatively legal-specific issue of whether *per se* or rule of reason standards applied. When the exclusions in medicine were shown to have been based on a concern for service quality, professional competence, or unprofessional conduct, the rigid *per se* standards, which deny the defendant an opportunity to explain the reasons for his actions, were not applied.

Under Sherman 2, issues of monopolization and conspiracies to monopolize dominate. In particular, a provider, or group of providers, is scrutinized when it has (or almost has) *monopoly power*, i.e. the ability to exclude competition and raise price above competitive levels, and is acting as if intending to use that power. When a group of competitors is involved, the issues are somewhat like group boycotts on a smaller scale. Normally, a group controls a resource, e.g. providing a specific service to a hospital, and forecloses another practitioner from having access to that segment of the market. Competitive restraint under these circumstances may, in general, be established if the following conditions are met: (a) providers with monopoly power control the facilities at which the foreclosure occurred, (b) the foreclosed competing provider is denied the use of the facilities, and (c) cannot find reasonable substitute opportunities; (d) the qualification of the excluded competitor would allow him or her to effectively function in the environment if not excluded.

Given these conditions, showing that competition (in contrast to a competitor) has been substantially harmed is often difficult. The hospital at which the exclusion occurs must be an essential resource for the claimant competitor to the extent that its facilities "cannot practicably be duplicated", even if the excluding hospital is the only one in the region.[16]. Thus, if there are other hospitals in the area that the potential competitor applicant could utilize, competition would not necessarily be substantially restrained with existing staff physicians at the hospital if privileges to a new potential competitor are denied. Thus, once again, the delineation of the relevant product and geographical markets becomes essential to the extent of determining whether or not the hospital denying privileges possesses any specific or unique features (location, prestige, completeness of facilities, etc) that would separate it into its own or more restricted market than if it would be included with the rest of the hospitals the in the area. In addition to the market power of the *hospital* in the relevant geographical market, the economic power possessed by physicians already on staff and part of the admitting decision making process may also essential, although could substantially complicate matters if the admitting committee at the hospital is made up of physicians not in the field of the applicant, hence are not actual or potential competitors. Finally, it helps if it can be shown that the applicant is a true potential competitor, that is, the economic status of decision making physicians on staff would or could substantially deteriorate if the new doctor would be granted privileges.

Price Fixing by Physicians - Maricopa County Revisited

Since the Socony-Vacuum decision, price fixing has been defined in rather broad terms. Indeed, any type of activity designed to directly or indirectly interfere with the market's pricing mechanism, regardless of whether aimed at maximum or minimum prices, or to eliminate price fluctuations and to stabilize prices, have been viewed as price fixing under Sherman 1, with the *per se* rule often invoked. This principle has been applied in medicine since the 1975 Golfarb decision, that is, since the professions were effectively opened to antitrust scrutiny. The Maricopa decision was briefly discussed in the previous chapter within the context of third-party payer conduct. Since the same case is often viewed as the classic price-fixing one in medicine, it will be dealt with in this section to a much greater extent. In fact, it can be postulated that having found the conduct in question a *per se* violation of Sherman 1, the Court may have rendered more disservice to competition in medicine than the benefits it hoped to achieve.

Let us now take a closer look at the factual background of the Maricopa decision[17]. Maricopa Foundation for Medical Care was organized by the Maricopa County Medical Society in 1969, with membership restricted to physicians, osteopaths and podiatrists, all in private practice as well as members of the Society. A goal of the Foundation was to set up maximum fee schedules by way of multiplying a "relative value" with a "conversion factor". Basically, "relative value" is a pure number assigned to each medical service unit or procedure, designed to compare various medical functions in terms of their intensity, difficulty, amount of training needed and applied, and amount of time involved. Relative value guides are utilized by third-party payers and government agencies in order to arrive at presumably fair fee structures paid to physicians. The fees thus derived by members of the Foundation would be the maximum charged for particular services and claimed from insurance carriers, with the latter having preapproved these fees. Physicians could bill patients under the maximum, and those involved with insurance carriers not affiliated with the scheme could be charged more. Complete coverage under the plan was guaranteed provided the patient used participating physicians and carriers. Non affiliated provider charges, in excess of the maximum set by the plan, would be covered by the patient.

A central question in the litigation was whether or not the arrangement constituted *per se* price fixing under Sherman 1. The State of Arizona alleged that the maximum fee schedule amounted to a price fixing conspiracy. The Foundation's response centered on the procompetitive effect of the plan, and on the fact that patients had access to alternative plans not participating in the scheme. At any rate, the health plans of the foundation availed patients a complete coverage, a choice of providers and lower premiums. In addition, the Foundation urged the court to consider the issues under the rule of reason approach, instead of as a *per se* violation, in view of the judiciary's lack of experience in the medical industry[18]. The Court rejected the proposition stating:

> Maximum and minimum price fixing may have different consequences in many situations. But the schemes to fix maximum prices, by substituting the perhaps erroneous judgment of a seller for the forces of a competitive market, may severely intrude upon the ability of buyers to compete and survive in the market[19].

At any rate, since the term "price-fixing" was applied to the Foundation's practice, and that is in fact what has transpired regardless the fact that maximum prices were set, traditional well established rules applicable price fixing practices should apply, namely the *per se* doctrine[20]. This was particularly the case since the plan involved

> price restraint that tends to provide the same economic reward to all practitioners regardless of their skill, their experience, their training, or their willingness to employ innovative and difficult procedures in individual cases. Such a restraint also may discourage entry into the market and may deter experimentation and new developments by individual entrepreneurs. It may be a masquerade for an agreement to fix uniform prices, or it may in the future take on that character[21]

It was further noted that the Foundation for Medical Care was

not analogous to partnership or other joint arrangements in which persons who would otherwise be competitors pool their capital and share the risk of loss as well as the opportunities for profit. In such joint ventures, the partnership is regarded as a single firm competing with other sellers in the market. The agreement under attack is an agreement among hundreds of competing doctors concerning the price at which each will offer his own services to a substantial number of consumers..[an arrangement that fits a] horizontal price fixing mold[22].

Additionally, it was suggested that in case of a real need for a fee schedule, instead of the participating providers themselves, outside entities such as state agencies, or even other insurers, could have prepared them.

While the majority of the Court considered the facts tantamount to *per se* price fixing under Sherman 1, the dissenting opinion had views which had seen the practice in a much more favorable light. If anything, the practice was seen as rule of reason issue, as questions were raised whether or not the issue really involved what traditionally could be viewed as price fixing. It was pointed out that Foundation providers could service uninsured patients and other carriers and charge any fee they wished. Physician membership in the Foundation was for one year, although renewable, terms, thus allowing providers to terminate their association with the plan for any reason they wished. They had no long-term commitment to the Foundation and were not obliged to provide their service exclusively through the Foundation sponsored insurance plans. In fact, the dissenters saw the arrangements in a procompetitive and cost containment light. They viewed the insurers as being essentially agents of their subscribers, the patients, hence representing the interests of the latter when signing the agreement involved in the challenged plan. This arrangement was seen as a marked improvement over the traditional UCR method of physician reimbursement[23].

There may be considerable merit in the views of the dissenting opinion, particularly as to the cost containment benefits of the plan. Within a traditional neoclassical economic context, agreements to fix prices inhibit competitive processes, and lower social welfare. However, medicine has not, and to a large measure still does not, fit the neoclassical market mold, and mold that was designed to accommodate nonmedical industries and markets. Upon an indicated or demonstrated need by the patients, providers allocated healthcare resources, and the consumer essentially relinquished both the responsibility for and the participation in much of the further decision making with profound impact on the costs involved. Furthermore, seeking medical services has largely been market neutral, cost irrelevant, emotion dominated, and profoundly influenced by lack of product knowledge and information. Much was predicated upon "trust", however acquired or solicited, by the provider. Consumers acted on an emotional basis in selecting providers without much understanding of what they need or, indeed, what they get. The patient was not in the position to control or depress healthcare costs by reducing physician fees. Healthcare costs containment efforts could not have been initiated by individual patients. Providers allocated resources to the treatment of the patients, and the patient was oblivious to costs if a third-party, such as an insurance carrier, paid the medical fees. And, so long as the third-party payer met physician payment requirements, the providers themselves had no vested interest in cost containment. Under these circumstances, and apart from social and political concerns, only one party was left with an incentive to control healthcare costs, the insurer.

A brief look at the Arizona health insurance market of that time is called for. This is particularly important since one prevailing view of the time was that the Foundations controlled prices only to forestall HMO development in the area, and to preserve the physician preferred fee-for-service payment system as well as the traditional practice autonomy which went along with it. In most states, Blue Cross has normally had a lion's share of healthcare policy holders. However, in Arizona at the time the Maricopa drama played out, commercial insurers covered more than three times the number of Blue Cross participants. Importantly, during the three year period, between 1975 and 1978, the HMO's market share almost tripled, having increased from just over 3% to over 8%[24]. This may mean that the maximum pricing strategy of the Foundations was either not designed to inhibit HMO development, or, if it was, the implemented pricing structure simply did not achieve its goal.

At any rate, questions can also be raised regarding the *per se* application of the Sherman 1 rule based on the proportion of patients serviced by Foundation affiliates. Although the Foundations' participating physicians accounted for some 70% of all practitioners in the area, they serviced no more than about 15% of all insured persons[25]. By any antitrust convention, 15% does not constitute monopoly power, unless no significant monopoly power may be called for by a Court dealing with conspiracies. In addition, a foundation participating physician may have patients involved with another reimbursement plan with no maximum fee structure, and those patients may also be billed directly by the physician. Thus, the modus operandi imposed on foundation participating physicians may have affected only a small proportion of their practice, as one out of seven patients in the area was in effect not even involved with the plan, and participating doctors had those patients potentially available to them as patients unrelated to the pricing rules involved in the Foundation's plans. In addition, the constrained pricing of the plan hardly inhibited HMO entry into Arizona healthcare markets, as the above figures clearly suggest.

Peer Reviews and Competitive Restraints

Peer review procedures, in a generic sense, are not uncommon. Perhaps, nowhere are they more relevant than in academia where peers are often called upon to pass judgment about their colleagues' performance, often with serious consequences involving promotions, tenure, financial status, and even entire careers. Although these processes may also be strongly influenced by competitive considerations between the evaluators and the evaluated, and factors other than authentic and pure evaluative in nature may enter into the picture, intra-institutional competition between the evaluators and the evaluated are of no concern to antitrust rules. Thus, elements of jealousy or internal politics do not bear upon society's interests to preserve competition in the market place. On the other hand, even under these circumstances scenarios may be posed where peer evaluation may have serious competitive implications in the market place. Thus, for instance, the blocking of the promotion of an academic by peer recommendations may solely be motivated by the peers' anticompetitive motives against the evaluated outside the institutional framework of the process, in a consulting environment where both the peer evaluators and the evaluated participate and compete.

The circumstances in medicine are similar although much more complex and multi-faceted. Peer reviews in medicine cover a wide range of professional activities, including formal and informal overviews of practice in a variety of environments such as groups and hospital settings. Furthermore, there community wide peer-reviews such those found in Maricopa, namely foundations for medical care that review claims for private insurers, and peer review organizations (PROs) mandated by federal law to oversee care to Medicare patients, although the later also performs review services for private third-party payers. Clearly, some of these review processes are of more interest to society than others, at least within the context of competition preservation. For the same reasons, some of these processes are of more interest to antitrust enforcers than other.

The antitrust implications of peer review procedures came into sharp focus with an Oregon case decided during and after 1984 where initially a jury found against eleven physicians and rendered a $2 million verdict for conduct performed within the context peer review. This case will be examined in detail later in this section[26]. The Patrick decision created a double-edged sword. Physicians and hospitals have become apprehensive about participating in peer review procedures for fear of exposing themselves to allegations of anticompetitive conduct. On the other hand, hospitals are socially, morally and legally constrained to have their staff's performance overseen by peer reviews, deemed essential for maintaining or improving the quality of provider care. In some form or another, peer reviews are required for licensing hospitals, certifying Medicare programs, and for hospital accreditation by the Joint Commission on Accreditation of Hospitals (JCAH) - since 1987 called the Joint Commission on Accreditation of Healthcare Organizations (JCAHC). A hospital's obligation in providing care entails not only selecting the staff but also to oversee their performance. Upon receiving indications of actual or potential physician performance problems, the hospital has the obligation to scrutinize the circumstances and make decisions as to the continuation of the involved physician's staff privileges. In order to perform these functions, the hospital requires the input of peers normally by way of a formal review process. The 1986 *Health Care Quality Improvement Act* recognized the importance of peer review functions[27], and provides limited immunity for reviews conducted in good faith.

In order to better understand the role of peer review functions, let us briefly examine the environment in which they are performed, that is, the structure of a "standard" hospital's medical staff, and where, how and why peer review functions are appropriate in that environment. In general, hospitals exercise considerable discretion in choosing their medical staff because the hospital's governing Board bears the ultimate responsibility for maintaining the quality of care at proper standards. As part of meeting its responsibilities to the Board, the medical staff monitors its own work by engaging in surgical ("tissue") reviews, review of pharmaceutic and therapeutic activities, examination of medical records, antibiotic and blood utilization reviews[28]. In addition, incumbent staff is responsible for verifying the credentials of applicants for staff privileges. In larger hospitals, members of existing staff perform these functions within the framework of formal committees, so called "credentialing committees". Upon collecting and evaluating credentials related data, the committee makes its recommendation to a staff executive committee made up largely of physicians, which, in turn, communicates with the Board for the latter's final decision. In addition to staff privilege related decisions, the credentialing committee" performs a number of functions on an on going basis, such as evaluation of staff member performance, technical skills and even meeting appropriate health requirements. This power of influence upon a final decision whether a physician will be retained on staff, or a new physician will be admitted to staff, constitutes the source of often alleged competitive restraints.

The main purpose of the peer review process is to maintain healthcare quality at appropriate levels, and to engage in a monitoring process technical enough in the field of medicine that the general public, the consumers, are not capable of performing. While the process is seen as protecting the interest not only of the patients but also of the providers (a type of self-policing effort), improperly conducted peer evaluation efforts can be conducted not in the interest of the evaluated, the hospital, or the patient, but in the competitive economic and selfish interest of the evaluators, and only of the evaluators, themselves. In situations like that, the only constraint upon the conduct of the evaluators may be the possibility of legal action based on the contents of their report. Yet, the same threat may interfere with an otherwise totally honest effort to evaluate one's peers in medicine, hence inhibit the process to the detriment of the profession and the patients themselves.

It is by way of attempting to overcome this potential hindrance to professional and honest peer evaluation efforts, that Congress passed the already mentioned Health Care Quality Improvement Act of 1986. As indicated before, the latter provides limited immunity to peer review committees, acting in good faith, against state and federal antitrust actions. Section 11101 of the Act sums up its general scope as follows:

(1) The increasing occurrence of medical malpractice and the need to improve the quality of medical care have become nationwide problems that warrant greater effort than those that can be undertaken by any individual State. (2) There is a national need to restrict the ability of incompetent physicians to move from State to State without disclosure or discovery of the physician's previous damaging and incompetent

performance. (3) This nationwide problem can be remedied through effective professional peer review. (4) The threat of private money damage liability under Federal laws, including treble damage liability under Federal antitrust laws, unreasonably discourages physicians from participating in effective professional peer review. (5) There is an overriding national need to provide incentive and protection for physicians engaging in effective professional peer review[29].

This immunity does not come without countervailing obligations, much by way of various reporting requirements. Insurance companies now must report all malpractice judgments to state licensing boards. State boards of medical examiners must report to state licensing boards all competence-related license revocations, suspensions, censures, or reprimands. Hospitals, in turn, specifically must request, and are availed to, all collected information about each applicant for staff privileges, and acting upon that information will likely immune them from antitrust action.

Earlier, I alluded to the Oregon case which centered on the issues of bad faith performance on peer review committees. At this juncture, I believe there is considerable merit in reviewing that case in some detail, and to see how these competitive dramas in medicine play themselves out in real life. The case also illustrates the changed atmosphere that has taken hold in medicine and within a large segment of the physician population. Physicians now often find themselves in a market place of a sort, having to compete with their peers for maintaining their statusquo and even livelihood.

The Patrick case centered on the issue of whether or not the state action doctrine protects physicians from federal antitrust liability for their conduct, actions, and decisions implemented on peer review committees. And, if so, will peer review committees be no more than instruments for eliminating qualified competition, instead of enhancing the quality of healthcare. The claimant, Timothy Patrick, MD. was a surgeon at a clinic as well as a hospital staff member. His employer, the clinic, wanted him to join in a partnership, however, he wanted to go out on his own to set up a competing practice. After Dr. Patrick started his own clinic, his staff colleagues at the hospital, also associated with his former employer clinic, began to shun him. After an unfortunate sequence of two abdominal operations performed by Dr. Patrick on the same patient, two operations which subsequently turned out to be uncalled for, as the patient had testical cancer, a surgeon, on the staff of the hospital as well as at Dr. Patrick's prior clinic, prompted a review of Dr. Patrick's hospital privileges. Alleging that Dr. Patrick's performance at the hospital was below the hospital's standards, a committee voted to terminate his hospital staff privileges. This is where the curtain on the antitrust drama rises.

Dr. Patrick claimed under Sherman 1 and 2 that the hospital credentialing committee's design was to curtail competition in healthcare rather than protect healthcare quality. As we noted earlier, the federal district court jury has in large measure agreed, and awarded Dr. Patrick, including treble damages, over $2 million. The verdict reverberated throughout the medical profession, particularly touching hospital and physician communities. After the appellate process commenced, major medical organizations such as the AMA, JCAH, and Oregon State physician and hospital associations filed their own briefs in support of the defendants' cause. Indeed, the Federal Circuit Court reversed the lower court's finding against the defendants on the grounds of state action immunity: members of the credentialing committee conducted their disciplinary action against Dr. Patrick pursuant to state law that requires just that type of peer review. State action immunity, if applies, even extends to bad faith and anticompetitive motives in the course of state mandated peer review processes. Dr. Patrick appealed to the US Supreme Court, arguing that the state action immunity did not apply. In the Court's view, the application of the state action immunity to peer reviews required two necessary and sufficient conditions: (a) it must be articulated and expressed state policy, and (b) it must be actively supervised by the state itself. The Court did not find the presence of active state supervision in the process, hence the immunity did not apply, and the members of the credentialing committee were, once again, found in violation of the Sherman Act. Peer review processes have become sensitive issues.

Nevertheless, peer reviews are essential in the interest of healthcare quality and that of the patient. How can one reconcile social benefits emanating from peer reviews with the potential private costs generated by successful antitrust actions brought against peer review committee members? How can peer reviews be conducted so as to perform their social role without competitive costs? How much competitive costs is society expected to tolerate in the interest of otherwise socially beneficial peer reviews? These questions are easier to ask than to answer. Some measures may perhaps be taken to reduce the risk of competitive restraints while performing a worthwhile process. Thus, physicians who have a personal and independent economic interest in the outcome may be excluded from the process. Additionally, demonstrated lack of personal bias, preoccupation only with professional competence, and consistency of peer review decisions by committees may help to answer some these questions.

Other Sources of Possible Competitive Concern

Since 1992 provider services for Medicare patients were compensated based on actual charges or statutory fees, which ever is lower. Three factors enter into the composition of statutory fees: (a) the relative value of the service performed, (b) a monetary conversion factor, and (c) geographic adjustments[30]. Factor (b) is designed to provide an incentive for physicians to limit current Medicare expenditures, in favor of future expenditures. If the ratio of actual to projected expenditures for a given year is less than 1, future reimbursements to physicians can increase, and vice versa. This may give rise to competitive restraints and antitrust concern among otherwise independent physicians if they agree among themselves to limit the dispensation of certain types of care to Medicare patients. Another source of competitive restraint in this context could also emerge if some providers agree to boycott another, inefficient or uncooperative, physician to protect future Medicare payments. However, these are hypotheticals, as no evidence of this conduct has so far been reported.

Another possible way for physicians to restrain competition is to impede the conduct of competitors by filing complaints against the latter with peer review organizations (PROs), or to insurance carriers. On the other hand, the Noerr-Pennington Doctrine, based on two landmark cases decided in this subject area some 30 years ago, appears to protect complaining physicians against antitrust liability[31]. The Doctrine applies to private entities in their efforts to generate or influence government legislation or regulation, even if motivated by anti-competitive intent, so long as they are not a mere sham to cover up anti-competitive activities. These protections are augmented by that of the 1986 Health Care Quality Improvement Act, already discussed.

A final area to be examined here for potential competitive restraint involving physicians is relating to the adoption of third-party payer guidelines. Although this may impact on competition among insurers more than providers, we will take a quick look at the issues here. In 1944 the Supreme Court determined that the business of insurance was part of interstate commerce, hence within the realm of antitrust enforcement[32]. Subsequently, by passing the McCarran-Ferguson Act, Congress exempted the insurance business from antitrust scrutiny, provided certain conditions are met: (a) the activity must constitute the business of insurance, (b) it must fall under state regulatory provisions, and, (c) no boycott, intimidation or coercion is involved[33]. The Supreme Court refined these conditions, by requiring that the activity must (1) have the effect of transferring or spreading policyholder's risk, (2) be an integral part of the policy relationship between the insurer and the insured, and (3) be limited to entities within the insurance industry[34]. Under these criteria, an insurance company's utilization of peer review committees to determine the reasonableness of provider fees did not qualify as business of insurance. Nor do criteria apply to collective agreements among insurers aimed at reimbursement policies[35]. Unilateral independent actions in this regard on the part of insurers by way of adopting practice guidelines for reimbursement would not likely have uncompetitive consequences.

References

1   Relman, A.S. "Antitrust Law and The Physician Enterprise" *The New England Journal of Medicine*, Vol. 313, No. 14, October 3, 1985, pp.884-5

2   "Attempts to Gain Access to Hospitals are Prevalent in Health Care Actions", *Antitrust & Trade Regulation Rep.* (BNA) No. 1150, Febr 1984, p.187.

3   Robinson v. Magovern 521 F.Supp 842 (W.D. Pa. 1981); Miller v. Eisenhower Medical Center 27 Cal. 3d 614 P.2d 258, 166 Cal. Rptr 826 (1980); Silver v. Quees Hospital 63 Haw. 430, 629 P.2d 1116 (1981)

4   Sarasota County Pub. Hosp Bd v. Shahawy 408 So. 2d.644 (Fla Dist Ct App. 1981); Pollock v. Methodist Hosp 392 F.Supp. 393 (E.D.La.1975); Holmes v. Hoemako Hospital 117 Ariz. 403, 573 P.2d 477 (1977); Shaw v. Hospital Authority 614 F.2d 946 (5th Cir. 1980)

5   15 U.S.C. PP 1,2,7 (1982)

6   Weiss v. York Hospital 745 F.2d 786 (3d Cir.1984), cert denied 470 US 1060 (1985);

7   Brunswick Corp v. Pueblo Bowl-O-Mat Inc. 429 US 477, 488 (1977); see also Flynn, L. "Antitrust Jurisprudence: A Symposium on the Economic and Social Goals of Antitrust Policy" *University of Pennsylvania Law Review*, Vol. 125, 1977, pp.1182-88

8   Hospital Building Co. v. Trustees of the Rex Hospital 425 US 738 (1976)

9   Cardio-Medical Assocs v. Crozer-Chester Medical Center 721 F.2d 68, 76 (3d Cir. 1983); Miller v. Indiana Hospital 562 F.Supp. 1259 (W.D.Pa.1983); Furlong v. Long Island College Hospital 710 F.2d 922 (2d Cir. 1983); Crane v. Intermountain Health Care 637 F.2d 715 (10th Cir. 1980)

10 Copperweld Corp v. Independence Tube Corp 467 US 769 (1984)

11 Weiss v. York Hospital 745 F.2d 786, 813 (3rd Cir. 1984)

12 Pontius v. Childrens Hospital 552 F.Supp 1352 (W.D. Pa. 1982)

13 Wilk v. American Medical Association 719 F.2d 207 (7th Cir.1983).

14 The rules lasted until 1980 when the AMA revised its published ethical standards, eliminating these items.

15 Weiss v. York Hospital 745 F.2d 786 (3d. Cir 1984); see also Balckstone, B. "The AMA and the Osteopaths: A Study of the Power of Organized Medicine" *Antitrust Bulletin*, Vol 22, 1977, p.405.

16 Robinson v. Magovern 521 F.Supp. 842, 913 (W.D.Pa. 1981)

17 Arizona v. Maricopa County Medical Society 102 S.Ct. 2466 (1982)

18 In another case, US v. Topco Associates 405 US 596 (1972), the Supreme Court indicated the need for considerable experience in pertinent business relationships before the *per se* approach could be applied in any case.

19 Maricopa at p. 2477

20 References were made, among others, to the Albrecht v. Herald Co. 390 US 145 (1968), Northern Pacific V US 356 US 1 (1958), and US v. Socony-Vaccum Oil Co. 310 US 150 (1940) cases.

21 Maricopa at 2175

22 Maricopa at pp. 2479-80

23 Maricopa at pp. 2480-84

24 *HMO Program Status Report*, May 1975, DHEW HSA (75-130 22A); see also Office of Health Maintenance Organizations, USDHEW, *National HMO Census of Prepaid Plans*, 1978.

25 Data from Ref# 24 indicates that Maricopa County had about 50% of the State's total insured of some 1.5 million, contrasted with Foundation's 100,000 enrollees.

26 Patrick v. Burget Civ. No. 81-260 LE (D.C. Or.Sept 11, 1984), reversed 800 F.2d 1498 ((th Cir.1986), reversed 108 S.Ct.1658 (1988)

27 42 U.S.C. S.11101. See also Darling v. Charleston Community Memorial Hospital 33 Ill. 2d 326, 211 N.E. 2d 253 (1965), cert denied 383 US 946 (1966) where the hospital's responsibility for good care to its patient was found to be independent from the same set of responsibilities owed by staff physicians to the patients.

28 JCAHO, *Accreditation Manual for Hospitals*, 1987.

29 42 U.S.C. S.11101

30 Omnibus Budget Reconciliation Act of 1989 (OBRA 1989)

31 Eastern Railroad Presidents' Conference v. Noerr 365 US 127 (1961); United Workers v. Pennington 381 US 657 (1965). See also California Motor Transport Co. v. Trucking Unlimited 404 US 508 (1972), and Garst v. Stoco 604 F.Supp. 326 (E.D. Ark. 1985).

32 US v. South-Eastern Underwriters Association 322 US 533 (1944)

33 Borsody, J. "The Antitrust Law and the Health Industry"*Akron Law Review*, Vol.12, 1979, pp.417-447

34 Union Life Insurance Co. v. Pireno 458 US 119 (1982); see also Group Life & Health Insurance Co. v. Royal Drug Co. 440 US 205 (1978).

35 Union Life p. 128.

Chapter 23
COMPETITION ENFORCEMENT IN THE HOSPITAL SECTOR

The traditional healthcare scene was not conducive for competition at most level, certainly not for price competition. Traditional forms of health insurance rendered any kind of price competition among physicians or hospitals irrelevant, at best. The incentives for efficient practice of medicine were not there. The US Department of Health Education and Welfare noted almost twenty years ago that

> Probably the principle factor contributing to inflation has been the predominant system of third party reimbursement based on what institutions spend and what physicians charge[1].

Physicians reimbursed at the "usual and customary" norm, and hospitals based on their reported "costs", issues of x-efficiency, and those of allocative efficiency within the healthcare sector, were of no concern to any single player, except for society as whole, with the latter having gone unrecognized for some time. The higher the cost reported by hospitals the greater has been the reimbursement, hence the revenue - and, importantly, vice versa. Prices and costs spiraled while resources were wasted.

A fundamental premise of the system has always been that physicians ordered the various services deemed necessary for the patients. Yet, the system released those physicians from all financial responsibilities associated with their service requisitions. Doctors simply did not have the incentive to seek out the cost-effective alternatives of equal or better quality. Presumably, in most cases physicians did not even know, nor perhaps care, about the cost of the services requested by them. Yet, over two thirds of healthcare costs may directly or indirectly be accounted for in terms of services requested by physicians[2]. Furthermore, the same syndrome applied to hospitals. Nonadmission, or early discharge, of patients, even if medically prudent and without jeopardy to the patient, simply reduced total hospital revenues.

Finally, covered by insurance, patients were oblivious and indifferent to costs, and had no incentive, nor adequate information, to seek out cost-effective care alternatives. The final result rewarded inefficient and extravagant providers on the expense of efficient ones.

Attempts to correct this predicament could be implemented in two fundamental ways: (a) government interference by way of regulations such as health planning agencies and hospital rate setting commissions, or, (b) reforming the medical market system by way of introducing competition, particularly competition in terms of price. The price variable in the competitive process was also recognized by the judiciary over half-century ago when the Supreme Court labeled it as the "central nervous system of the economy"[3]. In healthcare, the importance of implementing price competition among providers was also recognized over fifteen years ago by Dr. Ellwood, the leader of the "Jackson Hole Group" - a collection of healthcare professionals, frequently meeting in Jackson Hole, Wyoming, and presently considered by many as first line advisors to the Clinton Administration regarding the as yet forthcoming Health Reforms. Dr. Ellwood wrote back in 1978 that notwithstanding the traditionally existing non-price competition in provider markets, namely that hospitals have always been in competition with each other in terms of physician recruitment, reputation, and patients, but rarely if ever in terms of reduced cost or price.

> There is one awesome condition that hospitals and physicians must meet if the market is to work: .. doctors and hospitals have to compete with each other for consumers on the basis of price[4].

Provider price competition may, at least partially, be implemented in terms of direct entire or partial fees paid by consumers when receiving healthcare services, or in terms of insurance premiums. The latter prevails when patients choose among alternative insurance plans offering coverage at competing rates. However, in large measure, this competition involves insurers, and not direct providers, i.e. not between hospitals and physicians, although some types of coverage directly involves provider groups themselves, such as a staff model HMO. Existing plans overcome this "competition gap" by prompting providers to offer their services on a competitive basis - both in terms of efficiency and price, limiting the number of providers who may participate in the plans, thus generating a competitive bidding process among them. Thus, patients may exercise their "consumer sovereignty", their "dollar vote", in healthcare markets by way of market pressuring healthcare plans, and utilizing those plans' profit motives, to extricate lower service fees and more efficient services from providers, particularly when patients groups function through their own collective market power.

Competition Among Hospitals

It may be that, by traditional antitrust and industrial organization standards, more price competition among hospitals would improve efficiency and the quality of care. Yet, traditional standards cannot, at least could not, be applied to the healthcare sector. Healthcare is by-and-large what market researchers call an "experience good". Furthermore, it is highly consumer specific. The consumer, once again in a traditional sense, lacks adequate information for rational choice, and the procurement of the information is very expensive, and may not even be available in adequate quantity and quality directly to the consumer. To a large extent, the consumer must rely on "word-of mouth" sources of information. These sources include friends, family and other socially based sources most of the time[5]. In addition, the cost of information limits the field of providers with whom consumers become familiar. Prevailing insurance systems do not help either, for they make consumers largely oblivious to price differences among providers, and the elasticity of demand for healthcare in general low, allowing hospitals to raise their prices above competitive levels without risking significant reductions in patient admissions. The criteria for hospital choice in the mind of patients does not normally include price, but tend to center on perceived quality, nationally or regionally published ranking, and various other various amenities as well as marketing instilled subjective impressions. Once these perception have been imbedded, either by marketing or by the advisement of physicians involved, into the patients mind, no price changes or price differences will normally interfere with the decision.

Given the role of insurance, it may also be that a lack of price competition, and the predominance of non-price competition, among hospitals causes the quality of healthcare to be higher than if it were if consumers made their choice based on available price/quality information, as they do in non-healthcare markets. Thus, a lack of price competition among hospitals, and the emphases placed on non-price competitive factors such as increased portfolio of services offered or excessive levels of technology utilized, may substantially contribute to healthcare cost increases[6]. The fact that most hospitals are still nonprofit entities, does not alter this predicament. Most studies coping with the nonprofit dimensions of the hospital industry assumed that there is some sort of objective function which even a nonprofit hospital maximizes, whether it is prestige, quantity, quality, or, in the case physician controlled nonprofit institutions, physicians' income. Thus, their functioning in the market may not in the final analysis be different from profit seeking institutions[7].

In general, the literature reflects on three basic theories of hospital competition: (a) classical or modern oligopoly behavior; (b) excessive utilization practice; and, (c) information dilution conduct. *Oligopoly* theories by Stigler (collusive conduct), and those of the classics such as Cournot and Bertrand (interactive conduct) have been reviewed earlier in the volume. These and other contemporary theories by-and-large conclude that, at constant quality, there is a direct relationship between concentration and prices. We have also just noted that hospital markets tend not to display price competition even with lower concentration, probably due to the complexity of products supplied. Instead, cost-intensive non-price competition tends to dominate in the absence of collusion either of an endogenous nature (that is, by the hospitals among themselves), or via exogenous channels by way of regulation and health planning.

The *excessive utilization practice* is predicated upon the hospitals', particularly those controlled or heavily influenced by physicians, tendency to compete in non-price terms[8]. An underlying motive is to attract the best physicians to the hospital's staff. Physicians, in turn, have traditionally been attracted by conduct which has inevitably contributed to increased cost, although higher quality: increased and most up-to-date equipment, plenty of personnel, and the avoidance of over-crowded hospital rooms. Whether hospitals will or can increase price in the face of increased costs generated by increased non-price competition is not clear. To maintain profits, prices would clearly need to rise - or costs to fall, and the latter obviously does not occur. To a large extent, DRG based prices for Medicare patients allow for some increased costs. Cost shifting to private insurance payers, a vanishing breed, may allow for some of the other sources for at least maintaining the statusquo. Otherwise, hospitals may need rely on increased quantity, higher patient turnover, to remain afloat. Thus, the reasoning of this model may be extended by the practice of (a) keeping prices (or, in the alternative, profits, in the face of increasing costs) relatively constant, allowing society to benefit from increasing care quality emanating from non-price competition among hospitals, and (b) increase patient flow to maintain or increase total profit (in the face of a constant or only slightly increasing rate of profit); and (c) attempt to alleviate nonprice competition caused cost increases by other, jointly implemented programs, such as buying coalitions, retailing of wholesale acquired drugs, and the like, to be dealt with later in the chapter.

It may, of course, be that (b) would provide the impetus for this process to be self-reinforcing, since the competition for patients among hospitals was traditionally based on the same type of non-price variables as has already been noted to be the source of perennial cost increases. This may be labeled as the hospitals' "self-destructing competition by costs", and could be viewed as the major source of frequent hospital failures experienced during recent years.

In addition, the entrance of organized buying power by way of third-party alternative delivery systems will likely aggravate this predicament. Downward pressure on prices, in the face of increasing (or, at best, constant) costs will cause even more smaller or less efficient hospitals to depart or to be bought out, reinforcing trend toward greater concentration in the hospital industry. The latter will, in turn, countervail the buyer's price oriented market power, necessitating increased interference from regulators. A discussion of "managed competition", as a remedy for the healthcare cost spiral, follows later in this volume.

Finally, the *information dilution conduct* on the part of hospitals is predicated on the assumption that a major source of information to patients regarding hospitals come from other patients and individual experiences. It is further assumed that a patient needs repeatedly reinforced positive information regarding a given hospital before choosing that hospital for his or her own treatment[9]. If there is a proliferation of hospitals in any given community or region, the information that any potential patient receives regarding any given hospital will be diluted by the information received regarding the other alternative hospitals. Thus, if information regarding competing hospitals is thought to contribute to increased competition among those hospitals, information induced competition among many hospitals will in fact be lower, in spite of their larger number, due to the dilution, i.e. reduced intensity, of information received about any given hospital. Thus, in spite of their large numbers, some of the hospitals in this situation can increase prices and profits. This trend could be reinforced by the possibility that as the number of alternative hospital choices to patients increases, the cost of procuring information regarding each also increases, yielding reduced search intensity, and lower price elasticity of demand faced by hospitals.

A Closer Look at NonProfits

Nonprofits have goals other than profit maximization in a neoclassical micro sense. In fact, legal restrictions ban nonprofits from the distribution of profits[10]. Much of the nonprofits' operational success, however, may be attributed to standard neoclassical market failures. Assuming the consumers are aware of which institution is for profit and which one is nonprofit, nonprofit status breeds consumer confidence, and patients, for instance, do not have to be concerned with purely profit motivated procedures imposed upon them. Thus, imperfect information about product quality may be offset to an extent by confidence in the producer. The prevention of profits from being distributed among the owners themselves removes from the mind of the consumer, at least theoretically, the concern of quality being cut for the sake of lower costs and higher profits.

In healthcare, another type of market failure is attributed to consumer purchasing decisions made independently from the price and quality of the product, enhanced by the third-party payer system, insurance, lack of consumer and provider concern for cost, and the resulting moral hazard. It may be that the nonprofit status of many institutions involved, and the professional association based regulations to which they are subjected, breeds the trust necessary for at least retaining the economic statusquo.

While healthcare is fundamentally a private good, it may also be viewed as having substantial public good characteristics: the control of contagious diseases on the part of some ultimately benefits the rest of us at not cost. The benefits of costs and efforts incurred on behalf of those who actually pay, if they pay and whether or not they pay, cannot be restricted them alone - they accrue to the rest of society as well. Once again, nonprofits may be better suited for this type of situation, particularly since they are more willing to undertake socially beneficial services at low or no cost for some, benefiting the rest of society. In addition, presumably having a greater degree of trust from consumers, they are better able generate voluntary admission of true consumer preferences[11]. If nonprofits can alleviate some of the market failures, then it may be that any anticompetitive activities that they engage in are forgivable by society, hence they should not be subject antitrust enforcement. Thus, it is not surpassing that considerable confusion may be found even in the very few antitrust decisions pertaining to nonprofits organizations. The Sherman Act did not contain explicit exemptions of nonprofits, although it clearly targeted for-profit organizations. Over fifty years ago, the Supreme Court dealt with the issue by stating that "The end sought by the Sherman Act was the prevention of restraints to free competition in *business and commercial transaction...*"[12]. Thirty years later, the notion was reiterated by the DC Court of Appeals by interpreting the proscriptions of the Sherman Act as having been

> tailored ... for the business world not for the noncommercial aspects of the liberal arts and the learned professions. In these contexts, an incidental restraint of trade, absent an intent or purpose to affect the commercial aspects of the profession, is not sufficient warrant application of the antitrust laws[13].

Subsequently, the same principle was enunciated in a 1975 case where the court rejected an antitrust challenge against the NCAA by an athlete precluded from participating in his school's intercollegiate hockey program. A district court viewed the NCAA's eligibility rules as pertaining to amateurism and not to commercialism, so if any restraint of trade occurred, it was merely the unintentional result of pursuing legitimate amateur principles[14]. Yet, the exemption of nonprofits from the antitrust laws has still not become a recognized blanket principle. In the 1975 *Goldfarb* case, discussed earlier, the Supreme Court did not exempt the learned professions from antitrust enforcement. The Professional Engineers case appears to have confirmed this view, by indicating that if public service or public safety is involved the application of the *per se* rule may be suspended, but that does not obviate an evaluation of competitive restraints under the *rule of reason*. The Court rejected a ban on competitive bidding by engineers[15].

An interesting aspect of antitrust applications to nonprofits is in connection with the activities of nonprofit hospitals by way of maintaining *home health care* services. In this regard, the Robinson-Patman price discrimination rule is of relevance. Although discussed earlier, the basic principles of the Robinson-Patman Act (RP) may briefly be reviewed here. A 1936 Amendment to Section 2 of the 1914 Clayton Act, RP proscribes price discrimination, or discrimination amounting to or yielding price discrimination, among various *competing* purchasers of the same good where such discrimination results in restraint of trade. What makes the enforcement of this Act complex is not so much the interpretation of its proscriptions, but the inevitable application of its several built-in defenses: passing on actual cost savings; good faith meeting of competition; changing market conditions or marketability of goods; proportional availability of promotional or price concessions to all competing customers. Congress expressly exempted nonprofit institutions from RP by passing the 1938 Nonprofit Institutions Act: exempted the purchase of goods by a nonprofit institution for its own use. Section 13C exemption, as it is often referenced, states:

> Nothing in ...[the Robinson Patman Act]... shall apply to purchases of their supplies for their own use by schools, colleges, universities, public libraries, churches, *hospitals* (emphases added), and charitable institutions not operated for profit.

Thus, nonprofit hospitals could purchase drugs, for their own use presumably at the hospital, at a special discount. What if the drugs are used to treat the hospital's home healthcare (HH) patients? This issue was at the focus of a 1976 case[16]. The Portland Retail Druggists Association representing some 60 community pharmacies claimed that 13 drug companies price discriminated against the community pharmacies in favor of nonprofit hospitals by selling drugs to the latter at a lower price, arguing that exemption 13C applied to drugs used only for the hospitals' inpatients, and not for patients under the hospitals' HH program. The Supreme Court reinterpreted exemption 13C so as to apply in a much broader sense than the lower courts, and the original 1938 law, may have intended. Today's modern hospitals literally *deliver* healthcare to their patients, and the drugs acquired by hospitals at preferential prices for *their own use* includes the hospital's entire institutional care of its patients and not just the confines of the hospital's walls. On the other hand, if a nonprofit hospital establishes for-profit home healthcare subsidiaries, the 13C would probably not apply, and the hospital's use of its drugs acquired at preferential prices as a nonprofit institution in a for-profit setting, by reselling those drugs to the for-profit subsidiaries, would clearly be construed as a restraint on competition. A major task in circumstances of this type would entail a careful examination of the hospital's institutional structure.

A more recent case further clarifies and expands upon the Portland decision. Retail pharmacists in Oregon and California claimed that the Kaiser-Permamente Medical Care Program, a long established nonprofit HMO, has abused 13C exemptions by selling drugs, acquired at special nonprofit discount prices, to its members. The US Supreme Court refused to review a decision by the US Court of Appeals indicating that Kaiser HMO's purchases of drugs did qualify for 13C exemption[17]. In addition, the decision expanded the Portland doctrine beyond the institutional confines of a hospital to outpatient and ambulatory markets. Both the hospitals and the health plans that make up the Kaiser-Permanente Medical Care Program were considered as nonprofit institutions, and their use or dispensation of the drugs acquired at preferential prices was not vied as being contrary to 13C exemption from the Robinson-Patman Act.

Hospital Group Purchasing Organizations (GPO)

An extension of the issues discussed in the previous section involves similar conduct but implemented by way of different practice patterns. Medical products have routinely been priced discriminatory by lower prices charged to hospitals, and higher prices charged to other healthcare providers. The issues may involve vertical price fixing between the manufacturer and distributor, price discrimination, and agreements regarding the hospital's option to resell the products. For the practice to function, the manufacturer needs to control otherwise independent distributor pricing. The manufacturer must also circumvent commodity arbitrage (buy in the low market and resell in the high one). The latter two activities must be performed subject to vertical price and vertical nonprice antitrust constraints.

Medical products in this regard include bandages, syringes, IV solutions, sutures, surgical gloves, X-ray and other diagnostic equipment, surgical instruments, and so forth. Furthermore, the manufacturing industry, typically made up of hundreds of different product markets, is quite concentrated. Less than thirty of about 3000 manufacturers accounted for about 75% of sales in 1986[18]. Although some specialty items used in predictably high volumes are sold by the manufacturers directly to the hospitals, most products are distributed through some 2,000 intermediaries[19]. Since pressure upon hospitals to cut costs has been more intense than on other providers, particularly through the implementation of the Medicare prospective pricing system, hospitals have typically been more cost conscious, and more consistently request price concessions from manufacturers. A means to reduce costs, is to procure medical product efficiently; enter the GPOs, some of the large of which represent close to 1,000 hospitals[20]. In fact, while all hospitals belong at least one GPO, over half of all hospitals belong to more than one[21]. The hospitals' purchasing power obviously became a decisive factor for manufacturers in pricing their product. Furthermore, since historically much of the government's cost containment efforts focused on hospitals, non-hospital providers were less aggressive in seeking price concessions from manufacturers. In addition, these medical products typically represent a smaller proportion of non-hospital providers' costs than those of hospitals, contributing further to more passivity on the part of the former to reduce costs in this area. However, even if medical products were a substantial cost factor for non-hospital providers, their large numbers and relatively small size renders them less conducive for inclusion into GPOs. So, while a GPO with 800 hospitals may include some 10% of the hospital population, the same 10% of the non-hospital population in a GPO would need to include some 35,000 members, hardly a manageable number. The result is price discrimination in favor of hospitals, and on the expense of non-hospital providers.

Medical products are generally sold through distributors. The manufacturer seeks to assure that it gets a fair share of the profits. The task is to accommodate a lower priced hospital market and higher priced non-hospital market. Selling through distributors at a uniformly low price would access the hospital market, but cause profits to accrue from the nonhospital market to the distributors. On the other hand, attempting to capture the profits from the non-hospital market by charging a higher price to distributors would cut out hospital customers. Hence, in order to capture for itself as much of the profits as possible, the manufacturer needs to charge a different price to different distributor groups, depending upon their markets, i.e. whether hospitals or non-hospital providers. Additionally, the manufacturer must prevent commodity arbitrage by the hospital - the hospital reselling its cheaply procured supplies to non-hospital providers, thus ending up competing with the manufacturer in that market segment.

If it directly deals with GPOs or large hospitals, the manufacturer simply negotiates a lower contracted price. Distributors selling to non-hospital providers pay a higher. Those selling to hospitals and GPO will do so at a negotiated priced and get a rebate from the manufacturer. This type of arrangement may raise issues of vertical price fixing.

The competitive ramifications of manufacturer-hospital relationships was focused upon in a relatively old but rather educational case. A purchasing agreement was involved between a supplier of hospital goods and services and 29 nonprofit hospitals[22], and it was the first time that the antitrust laws were applied to shared purchasing agreements. It was found that both Sherman 1 and 2 were violated by the agreement and its implementation. The underlying fact situation is not atypical of many found in the industry. *American Hospital Supply Corporation* (AHSC) of Evanston, Il. is the largest manufacturer and distributor of hospital supplies in the US, with some 120,000 of products and services distributed. It serviced some 7,000 hospitals from a network of warehouses throughout the Country. AHSC agreed to sell a large volume of products to Voluntary Hospitals of America (VHA), along with agreeing to VHA getting volume discounts, price protection and other preferential services. The product and terms of each sale were negotiated with each VHA hospital who were not required to buy from AHSC, instead of blanket terms applying to all VHA hospitals. Nevertheless, the group discounts accrued provided that the hospitals collectively reached a certain purchase volume. Each hospital purchased at a flexible price up to the price cap, minus volume discount. Thus, the final price by each hospital was determined by the combined volume of all hospital purchases. VHA hospitals disclosed AHSC competitor prices so AHSC could match them, if it so desired. The complaint was filed by White & White Surgical Supply and a few of AHSC's other competitors who distributed to the same VHA hospitals, claiming conspiracy to fix price and to boycott between VHA and its individual hospitals on the one hand, and AHSC on the other, under Sherman 1. The complaint also included Sherman 2 and Clayton 3 counts for attempting to monopolize, tying and exclusive dealings, and Robinson-Patman counts for price discrimination. The court found conspiracy in restraint of trade, and attempted monopolization, in certain metropolitan areas.

Staff Privilege Related Problems Revisited

One side of this set of issues was examined in the previous chapter, focusing on the physicians' point of view. The same issues will briefly be reviewed here from the hospital's stand point. Clearly, some overlaps will occur, as basically the same issues are involved. However, I will concentrate on the hospitals' role and interests as much as possible in these controversies in contrast to those of the physician's involved.

It has already been noted that staff privilege cases are by far the single most common type of antitrust actions in the healthcare field[23]. They arise in a variety of fact situations: (a) Denial of an initial application for privileges or staff membership; (b) denial of allied health professionals' (typically nurses, midwifes, podiatrists, nurse anesthetists, and chiropractors) application for hospital privileges; (c) nonrenewal of existing clinical privileges; (d) granting of only partial privileges; (e) reduction, suspension or termination of privileges; (f) exclusive contract between the hospital and a group of providers (or an individual provider) to provide a given medical service at the hospital[24]. The average staff privilege related harm is claimed under Sherman 1 and 2 against the entire hospital as an institution, some of the medical staff, the entire medical staff as an entity, hospital administrators, and even members of the governing boards. If the dispute involves an *exclusive contract* between the hospital and a group of providers, in addition Sherman 1 conspiracy and Sherman 2 claims, the claimant normally includes other noncompetitive provisions under Sherman 1, such as exclusive dealings and tying contracts[25]. In cases with an *absence of exclusive contract issues*, the disputes normally center on conspiracies among medical staff members, and between the latter and the hospital[26]. If in the latter cases Sherman 2 issues added, they point to monopolization, attempted monopolization, or conspiracies to monopolize in particular medical service market where the claimant sees himself or herself to be an actual or potential competitor. In general, however, if Sherman 2 issues dominate, the relevant market and market power that becomes of prime concern is that for the hospital, specifically whether or not the hospital constitutes an indispensable opportunity for the claimant to compete, i.e. the hospital is an "essential facility" for the individual provider to survive or succeed in the market place.

The courts do not appear view staff privilege cases as their favorite type of disputes calling for resolution. These cases tend to be expensive and often prolonged. The defendants win an overwhelming majority of the cases. In addition, the courts do not welcome the need to second guess hospital and medical staff staffing decisions, which are often imbedded in technical as well as intra-institutional political considerations[27].

Cases involving staff privilege exclusion disputes, in the *absence of hospital-physician exclusive contracts*, often need to resolve whether or not there is a *possibility* of conspiracy among the defendants in the first place. Can a hospital conspire with its own staff, when the both constitute one single entity, and one entity cannot conspire with itself. If the involved staff members have their own independent economic interests, separate from that of the hospital, there may be a plurality of actors, hence conspiracy plausible[28]. The *fact* of conspiracy is difficult to establish, as it may not be construed to rest with the decision of a hospital to accept a medical staff's negative recommendation regarding the fate of an existing or potential staff member[29]. In one case, the court simply suggested that the claimant was unable to prove and agreement to reduce his privileges. In another case, the hospital's decision to close a department was attributed to an outside consultant's recommendation and not to a conspiracy. Even where a hospital department head repeatedly suggests negative views to the hospital's administration regarding a claimant, no conspiracy was found where the department head and the hospital reached their decisions independently[30]. Thirdly, a legal issue, but with far reaching economic consequences, is the litigation standard to be applied in a conspiracy case: *per se* or rule of reason. The first one terminates the litigation at the lower court level with the granting of the claimant's summary judgment, sparing further time, litigation expenses and expert witness participation. The latter seeks to ascertain the alleged conduct's impact on the market, and on competition. Thus far, medical privilege decisions appear to have largely been predicated upon rule of reason standards.

Conspiracies run afoul with antitrust rules only if they are undertaken with anticompetitive intent and purpose, or if they result in unreasonable restraints in competition. However, most of the cases, however, tended to rely on intent[31]. Perhaps the most likely reason for that has been to avoid pursuing complex and expensive market analyses which at times run into serious data and measurability problems, and may nevertheless yield highly subjective results. If pursued, two relevant product markets and two relevant geographic markets would need to be measured. That for the hospital, and another set for the claimant physician's services. In general, a hospital would have no difficulty showing that its exclusionary decision in fact has pro-competitive effect for its own market. Hospitals do compete in terms of their proven competence in certain fields of endeavor, which, by precluding physicians not in that field, can be relied upon. They may want to develop specific educational and research programs, once again not congruent with the excluded physician's qualifications, and so forth[32]. The restraint on competition, if any, is often more convincingly demonstrable in the involved physician's services markets. Thus, if access to the hospital's facilities are indispensable or even essential for carrying on the physician's practice, the exclusion could wipe out a competitor in the relevant geographical market, with the questions still remaining as to alternative facilities available to the excluded physician, and the magnitude of competitive restraint generated even if no alternative facilities are available to him or her[33]. Finally, a trade-off may need to be dealt with; do the *pro*competitive effects in the hospital's market outweigh any possible *anti*competitive effects in the physician markets? The formulation of an opinion regarding this issue is not much different from, and certainly not easier than, contrasting the efficiency impact of a merger with the "dead-weight-loss" of the emerged monopoly[34].

The discussion in this section thus far assumed the *absence* of an exclusive contract between the hospital denying privileges to a physician and some other physician or a group of physicians. Another frequently occurring situation involves the *presence of an exclusive contract* between the hospital and another physician, or group of physicians, to perform a specific range of services for the hospital, often involving radiology or anesthesiology. The contract may be implemented in various forms. Thus, the exclusive arrangement may involve a physician on salary with the hospital, the two constituting one entity incapable of conspiring with itself, as was noted earlier. A tying claim under those circumstances may be plausible since the hospital ties the services of the physician to its general range of inpatient services. If the physician is an independent contractor with the hospital, a claim of conspiracy is plausible, except if the physician bills separately, and the hospital (the source of the tying product) derives no specific economic gain from having that physician perform the services (the tied product) on its premises, the notion of "tying" may be difficult to sustain[35].

Recent case history in this respect does show some view transformations. A court in the mid-1970s simply did not see the justification for involving the Sherman Act in matter where a radiologist had an exclusive contract with a hospital. In fact, the judicial attitude did not change for at least five years[36]. In an early 1980s case, a district court found an exclusive contract between a hospital and an anesthesiologist to be in restraint of trade under Sherman 1, based on the notion that the hospital's patients were the relevant buyers at that specific hospital, hence that hospital was the relevant geographic market which was foreclosed to alternative providers of anesthesiological services. If the purchasing camp is changed from the hospital's patients to the hospital itself, that is, the hospital is seen as the purchaser of these services, then the reasoning changes: the geographical market must be viewed for the hospital in competition with other hospitals, expanding the relevant market to include other competing hospitals, thus adding competing hospitals to the foreclosed anesthesiologist's options and reducing the restraint on competition. Indeed, ultimately this view was adopted upon remand to the district court, the geographical market for anesthesiologists was seen as the entire country from where the hospital can secure its anesthesiology needs[37]. In a 1983 advisory opinion, the FTC suggested certain factors which need to be considered under the rule of reason in order to assess hospital based exclusive contracts with specific providers: (a) the manner whereby the hospital arrived at the decision to enter into exclusivity - unilaterally or in conspiracy with the staff, (b) the relevant market and the hospital's market power, (c) the duration and purpose of the contract, (d) possible and significant procompetitive effects[38].

The issues were substantially confronted in a 1984 case, that has become a landmark decision of a sort in the area of exclusive contracting between a hospital and individual providers[39]. East Jefferson Hospital in New Orleans contracted with a group of anesthesiologists for services in its operating rooms. The hospital's inpatients had no alternatives to hospital provided anesthesiological services. Dr. Hyde, another anesthesiologist, was excluded from providing those services at the hospital. He claimed that the hospital engaged in tying practices (with the hospital's inpatient, particularly surgical, facilities being the tying product, and the contracted physicians' anesthesiological services the tied product), and illegal exclusive contracting. The hospital billed the patients for all services rendered in the operating rooms, and split the revenue with the contracted doctors.

The New Orleans metropolitan area had about twenty hospitals, and some 70% of the patients located in East Jefferson's immediate area (Jefferson Parish) went to hospitals other than East Jefferson. The Supreme Court found the arrangements *not* in violation of the Sherman

Act, although there was considerable disagreement whether or not and to what extent the *per se* rule should apply, and the Court was not willing to abandon the long established applicability of the *per se* rule to illegal tying agreements. It was also recognized that no significant anticompetitive effects can occur if the seller has no market power in the *tying* product and the market for the *tied* product is not concentrated and nor is it protected by entry barriers. As to the *exclusive dealing* aspects of the Hyde case, the major dimensions of an investigation would need to ascertain (a) the ultimate purchaser of the services involved, i.e., is it the patient or the hospital; (b) the relevant geographic market; (c) the extent of competitive restraint in the delineated markets; (d) possible benefits that may accrue to society (the patients) from the arrangements.

References

1   HEW, *Forward Plan for Health: Fiscal Year 1980-82* (1976)
2   Egdahl, E. "Fee For Service Health Maintenance Organizations" *JAMA* Vol. 241, 1979, p.588
3   United States v. Socony Vacuum Oil Co. 310 US 150, at p. 224 (1940)
4   Ellwood, P. "The Importance of the Market" *Journal of Health Policy, olitics and Law* Vol. 2, 1978, p. 447₁
,   ancur, O. "Commentary: Organization and Financing of Medical Care" *edical Care*, Vol. 23, No. 5 May 1985, pp. 432-37₁
,   ooth, A. Babchuk, N. "Seeking Health Care From New Resources, *Journal f Health and Social Behavior*", Vol. 13, No. 1, March 1972, pp. 90-99. See also Wolinsky F.D. and Steiber, S.R. "Salient Issues in Choosing a New Doctor", *Social Science and Medicine*, Vol. 16, No.7 1982, pp.759-767
6   Mancur, O. "Commentary: Organization and Financing of Medical Care" *Medical Care*, Vol. 23, No. 5 May 1985, pp. 432-37
7   Pauly, M.V. "Behavior of Nonprofit Hospital Monopolies: Alternative Models of the Hospital" in Havinghurst, C.C. (ed), *Regulating Health Facilities Construction*, American Enterprise Institute, Washington, DC 1974, pp.143-63; and, Pauly, M.V. Nonprofit Firms in Medical Markets, *American Economic Review*, Vol. 77, No. May 1987, pp.257-62.
8   Salkever, D. D. "Competition Among Hospitals" in Greenberg, W. (ed) *Competition in the Health Care Sector, Past, Present, and Future*, Aspen Systems Corporation, Germantown MD, 1978, pp.159-62.
9   Satterwaite, M.A. "Consumer Information, Equilibrium Industry Price, and the Number of Sellers" *Bell Journal of Economics*, Vol. 10, No. 2, 1992, pp.483-504
10 Oleck, O. "Nature of Nonprofit Organizations" *University of Toledo Law Review*, Vol. 10, 1979, pp. 962-68.
11 See Demsetz, H. "The Private Function of Public Goods", *Journal of Law and Economics*, Vol. 13, 1970, p.293. However, see also Oakland, K. "Public Goods, Perfect Competition, and Underproduction" *Journal of Political Economy*, Vol. 82, 1974, p. 293.
12 Apex Hosiery Co. v. Leader 310 US 469, at p.493 (1940)
13 Marjorie Webster Junior College Inc v. Middle States Association of Colleges and Secondary Schools 432 F.2d 650, at p. 654 (DC Cir. 1970).
14 Jones v. NCAA 392 F.Supp 295 (D.Mass 1975)
15 National Society of Professional Engineers v. US 549 F. 2d 626, at p. 632 (9th Cir. 1977)
16 Abbott Laboratories v. Portland Retail Druggists Association 425 US 14 (1976).
17 DeModena v. Kaiser Foundation Health Plan 743 F.2d 1388 (9th Cir.1984)
18 "Twenty Med-Surg Companies Control Half of the US Market" *Hospital Material Management*, July 1989, p. 1.

19   "Group Purchasing Proliferation: Do Benefits Exceed Costs?" *Hospital Purchasing Management*, May 1984, p.3-5

20   Wagner, A. "Group Purchasers Want Commitment" *Modern Healthcare*, May 5, 1989, p.34

21   Wetrich, J. "Group Purchasing: An Overview" *American Journal of Pharmacy*, Vol. 44, 1987, P. 1582

22   White & White Inc. v. American Hospital Supply Corporation 540 F.Supp. 951 (W.D.Mich 1982).

23   National Health :awyers Association, *Press Release*, Janury 23, 1985.

24   Robinson v. Magovern 521 F.Supp. 842 (W.D. Pa., 1981); Nurse Midwifery Associates v. Hibbett 577 F.Supp. 1273 (M.D. Tenn. 1983); Ghan v. NME Hospitals 772 F.2d 1467 (9th Cir 1985); Cooper v. Fortsyth County Hosp Authority 604 F.Supp. 685 (M.D.N.C., 1985); Kaczanowski v. Medical Center Hospital of Vermont 612 F.Supp 688 (D.Vt.1985); Feldman v. Jackson Memorial Hospital 571 F.Supp.1000 (S.D. Fla. 1983); Wilk v. American Medical Association 719 F.2d 207 (7th Cir.1983); Pontius v. Children's Hosp 552 F.Supp. 1352 (W.D. Pa. 1982); Cardio-Medical Associates v. Crozer-Chester Medical Center 721 F.2d 68 (3rd Cir. 1983); Hayden v. Bracey 744 F.2d 1338 (8th Cir. 1984); Seidenstein v. National Medical Enterprises 769 F.2d 1100 (5th Cir. 1985); Jefferson Parish Hospital District No. 2 v. Hyde 104 S.Ct. 1551 (1984); McMorris v. Williamsport Hosp 597 F.Supp. 899 (M.D. Pa. 1984).

25   See Jefferson Parish case

26   See Weiss v. York Hospital 745 F.2d 786 (3d. Cir. 1984)

27   Marrese v. Interqual Inc. 748 F.2d 373, at 391-2 (7th Cir, 1984); Pontius v. Children Hospital at p.1361; Cardio-Medical Associates v. Crozer-Chester Medical Center, at p.1069; Robbins v. Ong 452 F.Supp. 110, at p.115 (S.D. Ga 1978);

28   Note, "Conspiring Entities Under Section 1 of the Sherman Act", Harvard Law Review, Vol. 95, 1982, p. 661

29   Monsanto v. Spray-Rite Service Corp 104 S.Ct. 1464 (1984)

30   Robinson v. Magovern 521 F.Supp. 842 (W.D. Pa. 1981); See also, McMorris v. Williamsport Hospital 597 F.Supp. 899 (M.D. Pa. 1984), and McElhinney v. Medical Protective Company 549 F.Supp. 121 (E.D. Ky. 1982)

31   Kreuzer v. American Academy of Periondontology 735 F.2d 1479, at p. 1492-94 (DC Cir. 1984); see also Jefferson Parish, p. 1565; Robinson v. Magovern, p. 1006; Smith v. Northern Michigan Hospitals 703 F.2d 942, p. 949 (6th Cir. 1983); and Pontiun v Childrens Hospital, at p. 1372.

32   Stone v. William Beaumont Hosptal 1983-2 Trade Cas (CCH) (E.D. Mich 1983); Robinson v. Magovern; Weiss v. York Hospital.

33   Trepel v. Pontiac Ostheopatic Hospital 599 F.Supp 1484 (E.D. Mich 1984)

34   Williamson, O. "Economies as an Antitrust Defense:The Welfare Trade Offs" *American Economic Review*, Vol. 58, 1968, p.18.

35   McMorris v. Williamsport Hospital 597 F.supp 899 (M.D.Pa. 1984)

36   Harron v. United Hospital Center 522 F.2d 1133 (4th Cir. 1975), and Capili v. Shott 620 F.2d 438 (4th Cir. 1980).

37   DosSanton v. Columbus-Cuneo-Cabrini Medical Center 684 F.2d 1346 (7th Cir. 1982).

38   Berman, B.I. Acting Secretary, Federal Trade Commission, Letter - Burnham Hospital Advisory Opinion to Robert E. Nord, February 24, 1983.

39   Jefferson Parish Hospital District No.2 v. Hyde 104 S.Ct. 1551 (1984)

Chapter 24
STRUCTURAL AND REGULATORY CONSTRAINTS ON HOSPITAL COMPETITION

Hospitals are in a much increased competitive environment, brought about largely by the intensified cost consciousness on the part of the various buyers of hospital services. Healthcare buying coalitions formed by various purchasing groups, businesses, large employers, and the like, are designed to cap or at least restrain healthcare costs. Healthcare buyers prompt hospitals to compete in various terms, but particularly in terms of price. In fact, concerted actions on the part of purchasers even received governmental blessings[1]. A direct result of spiraling hospital healthcare costs was the Medicare prospective reimbursement payment system based on DRGs, paying hospitals fixed sums based on patient diagnosis, instead of retrospectively reimbursing hospitals for their costs. It appears that the DRGs have intensified hospital competition for patients in order to fill capacity; they prompted hospitals to enter into joint cost saving arrangements such as joint ventures in order to benefit from economies of operational scale and scope; and, it also prompted hospitals to diversify into areas traditionally not considered typical inpatient related hospital endeavors.

Healthcare cost related concerns also contributed to establishment of alternative delivery systems, HMOs, PPOs, and medical plans competing with traditional Blues based arrangements, and other commercial health plans. Hospitals compete with each other by being increasingly participating members in these plans, by founding these plans, or by contracting with such plans to provide services for them[2]. We have already noted the impact of the more increasingly competing, but declining number, of hospitals on the increasing physician population, and their often troubled efforts to gain or retain hospital staff privileges. Hospital have become, and could become, quite choosy. They will likely pick physicians not only based on their stature and competence, but also on their practice patterns and utilization intensity. Physicians who overutilize, assuming other factors constant, are not welcome. Finally, to complicate the competitive scene even more, hospitals have established off-site ambulatory centers in competition with physicians, while physicians are increasingly setting up and owning diagnostic radiology, outpatient surgery, and emergency care centers, in competition with hospitals. The American healthcare web has gotten intricate, complex, and, in a global sense, largely unmanageable. In this chapter we will take a look at some of the structural and regulatory areas where hospital based competitive concerns, and antitrust issues, may be found.

Hospital Mergers

Earlier in the volume we extensively examined the economic and general antitrust issues relating to mergers, the types of mergers, the motives for mergers, and merger guidelines. While referred to, these issues will not be analyzed to any significant extent in this chapter. Our concern here focuses on hospital mergers, their impact on competition, and competitive (antitrust) implications.

Hospitals, for-profit and not-for-profit, merge to protect their long-term economic interests. Mergers in the hospital sector are largely similar to those in the non-hospital sector: excess capacity, lack of profitability, increasing capital costs, and simply to cope with future uncertainty. Mergers also expand market share, and the increased size may constitute a better bargaining or market position against third-party payers. Hospital mergers have for some time escaped serious antitrust attention largely because of the size of the merging parties involved. The Hart-Scott-Rodino Act of 1976 requires merging companies to report their plans to the government if one company has more than $100 million and the other more than $10 million in assets. Until recently, it appears that most non-profit hospitals, which, in turn, constituted a majority of hospitals, did not meet this threshold. By 1985, however, the FTC's decision against a merger involving the Hospital Corporation of America constituted the third signal that mergers in the healthcare field are viewed in the same manner as those on the non-healthcare scene[3]. Nevertheless, there appears to be a conflict between the Health Planning Act of 1982[4], and the emerging mood in the hospital market place. The Act, for purposes of cost saving, explicitly encourages consolidations among otherwise competing hospitals. In addition, the prospective reimbursement system itself encourages hospital mergers by mandating efficiency enhancing measures, such as mergers.

When challenging hospital mergers, and scrutinizing their competitive impact, the same considerations and analyses are needed as in merger cases involving non-hospital entities. The relevant market has to be delineated. The pre-merger market shares of the parties must be considered, and the post-merger market power of the new entity is assessed. These issues will not again be reexamined here, as they were extensively dealt with earlier in the volume. However, let us take a look at some hospital merger cases of major historical significance, in order to illustrate how the issues are dealt with in hospital market contexts. Within the context of these cases, standard issues relating market definitions and market power measurements will be reiterated. A 1977 case focused on product market definition[5]. In particular, the issues centered whether Humana's take over *Medicorp* would constitute a restraint of trade in a product market that was delineated in terms of the acquisition, development and management of hospitals, and a submarket defined as these activities carried on by investor-owned companies controlling three or more hospitals. Medicorp, resisting the takeover, argued that investor owned hospital chains, like Humana, in effect compete by setting up hospitals in communities where other hospitals already exist. If allowed, Medicorp's acquisition would result in a 29.5% share in that market for Humana. The court declined to accept this market context, indicating that for a market to exist there must be a buyer, seller, and an exchange of payments for goods or services between them - none of which was literally present in this situation. Nor were there special attributes that would have justified the presence of a submarket. The relevant product market was defined by the court as the delivery of short term acute care community hospital services for doctors and patients. The geographic market was found to be Bluefield, West Virginia, where Humana would have controlled 100% of the beds after the merger. Nevertheless, viewing the consequences as minimal, the court did not grant a preliminary injunction against the merger sought by Medicorp.

The first federal antitrust challenge to a hospital merger occurred in 1980 in the US. v. *Hospital Affiliates International (HAI)*, Inc[6], under Clayton 7 and Sherman 2. The government succeeded in preventing a private psychiatric hospital in New Orleans from acquiring another similar facility while owning 50% of a third one in the same city. The claimed relevant geographic market was an eleven county health services area including the City of New Orleans, where inpatient psychiatric services (the claimed product market) were provided by three private psychiatric hospitals, a state psychiatric hospital, and the psychiatric units of seven acute care hospitals, as well as two federal hospitals and two state hospitals. The Justice Department claimed that the psychiatric wards of the government hospitals should not be included in the relevant market because of their different requirements for admissions and staffing. In addition, the Department proposed the existence of a submarket made up of services rendered by private psychiatric hospitals. Data indicated that, if allowed, the merger would have increased HAI's market share from 32.5% to almost 73%, approaching monopoly levels. Hence, without considering whether a submarket was in fact present, or that a Sherman 2 violation may have occurred, the merger was enjoined.

The degree and depth of market analysis increased in a mid-1984 decision by the FTC, shortly after the introduction of the 1984 Merger Guidelines, involving *American Medical International's (AMI)* attempt to acquire the 138 bed French Hospital in San Luis Obispo (SLO), California[7]. The City had two hospitals, in addition to French: Sierra Vista 172 bed facility also owned by AMI, and SLO General Hospital with 78 beds, owned by the County. SLO County, outside the City had two other hospitals: fifteen miles south of the City, Arroyo Grande with 79 beds, owned by AMI, and twenty miles to the north an 84 bed facility, Twin Cities Community Hospital, owned by National Medical Enterprises. Furthermore, within an 80 mile radius of the City of SLO, in Santa Barbara County two hospitals with 48 and 125 beds could be found, and in Monterey County a 42 bed facility existed. The administrative law judge found a product market containing a *cluster* of acute care hospital services, affirmed by the entire Commission. AMI's argument that the relevant market should include all non-hospital providers who offered services also provided by the hospital was declined:

> although each individual service that comprises the cluster ... may well have outpatient substitutes, the benefit that accrues to the patient and physician is derived from their complementarity. There is no readily available substitute supplier of the benefit that this complementarity offers on patient and physician[8].

In essence, patients were seen as purchasing not just the individual service they actually receive but also the availability of all ancillary services offered by hospitals but not by non-hospital providers.

Patient origin data, showing patient inflow and outflow patterns, were used by the Commission to determine the relevant geographic market. Less than 10% of the patients admitted to hospitals in SLO County resided outside the County, and, no more than about 15% of the County's residents went to hospitals located outside the County. Thus, the small cross-county line migration of patients in either direction prompted SLO County itself to be considered as the relevant geographic market. The City of SLO was also examined as being a relevant geographic market, although the picture in some respect was not quite as clear. For instance, only about 50% of City hospital admissions originated from within the City itself. Yet, among the residents of the City, very few patients used hospitals outside the City, as shown by the patient origin data for hospitals outside the City. In addition, some 98% of the admissions in City hospitals were referred by physicians with offices in the City, and hospitals there perceived the City as being a separate geographic market. Hence, the Commission also found the City of SLO to be a relevant geographic market. The acquisition increased AMI's market share, in terms of inpatient days, from about 56% to some 75% in the County, and from 58% to 87% in the City. The changes in the HHI were from 3818 to 6025 in the County, and from 4370 to 7775 in the City. Additionally, high entry barriers, hence unlikely new entrants, were seen by way of CON laws and existing excess capacity.

AMI's defense was based on three premises. (a) The Health Planning Act in effect provided immunity to hospitals when attempting to merge. However, the merger was seen as completely voluntary not mandated, prompted or even recommended by health planning or other state agency. (b) The merger would not significantly impede competition because there was minimum competition among hospitals anyway due to the dominance of the then prevailing cost-based and other third-party reimbursement plans. However, while admitting that these plans may have significantly reduced price competition among hospitals, for that reason alone the Commission wanted to protect whatever little price competition among hospitals may have remained:

> ....assuming that the limited price competition that does exist in these markets may produce only marginal benefits in terms of overall consumer welfare, the antitrust laws will endeavor to protect it.... for if nothing else, the hope of price competition will be enhanced[9].

Indeed, with the implementation of the PPS by way of DRGs, price competition may have further diminished in hospital markets. However, we have indicated already that inter-hospital competition may at any rate be more intensive in terms of non-price variables than in terms of price. Thus, competition among hospitals for competent physicians, and for patients by way of improved quality of service and prestige should be viewed as having attained greater importance, particularly in view of the reduced intensity of price competition. (c) Efficiencies and cost savings emanating from larger size attained through a merger. AMI produced no data or proof otherwise to the effect that such efficiencies would in effect occur pursuant to the merger, or that such efficiencies would offset the anti-competitive impact of the merger, or that any cost savings would in fact be passed on to patients.

In the HFI and AMI cases the post-merger market shares were large enough to clearly suggest competitive consequences, thus providing minimum guidelines as to the application of government merger policies to the hospital industry. A 1985 case appears to have contributed to clearing any doubts about standard merger policies being applied to the hospital industry with the same rigor as to any other industry. In *Hospital Corporation of America* (HCA)[10], the FTC found substantial competitive restraints in mergers that resulted in market shares only a small amount larger than prescribed by the then prevailing guidelines. HCA made two acquisitions in Chattanooga TN., where it already owned a hospital. By acquiring Hospital Affiliates International with its five owned or managed hospitals, HCA would have managed or owned six of the fourteen area hospitals. In the relevant geographic market (the Chattanooga urban area), the merger gave HCA control over four out of eleven hospitals. The concentration became intensified when a few months later HCA acquired another hospital (Health Care Corporation - HCC) that owned one hospital in the same area, increasing HCA's control to over half of the hospitals in the Chattanooga Metropolitan Statistical Area (MSA). The FTC challenged both mergers.

The relevant *product market* suggested by the FTC was to exclude out-patient services - and the non-hospital providers offering those services, and was to include only the cluster in inpatient services provided by the hospitals. HCA, attempting to reduce its market share to judicially harmless levels, argued to the contrary, namely that the relevant market should include not only the cluster of typical hospital inpatient services, but also all other ambulatory services offered by hospital and non-hospital providers. Although the administrative judge at the FTC included all services, ambulatory and inpatient, in the relevant product market, only those services were counted that were offered in a hospital environment, needed by acute care patients, not those offered by non-hospital providers. The full Commission indicated that the outpatient and inpatient services probably constitute separate product markets, where all providers, including physicians' offices may be considered as players in the former, but only acute care hospitals in the latter. In hospital merger cases, however, the relevant product market will likely be viewed in terms of the cluster of *inpatient* services, probably much more concentrated that all offered services combined.

There was also some dispute in this case regarding the relevant *geographical* market. Using patient origin data (depicted as "shipment patterns" in earlier studies[11]), HCA viewed the market as comprising the SMA, or that plus one county. The claimant, on the other hand, relied on patient origin data plus physician admitting patterns, and suggested a smaller four county urban area. The original "shipment pattern" method simply defined the relevant geographic market as that smallest area from which no more than 10% (in case of a "strong market"), or 25% (in case of a "weak market") of the patients seek hospitalization *outside* the area. Furthermore, similarly used 10% and 25% factors are applied to patients flowing *into* the area from outside regions. In another words, a strong geographical hospital market will see no more than 10% patient migration in or out, with that number 25% for a weaker market. A dynamic version of this analysis simply takes into consideration the patient migration consequences of potential changes in price and/or service quality within and outside the immediate market area.

The impact of the merger on concentration could be measured in terms of at least three variables: (a) bed capacity, (b) inpatient days, (c) net revenues. There was little variation found among the three, so it did not matter which one was used. The pre-merger HHI already showed a relatively highly concentrated market with an index of 1932. HCA's market share increased from 13.6% to 22.9% as a result of its acquisition of HAI, and the HHI went up to 2242 from its previous 1932 level - using approved number of beds. The second, HCC, acquisition increased HCA's market share to 26.7%, and the HHI to 2416 - suggesting to the FTC an increase in concentration to the point where collusion was much more likely. As to any notions that the hospital industry may be unique in terms of the competitive evaluation of mergers, the Commission clearly stated that:

merger analysis in this industry need be no different than in any other case; market share and concentration figures, evidence of entry barriers and other market evidence taken together appear to yield as accurate a picture of competitive conditions as they do in other settings[12].

The different nature of the hospital industry due to the already discussed differences in terms of the main competitive variables, i.e. diminished price competition augmented by quality-based rivalry for patients and physicians, and the fact that the ultimate consumer is not the one who makes final consumption choices, do not mandate, or even warrant, merger analyses any different or more lenient from those conducted in other industries.

Joint Ventures

Hospitals have long participated in various ventures jointly with other hospitals and institutional healthcare providers. Recently, market and competitive factors intensified the activity. The prospective payment reimbursement regime (DRGs), contributed to increased hospital joint venture activities at least through two channels: (a) fixed per-patient DRG-based revenues prompted cost cutting and increased efficiencies, often achievable only through joint ventures; (b) the same fixed per-patient DRG-based revenue prompted a drive for increased patient flow, higher market penetration, protection of already achieved market shares, all of which could be facilitated by certain types of joint venture. And, increasingly competitive environments may be made more lenient and bearable by using joint ventures as a means to reduced competitive ends.

Joint ventures in the antitrust arena have often been somewhat of an elusive target. A noted antitrust scholar and authority, for instance complained that "joint venture.... [is] ... an expansive notion without definite meaning or antitrust consequence"[12]. Joint ventures can entail any kind of cooperative activity which otherwise would call for competition. A "joint venture" is consummated whenever two entities do anything together. The number and variety of activities involved can be large, calling for different types of antitrust analysis. The participants may have a variety of market relationship with each other prior to or during the joint venturing, horizontal, potentially horizontal, vertical, or conglomerate, again calling for different types of antitrust consideration. In addition, the degree of economic integration involved in the joint venture can vary over wide ranges and degrees Nevertheless, the antitrust questions need to boil down to the extent to which competition is restrained in a product and geographical market as result of the joint venture.

In dealing with the anticompetitive impact of a joint venture, a number of major issues need to be examined. If a firm chooses to expand by way of joint venturing, instead of internal expansion, it may choose a variety of methods. The integration may be loose and informal at one end, or it can take the form of a formal merger or the creation of a new entity, at the other extreme, or somewhere in between. A widely accepted definition of joint venture for antitrust purposes in this regard suggest that

> [it] is an integration of operations between two or more separate firms, in which the following conditions are present: (1) the enterprise is under joint control of the parent firms, which are not under related control; (2) each parent makes a substantial contribution to the joint enterprise; (3) the enterprise exists as a business entity separate from its parents; and, the joint venture creates significant new enterprise capability in terms of new productive capacity, new technology, a new product, or entry into a new market[13].

The query is often directed to whether or not there is an economic need (e.g. increased efficiencies) to establish a new enterprise in order to carry on the operation, whether the firms could have or would have entered the enterprise independently from each other hence become competitors in that area as well, or whether any one of the firms would have entered the enterprise alone, with the other simply remaining outside as a potential entrant, keeping the entered firm's conduct under potential competitive check. In addition, a fundamental issue may be whether we are in fact dealing with a joint venture, destined to increase output, or do we have a *cartel* aimed at reducing output and raising price. Thus, earlier we have seen in the *Maricopa County Medical Society* case that independent and otherwise competing physicians formed a foundation aimed at joining their contracting activities with outside health insurers, and setting a maximum price level charged to policy holders. The court found this arrangement to be a *per se* price fixing arrangement under Sherman 1, an arrangement which offered no new product to consumers but only a new system whereby old products were sold to consumers. The possible pro-competitive impact of the arrangement through likely efficiencies in maximum reimbursement settings by the physicians rather than by the insurers was seen to be more than offset by the potential competitive restraints which the arrangement was capable of achieving.

An important basis for recognizing anticompetitive potentials for a joint venture is its *production portfolio*. Input producing or procuring joint ventures may in general be viewed as having less anti-competitive potentials than those that deal in output. In healthcare, an input producing venture would, for instance, involve group purchasing arrangements or shared catering or laundry services. On the output side, the same hospitals may jointly operate diagnostic imaging facilities such as MRIs, or ultrasound. Input producing/procuring ventures may yield competitive restraints by excluding competitors from the arrangement, therefore from its benefits, or if the included participants generate through their market power substantial cost benefits for themselves which excluded competitors cannot obtain. The analysis of differences and implications of these various arrangements is made more complex by difficulties that one may encounter attempting the determine whether a joint venture is an input or output oriented one in the first place. Thus, a venture involving radiologists and a hospital aimed at acquiring, say, radiological diagnostic facilities, may be seen as an output venture by the hospital, but an input venture on the part of the physicians who use those facilities to arrive at their diagnosis.

The economic status and relationship of the parties in the venture may be significant. Thus, ventures formed by entities that were or are horizontal competitors with each other harbor more potential competitive harm than those in vertical or no prior competitive relationship to each other. Yet, whether or not the parties to the venture were competitors prior to the formation of the venture, the potentially negative impact on competition depends on the likelihood of their entry into the competitive arena where the venture is being formed; that is, how effective potential competitors, threat, to each other they would have become, which in turn depends on prevailing entry barriers.

Structural Issues in Reimbursement Negotiations

Hospitals often negotiate jointly reimbursement terms with third-party payers. In situations such as that, the issues often center on whether this type of conduct can be viewed as horizontal price fixing, and whether the collective market power of the negotiating group is used to enforce the negotiated terms by way of group boycotts. The latter presents particularly antisocial consequences. A group of hospitals, for instance, collectively choosing not to participate in a payment plan due to it being deemed as inadequate, can have severe competitive and antitrust consequences. Thus, a 1978 matter involving four nursing homes and their trade association agreeing not to accept Medicaid patients unless Medicaid reimbursements were increased was seen as a *per se* Sherman violation and attempted monopolization under Sherman 2[14]. Similar actions were subsequently taken by the Justice Department involving concerted actions on the part of providers not to participate in payment plans unless the reimbursements were increased[15].

A noted case involved the Michigan State Medical Society[16]. Members of the Society agreed to negotiate fees with Medicaid and Blue Shield plans, and engaged in group boycotts to increase fees. The Commission did not view the matter as a *per se* violation of Sherman 1, although indicated that no actual effect on fees need to be registered in order to find a strong potential for restraining price competition among physicians. The Society's argument that the arrangement was necessary in order to offset unfair third-party payer market power such as that could be found for the Blues was seen as one needing legislative or regulatory remedy, instead of one by way of boycotts in the market. Indeed, the Commission found no social or economic mitigating factors for the conduct, although it did note a need for fees-related informational interaction between providers and third-party payers, provided no coercion is used.

Vertical Integration

Regulatory and market based competitive factors have compelled hospitals to diversify into new product and service areas such as ambulatory care, home health programs, nursing homes, and even the insurance business[17]. Vertical integration by hospitals may be implemented in variety ways: sole ownership, joint venture with another party, or, by way of a contractual agreement with an existing entity. The hospital's economic interests are served if it channels its patients needing services provided by the integrated provider to that provider. Thus, discharged patients may be referred by the hospitals to home healthcare systems owned by, or affiliated with, the hospital, or patients simply would not be informed of existing alternative home healthcare facilities. The competitive concerns that emanate from this type of practice rest largely with the exclusion of non-affiliated but competing home healthcare providers from the discharged patients' consideration[18].

The extent and volume of foreclosure depends on the hospital's inpatient and referral market share in the region. A major medical center affiliated with a home healthcare facility of substantial capacity can foreclose a large proportion of the rest of the home healthcare market in that region. If the home healthcare facility is not owned by the hospital, excluded competitors may see the practice as the implementation of an *exclusive contract* agreement between the hospital and utilized home healthcare facility. If there is an ownership relationship between the referring hospital and the home healthcare facility, then the referrals may invoke competitive restraint perceptions by way of *tying* agreements. In either case, the hospital's market share in the inpatient, hence potentially referral, market is the key factor in considering the ultimate restraint in competition. Competitive restraints in this context may be seen to vary directly, if not proportionately, with the hospital's market share.

In connection with *exclusive dealing* contracts, two factors appear to be significant: whether or not the hospital informed its discharged patients of the existence of alternative home healthcare facilities in the area, and the proportion of the hospital's discharged patients being serviced at the specific home healthcare facility. These issues weighted heavily in a case that was settled before trial, but nevertheless gave expression of prevailing judicial sentiments[19]. The only hospital and a home health agency in a region of Washington State had a close relationship for many years, although no exclusive contract was ever signed. The claimant, a competing home healthcare facility, asserted that the hospital's discharge planning was constructed so that a majority of patients were channeled to the defendant agency, and that the hospital did not even inform he patients that an alternative facility existed. The arrangement was seen as if an exclusive contract existed between the hospital and the favored agency, and the hospital's market share as a major source of referral was a decisive factor. Indeed, the extent of the foreclosure is determined by the percentage of *all* patients needing home healthcare services in the region that come from the hospital under scrutiny.

When formal affiliation, such as partial or complete ownership, exists between the hospital and a home health agency, the possibility of *tying* arrangements surfaces. The tying product being the hospital's cluster of inpatient services, and the services of the home healthcare agency being the tied product. However, once again, circumstances surrounding the hospital's conduct play an important role. Thus, in a 1985 case, no tying agreement was found to exist unless the hospital was found to require all of its patients, and not just those that needed them, to use the hospital CAT scan facilities:

> All patients who use the hospital's services are not required to use its CAT Scan equipment. Thus, there is no tying product... would constitute a tying agreement only if all patients sought the hospital's services were required to undergo a CAT Scan[20].

Furthermore, it does not appear likely that a tying is seen as consummated if the hospital merely recommends its discharged patients that they use the hospital's affiliated facilities. On other hand, patients lacking medical market information as they often do, even a recommendation, along with not advising patients of available alternatives, may be viewed as implicit coercion to use the hospital's own facilities.

Competitive Restraints by Regulation

In 1974, Congress enacted the National Health Planning and Resources Development Act, placing the healthcare industry into regulatory confines, and setting up provisions for federal funding of state and local health planning activities and state Certificate of Need (CON) programs. Subsequently most states adopted CON laws in accordance with the Act[21]. As soon as these laws were enacted, considerable potential conflict was noted between them and the federal antitrust laws, particularly since these regulations were essentially designed to restrict output and allocate resources by administrative means instead of via the market forces[22]. Thus, the CON laws were meant to avoid capacity duplications and unnecessary service production by mandating state pre-approval of major expansionary capital projects. Health System Agencies (HSAs), local nongovernmental planning bodies, on the other hand, are designed to continuously study the healthcare scene in a region, develop health system plans, and attempt to implement them by interacting with appropriate healthcare providers. In essence, the conflict between healthcare regulation and the federal antitrust laws may be perceived as an inherent conflict between two sets of federal regulatory laws, the former constraining competition by restricting entry and otherwise interfering with market forces, the latter attempting to at least preserve if not enhance competition in particular, including healthcare, markets. In 1979, Congress passed the Health Planning and Resources Development Amendments to the 1974 Health Planning Act[23]. However ,the Amendments appear to concentrate on the applicability of antitrust laws to the actions of the health planning committees, and not to the actions of private providers even when the latter act is in response to HSA recommendations.

An area of health planning where competitive restraints may be found, involves the very purpose of the Act, having providers abide by its spirit and provisions. HSA generated plans recommend the type and volume of healthcare services in particular regions. Thus, an HSA may suggest that certain hospitals be closed; or, that some services be terminated at a given hospital and the same service be concentrated in the area's other hospital, or hospitals. These recommendations directly interfere with the functioning of market forces by way of efficient resource allocation, for they solicit agreements, voluntary compliance, between and among providers not to compete with each other in specific service markets. While, at least to date, there does not appear to be any major piece of antitrust litigation that addressed these issues to any significant extent, the Justice Department's response to a business review letter request by a Virginia health planning agency may shed some light on enforcement posture, at least of that time. The Virginia health planning agency intended to perform functions such as reviewing CON applications and making recommendations to state agencies regarding their merits; review and assess federal grant applications; assess existing health services in terms of their volume, composition and distribution; and, implement its health systems plans with the voluntary cooperation of providers in terms of the allocation of new or existing services and facilities. In its response, the Justice Department appears to have cleared the way for the performance of the first three functions, without endorsing the fourth type of activity. In particular, the Department stated:

> .. agreements among competing hospitals limiting the number of patients they could serve or the kind of services they could offer in the absence of conscious and explicit authorization and supervision by the State are probably not contemplated by the [federal health planning] Act nor exempt from the federal antitrust laws[24].

Although much of CON application activity in most states have now receded, let us say a few words about that regulation's implications for competitive restraints. Furthermore, under certain provisions of the presently expected regulatory reforms CON-like activity may once again be utilized in some form or another. We may note again that the CON process entailed hospitals and other healthcare facilities requesting approval from a state agency, normally a state Health Department, of major capital expenditures. Local HSAs, involving patient and provider representatives, reviewed the application to assess the need for the anticipated expenditure in the community, and made recommendations to the petitioned state agency. The normal administrative hearings conducted by the agency, if yielding negative results for the applicant, have often been followed by administrative and judicial appeals. And the drama has not stopped there.

Much of antitrust activity thus far relating to health planning involved CON application controversies[25]. Most applications carried substantial stakes with them. These stakes involved the applicant's prosperity, or survival, prestige for the institution and for the physicians with staff privileges at the institution, introduction of new services, expansion of existing services, market penetration, preemptive competitive gestures, and so forth. The complaints alleged activities such as competing hospitals attempting to block market entry by procedurally delaying the processing of applications, by filing similar competing applications, and placing opposing representatives on planning agencies. Sherman 1 and 2 by way of group-boycotts, conspiracy to restrain trade, monopolization and attempted monopolization were all often alleged in these cases, notwithstanding the fact that health planning laws contemplated the involvement of providers in the CON assessment process. Thus, the issues centered not on whether provider participation was socially desirable, but rather on the extent and nature of that participation. In general, the examination of the issues as to whether the Noerr-Pennington, state action, or implied repeal immunities applied far overshadowed substantive competitive issues traditionally examined under the Sherman Act.

The 1993 Antitrust Enforcement Reforms[26]

The US Justice Department and the FTC issued six new policy statements regarding their enforcement intentions in the area of joint activities in the healthcare field. These address hospital mergers, hospital joint ventures involving high-tech or costly medical equipment, physician dissemination of information to purchasers of healthcare services, hospital participation in exchanges of price and cost information, healthcare group purchasing agreements, and physician network joint ventures. The intent of these policy statements is to guide healthcare providers through the antitrust maze in view of the possible implementation of some or most of the Clinton healthcare proposals, and the resulting changes that may emanate from those proposals on the healthcare scene. In particular, the statements are intended to call attention to the fact that activities on the part of healthcare providers that are not seriously anticompetitive and are aimed at reducing costs by likely increases in efficiency will not be challenged under the antitrust laws.

The statements present so called "antitrust safety zones", that is, fact situations in which the enforcement agencies, the US Department of Justice and the FTC, will not challenge under the antitrust laws conduct or structural changes that providers may implement in the interest of efficiency and cost savings. By delineating these safety zones, the statements also indicate some of those situations which are likely to fall outside the safety zone. Furthermore, providers may get some prompt advance opinion from enforcement agencies within 90 days of having submitted facts and information to them - "expedited business review" from the Justice Department, and an "advisory opinion" from the FTC - in order to reduce antitrust uncertainties and risks during times of dramatic changes on the healthcare scene.

Regarding *hospital mergers*, antitrust enforcement has, in fact, not been rigorous even thus far. Of the 200 hospital mergers that occurred during past five years, only eight were challenged[27], with most of the rest having involved hospital units without significant competitive power prior to the merger. Even where significant increases in concentration took place pursuant to the merger between two hospitals, they were often viewed as a source of operating or administrative efficiency leading to substantial cost savings.

Pursuant to the new statements, an antitrust safety zone comes in to effect in connection with hospital mergers when at least one of the merging hospital units has less than 100 licensed beds, and an average daily census of less than 40 patients. This policy particularly affects small rural hospitals who may need to merge in order to survive but may have in the past been concerned with potential antitrust exposure and related expenses. Once again, hospitals may receive reassurances, or otherwise, as to whether or not they are in the safety zone by way of an expedited 90 review procedure.

Joint ventures among hospitals to acquire and operate high-tech and high priced capital equipment have never been challenged by enforcement agencies. The general view has always been that whatever potential or actual competitive restraints may emanate from such a practice, they are likely to be outweighed by the cost savings that accrue from this type of joint purchasing efforts, and the increased efficiency due to full capacity utilization of the acquired equipment if more than one hospital utilizes them. At any rate, for future reference, the antitrust safety zone for joint ventures of this type would be determined based on an assessment whether or not the joint venture is reasonably necessary to recover the capital equipment's purchase price, along with the cost of its operating, and the expenses involved in the marketing of the services it provides. The other condition for immunity in this context is the finding that the venture does not include hospitals that could have procured the equipment by themselves and thus could have provides services competing with the hospitals involved in the venture. Acceptable examples cited in the statements include jointly acquired and operated MRIs in rural hospital settings, or the acquisition and operation of helicopters by a group of community hospitals.

Another area of safety zone covers the *collective dissemination of non-price information by doctors* to healthcare purchasers, which is viewed as having potential pro-competitive effects and a positive impact on healthcare quality. These activities may include the collective provisions of underlying medical data and collective efforts as developing practice parameters. This, however, would not allow physicians to threaten or actually implement a boycott against healthcare purchasers should the latter not concur with physician proposed terms regarding the provision of services. Importantly, this safety zone does not exempt most types of collective activity on the part of physicians regarding fee-related information.

Various independent entities, such as healthcare consulting firms, often engage in the *collection and dissemination of various healthcare cost data*, including hospital service prices, and data of interest to hospital service personnel such as wages and benefits. Such surveys may be viewed as falling into the antitrust safety zone if they are conducted by third-party entities, the collected data is more than three months old, and the collected price and cost data cover at least five hospitals, presented in a manner aggregated enough so as not reveal any hospital-specific data.

Agreements among healthcare providers aimed at the *joint procurement of inputs* (such as laundry and food services, computer services, prescription and other pharmaceutical products) may be viewed as competitively harmless, hence will likely go unchallenged, as they usually have in the past. These agreements are seen as efficiency enhancing and cost reducing efforts, in the long-term benefit of the patients. The chance of antitrust challenge to such agreements becomes real and increases, however, if the purchases made pursuant to the agreement exceeds 35% of the total volume of transactions in the products and services involved in the region, and the cost of the jointly procured product or service is greater than 20% of the total revenues generated from the *sale* of all products and services by each of the joint purchasing agreement's participants.

Finally, *physician network joint ventures*, controlled by physicians, that jointly market member physicians' services, collectively provide information to healthcare purchasers, and even collectively negotiate contract terms with healthcare purchasers, are viewed as potential sources of cost savings as well as competition. A joint venture of this type is considered to be in an antitrust safety zone if it includes no more than 20% of the physicians for each specialty, in each relevant geographic market, and where the members bear a substantial financial risk for the success of the joint venture.

Reference

1 Favorable business review letters were issued by the US Department of Justice regarding coalitions designed to collect and disseminate hospital pricing information in certain regions of the country. See Business Review Letter from Rule, C.F., Acting Attorney General, Antitrust Division to the Stark County, Ohio, Health Care Coalition, August 30, 1985. Similarly favorable review was issues in 1982 by then Assistant Attorney General William Baxter, Antitrust Division, to the Maryland Health Care Coalition on February 19, 1982.

2 Refer to our discussion of theses plans earlier in the volume.

3 3 Trade Reg. Rep. (CCH) #22,301 (FTC Oct. 25, 1985). The first two involvedAmerican Medical International, 3 Trade Reg Rep. (CCH) #22,170 (FTC July 2, 1985), and US v. Hospital Affiliates International 1980-81 Trade Cases (CCH) #63,721 (E.D.La. 1980).

4 National Health Planning and Resource Development Act, 42 U.S.C. #1320a-1, Sect 1122 (1982).

5 American Medicorp Inc. v, Humana, Inc. 445 F.Supp. 589 (E.D. Pa. 1977)

6 1980-81 Trade Cas (CCH) at 77,853-54

7 FTC v. American Medical International 3 Trade Reg Rep. (CCH) 22,170 (FTC July 2 1984).

8 AMI at 23,040

9 AMI at 23,046

10 3 Trade Reg Rep. (CCH) 22,301 (FTC October 25, 1985)

11 Elzinga, K. and Hogarty, T. "The Problem of Geographic Market Delineation in Antimerger Suits" *Antitrust Bulletin*, Vol. 18, 1973, p. 45, and by the same authors "The Problem of Geographic Market Delineation Revisited: The Case of Coal" *Antitrust Bulletin* Vol. 23, 1978, p.1

12 Areeda, P. *Antitrust Analysis: Problems, Text, Cases,* Little Brown and Co. 3rd Ed. Boston, MA. 1981, p. 471.

13 Brodley, A. "Joint Ventures and Antitrust Policy" *Harvard Law Review,* Vol. 95, 1982, pp.1521-6.

14 DeGregorio v. Segal 443 F.Supp. 1257 (E.D. Pa. 1978)

15 US v. Montana Nursing Home Association 1982-2 Trade Cas (CCH) 64,852 (D.Mont.1982); US v. South Carolina Health Care Association 1980-2 Tradce Case (CCH) 63,316 (D.S.C. 1980).

16 FTC v. Michigan State Medical Society 101 FTC 191 (1983)

17 Moore, J. "CEOs Plan to Expand Home Health, Outpatient Services" *Hospitals*, January 1, 1984, p.1.

18 These antitrust concerns do not include the proscriptions of state and federal laws which refer to the receipt of rebates or kickbacks in return for the referral of patients - often referred to as "fee-splitting".

19 Beacon Medical Care Inc.v Sound Home Health Services Inc. No. C84-478T (W.D.Wash, filed August 9, 1984)

20   Coastal Neuro-Psychiatric Associates v. Onslow Memorial Hospital 1985-
     1 Trade CAs. (CCH) 66,432 (E.D.N.C. 1985)
21   It should also be noted that by 1992, at least half of the states have parted
     with the practice of requiring CON applications from hospitals planning
     major capital expansions.
22   Miller, K. "Antitrust and Certificate of Need: Health Systes Agencies, the
     Planning Act, and Regulatory Capture" *Georgetown Law Journal*, Vol. 68,
     1980, p.873; Note, "Antitrust and Health Planning Under the 1974 NHPRD
     Act, *Journal of Corporate Law* !982, p.311.
23   Public Law 96-79,93 Stat,592 (1979)
24   Letter from Sanford M. Litvack, Assistant Attorney General, Antitrust
     Division, to William G. Kopit (May 6, 1980).
25   Huron Valley Hospital v. City of Pontiac 612 F.Supp.654 (W.D. Mich.1985);
     St. Joseph's Hospital v. Hospital Corporation of America 1985-2 Trade
     Cas. (CCH) 66,784 (S.D. Ga.)
26   This section is based entirely on US Department of Justice and the Federal
     Trade Commission, *State of Antitrust Enforcement Policy in the Health
     Care Area*, Washington, DC. September 15, 1993.
27   See discussion on hospital mergers in Chapter 24.

PART FIVE

HEALTHCARE COSTS, POLICY AND PROGNOSES

Chapter 25
THE ECONOMIC CONTRIBUTION OF THE HUMAN IMMUNODEFICIENCY VIRUS - HIV

HIV infections and related diseases have now captured the imagination of the public and the media. Initially, the preoccupation was based on the perceived romantic images of those celebrities who were first publicized as having been inflicted with the diseases, and who subsequently passed away. These included famous movie stars, and sports heros. Subsequently, and to an extent concurrently, the problems began to hit home, particularly in segments of the gay community, their friends, and families. In addition, the statistical conveyance of the disease as being that of the poor, the drug addict, and the inner-city minority, all tainted and continue to water down our complete appreciation of the epidemic at hand from a social, political and even psychological points of view. The arrival of "AIDS", if indeed that date can be reliably ascertained, was also poorly timed. The first reported cases date back to about 1981, just about the time when the new Reagan administration was setting out to cut healthcare costs by reducing federal healthcare spending, and also reducing the funds available to states to finance their respective programs. Yet, by the mid-1980s, the disease was notably spread among minorities in the metropolitan areas of New York, New Jersey, California, and Florida, and became a serious social, economic and medical concern in other part of the country. So, by the late 1980s, attention was redirected to the disease on a much broader scale. Due to the *potential* social, medical and economic consequences that can be associated with AIDS, HIV caused infections have now become known as chronic diseases, and receive perhaps more attention than other major health related maladies such as cancer, alcoholism, and automobile injuries, although the latter even individually still claim a much larger number of mortality victims, and command higher social and economic cost, than HIV infections do at least at this stage. These circumstances have been augmented by rather vocal political groups, such as gays, often viewed as more vulnerable to AIDS than others, claiming social negligence and even discrimination by governments and other power groups not paying adequate attention through insufficient resource allocation to this problem.

The HIV caused epidemic is now often compared to other health problems of plague magnitude. Thus, we hear analogies to black death, yellow fever, small pox, polio, and other health problems of major historical significance, although the fear is also expressed that while these other historical plagues have receded into oblivion by themselves or due to medical advances, AIDS is not likely to be an easily met challenge[1]. It has been around too unrecognized for too long. It has been spreading around the world for many years ununderstood and even unnoted, and has been incubating unnoticed for possibly over a decade. Thus, AIDS may in fact not be a "normal" chronic disease, but one that requires special political, medical and economic attention. Furthermore, its social gravity is increased by the fact that many of the victims were of limited or no economic means, had no insurance to cover the treatment, have been too young to be covered by Medicare, and passed away before they could become eligible under Social Security. They could be seen as initially unsuspecting victims of a problem that sneaked up on them, uncared for by a largely uninformed and even prejudiced society, to be mercilessly allowed to drown in the ravages of a largely unknown and unforgiving disease.

The US Healthcare Financial Environment and the HIV

This section will first reiterate briefly some of the basic premises of the US healthcare system, in order to show how it may be suitable, or unsuitable, for dealing with the HIV epidemic. We have noted a number of times in the volume that the financial sources for healthcare delivery rest with Medicaid, Medicare, private/commercial health insurance, the patients' own pockets, and the delivery of uncompensated services by providers. Over half of the US population is covered by privately underwritten group plans, administered through the *employer* who would normally purchase the coverage for their employees from commercial insurers and the Blues, although lately employers often finding it more economical to pay their employees' healthcare costs from their own pockets (self-insure) not sharing the risk with an insurer. Under COBRA, employers also offer an 18 month continuation policy to those who lose their jobs. The federal government normally finances between 50% and 80% of state administered and implemented *Medicaid* plans, that cover aged and disabled people with incomes and assets below state prescribed levels; because of stringent qualification requirements, Medicaid often covers no more than about 40% of the poor. Once diagnosed, an HIV infected patient is normally considered "disabled", and eligible for Medicaid after the necessary asset and income "spend-down".

The federal government's payroll taxes, special premiums and general revenues finance *Medicare*. Eligible are the elderly and those disabled for at least two years. Since most AIDS patients are under age 65, and relatively few survive beyond two years after being diagnosed, Medicare's share of HIV related costs has been relatively small. Beyond the above, about 37 million members of the US population are covered neither by Medicare nor by Medicaid, nor by the private or commercial insurers. They are simply *uninsured*, and many more are inadequately insured due to copayments, deductibles, premiums and drug charges. They are expected to pay all or most of their healthcare costs. The voluntary contribution of healthcare services by providers normally comes about by way of treating uninsured persons in a hospital environment on an emergency basis. While they normally attempt to, and often do, shift the cost of such care onto privately insured or traditional fee-for-service patients, to the extent that they cannot succeed at doing so, they in effect provide an alternative form of "healthcare financing" by way of healthcare service "donation". HIV infected people are normally covered by private insurance, if they participate in the plan, although once diagnosed with aids, they may soon fall into the "disabled" category. While those infected through intravenous drug consumption are generally poor, most may not meet other Medicaid constraints, nor benefit from free care in emergency room situations because of a lack need for that kind of service at the beginning stages of the disease. Of course, once AIDS is diagnosed, technical disability sets in. The victims often become unemployed, although their employer sponsored coverage may continue for 18 months. After the 18 months, they exhaust their own financial resources whether in the form of income or assets ("spend-down"), so that they become sufficiently poor to meet specific state requirements for Medicaid. After twenty-four months, if they are still alive, they become eligible for Medicare. Uninsured people diagnosed with AIDS move directly into the "spend-down" stage, and benefit from Medicaid as soon as they become poor enough. The "spend-down" process, and, subsequently, Medicaid covers a certain proportion of AIDS related healthcare costs. The proportion may range from zero (in the case of unpaid bills) through some higher proportions covered Medicaid. The proportion is rarely 100% of the healthcare costs incurred throughout the entire care period of an AIDS patient. The difference between the amount or proportion covered by the "spend-down" or Medicaid and the *actual* healthcare cost incurred during the entire treatment period, may be labeled as *"unrequitted transfer care"*, or simply just *"transfer care"*, that is, care donated by the providers themselves.

While specific and more detailed accounts of costs, cost and case projections will be presented a little later, let us here take a bird's eye view of some of the numbers involved with the HIV epidemic. Back in 1988 the Center for Disease Control (CDC) indicated that some 100,000 people in this country were diagnosed with AIDS (i.e. HIV caused clinical symptoms), with about 50% of them having died within two years thereafter. CDC also projected that there would be 170,000 AIDS patients alive in 1992[2]. The average lifetime cost of treating patients was estimated in the late 1980s somewhere between $30,000 and 140,000, having proven to be on the low end rather than high[3]. Once again, these numbers refer to the treatment of the syndromes, i.e. the serious medical problems developed as a result of a likely long-time presence of the HIV, i.e. the setting in of what is commonly known as the Acquired Immunodeficiency Syndrome, or "AIDS". The costs associated with pre-AIDS stage care is probably much lower, and much more difficult to even estimate. However, even in this regard some fundamental relationships prevail. The emergence of some drugs (e.g. AZT) does appear, according to some studies by NIH, to delay the on-set of full fledged AIDS, thus adding years to a patient's life. On the other hand, the added years also add the substantial costs of utilized medication, particularly AZT. This situation however does allow focusing in on the main cost factor prior to the on-set of full AIDS, namely the drug. If clinical trials suggest effectiveness with lower doses, and the manufacturer (Burroughs-Wellcome) lowers the price of the drug, considerable cost savings may be attained at the early stages of the infection, given the number of patients remaining constant. However, as we will see later in this chapter, that is not likely to be the case. Although the projected numbers increase, there is no consensus as to by how much and to what levels. The projected range is between half-million to 1.5 million people carrying the HIV[4]. Yet, measurements are difficult if not impossible to implement. For the first few years, many infected people may not even be aware of their pending predicament. Some who may be aware, do not seek medical treatment until the first serious symptoms appear, several years later. Finally, as we suggested earlier, others who may be aware of their disease, and already encounter serious symptoms, do not get treated because they cannot afford it, hence remain statistically unaccountable, until the emergency stage arrives, with very limited life expectancy, and incurred costs, thereafter.

The Cost of AIDS - A Closer Look

The cost of treating AIDS patients may be grouped into two major categories, direct and indirect costs. The former would by far be weighted heaviest with costs incurred in connection the clinical treatment of the patient in a hospital inpatient environment, but would also include community service and voluntary costs. Indirect and social costs entail mostly time, efforts and some moneys expended by way of information dissemination, counseling, education campaigns, and blood supply protection, to mention a few items.

Direct cost estimates have focused almost exclusively on inpatient hospital environments, almost entirely disregarding pre-AIDS treatment costs. In addition, substantial variation was noted among individuals in terms of their needs for care, treatment, and incurred costs. Different patients require different number of hospital admissions, various intensities of social and psychological support, and these, in turn, also vary by treatment methods and by provider. Assuming some 168 days of hospital inpatient treatment per patient, one study estimated the lifetime cost of AIDS at $147,000[5]. Subsequent studies viewed the 168 days length of stay (LOS) too high, and yielded lower estimates by way of a mean lifetime cost of about $28,000 incurred by those treated in San Francisco General Hospital and died by 1984. The average admission needed 11.7 days of LOS, with the total number of LOS days over an average patient's lifetime, not exceeding about 35 days[6].

Another study conducted about the same time, and based on a cross-section of patients during a period of one year, suggested an average lifetime cost of about $50,000 for AIDS inpatients in Massachusetts hospitals, with a lifetime average per patient LOS of 67 days[7]. A British study, following specific patients to the stage of their death, found an average LOS per admission of 17.2 days, and 50 days over the patient's lifetime. The same British study found an average lifetime hospital (inpatient and outpatient) cost of some $10,000 incurred on a general medical ward of a National Health Service Teaching Hospital[8]. It was further found that drug users' treatment was much more inpatient intensive than those required by gays, due presumably to further complications brought by drug usage[9]

The studies further point to LOS as being the most heavily weighted determinant of the incurred cost levels because over 80% of hospital costs are incurred by way of in patient case, a predominant portion of the latter being basic room (lodging) charges. Thus, a reduction in LOS by replacing it, wherever possible, with community or outpatient care may mitigate AIDS related healthcare costs. Furthermore, studies even suggested that inpatient care of an average AIDS case does not necessarily generate better results than outpatient or community care. Thus, considerable costs savings were found in San Francisco by reduced length of stay, the utilization of hospices, hostels, home care, and the voluntary contributions of social and community services[10]. It is also apparent that as the disease becomes better understood, new, bolder and more innovating treatment methods will be developed outside the expensive hospital inpatient environment.

This is not to say that community services constitute a free good. Two community based projects in San Francisco providing housing, hospice and community healthcare support to AIDS patients, spent some $1.6 million during 1984-85. This does not include donated services estimated at a value of some $800,000. Nevertheless, these expenditures were substantially lower than inpatient hospital costs would have been during a comparable time period, with results not shown to be inferior in any respect to those attained in a hospital inpatient environment. In fact, it was shown that the cost of home-based per average patient-day in San Francisco was $94, a little over 10% of the cost of contemporaneous hospital care[11].

Estimating the direct cost of HIV diagnosed but not AIDS patient treatment is more difficult. One study of a group of gay men in San Francisco indicated that there is an approximate ratio of 9:1 between having the HIV and those in the sample who had full blown AIDS[12]. Although the formers' need for inpatient or institutional care may be relatively small, their sheer volume may add substantially to the overall cost of dealing with the HIV virus, particularly due to relatively expensive drug applications. Furthermore, much of the above discussion was conducted in terms of *average cost* per patient. And, in many instances it may be a more useful yardstick of cost measurements than marginal cost, especially if existing facilities can accommodate new patients. However, as the number of new cases, particularly at the later stage of the disease, continues to mount, obvious questions relating to *marginal cost* associated with facility expansions will likely surface. In addition, treatment hours and resources devoted to AIDS patients could have - particularly in the most relevant metropolitan areas of New York, San Francisco, and Southern Florida - likely and large part been devoted to non-AIDS patients. Hence, the explicit direct cost of AIDS must be augmented by the relevant *opportunity costs* involved. Either more hospital beds and other treatment facilities will be needed, or those that would have been closed down will now need to be kept open. These are real and direct costs, although not explicit, and must be included in any reliable estimates of the total direct cost of the disease.

Indirect costs may be noted by way of the impact of AIDS not only on healthcare expenditures but also on the victim's own personal life, including employment and family, although their measurement may be a problem. These costs may be proxied to an extent by using such relatively measurable variables as lost productivity due to the disease and the various benefits that may be paid to the victim. Thus, costs attributable to lost productivity as a result of the first 10,000 cases of AIDS in the US was estimated at some \$4.6 billion[13], and the indirect cost of the first 540 cases in the UK was estimated at some 150 million pounds[14]. These estimates are, of course, based on certain assumptions which may or may not hold true at any time, such as loss of productivity due not only to the illness itself but also to prevailing adverse economic conditions, i.e. the victim would have been out of work regardless of the disease.

The indirect cost category should also include programs such as counseling those with the HIV virus as to desirable social and personal conduct, advising persons in high risk groups as to proper precautions against being infected, the implementation of preventive counseling and services for drug users, and services of a similar nature often provided at local levels. In addition, costs are incurred by the various means used to protect the healthcare providers and their staff, such as protective supplies, educational and counseling programs, preparation and dissemination of guidelines, and the like. Blood donors need to be tested, and donated blood screened. Although it may be an important cost related issue, there does not seem to be studies in the US indicating how many infections were actually or potentially prevented by these costly screening procedures. Of course, the argument that even if one infection is prevented it is worth it, may also be difficult to refute at least on emotional, social and political grounds. However, a more valid query may address the amount of *direct* costs that are avoided by incurring the *indirect* costs in the preventive areas. Thus, it would be economically impossible to refute an argument that substantial direct economic costs, and some indirect ones due to not incurred losses of productivity and social costs, are avoided by incurring certain types of preventively related indirect costs. Unfortunately, there are not enough data processed or studied to arrive at some definitive answers in this regard.

Economic Forecasts of the Disease

There have been some studies attempting to map the future tracks of AIDS, both in terms of the number of cases and in terms of the costs involved. A recent study from two Columbia University economists suggest that past projections of the *number* of AIDS tend to exaggerate the future extent of the epidemic, particularly among gay/bisexual males and other high risk groups. Not finding evidence that the overprojection may have been significantly due to the use of AZT, or to the implementation of other medical treatments, the authors believe that substantial reductions in the number of newly infected gays commencing in 1983-85 may account for the upward bias[15].

The authors constructed crude projections of their own for AIDS cases to be reported to the CDC in 1994 and 1995, using two different statistical techniques, within major transmission categories such as blood transfusion and product utilization, homosexual/bisexual men, and intravenous drug users. The data used for the projections were based on those AIDS cases that were reported to the CDC between 1982 and 1990. They then combined their own method with those used in the past to generate a "composite projection"[16]. The results indicate that traditionally projected AIDS frequencies are much higher, in all transmission categories, than their own, or those of the composite projection results. The traditionally used methods yielded 72,000 new cases in 1994 and 79,000 new cases for 1995, while the method that combined the authors' with the traditional one resulted in 55,000 and 57,000 new cases respectively. For the two transmission categories (gays/bisexual, and blood products categories), the authors' own projections have dropped substantially bellow those of traditional studies (for gays/bi's 15,000 v 32,000 in 1994, and 11,000 v.34,000 in 1995). The traditional method projected a 72% increase in the number of new cases between 1991 and 1995 (a +10% change between 1994 and 1995 alone). Their composite method yielded a relatively low increase of 24% between 1991-94 (a +4% change between 1994-95). Finally, with significant implications for social policy and resource allocation decisions, traditional methods suggested gays/bi's as the dominant transmission category during 1994-95, while the authors' composite projection pointed with greater emphases on iv/drug users[17].

A study, focusing on projecting the *direct costs* (hospital inpatient care, physicians, drugs, nursing homes, and home health care) of AIDS, was published recently, although it also ventured into forecasting the number of AIDS cases for the immediate future[18]. This study did not consider more indirect cost factors such as testing, education, social support services, transportation. Furthermore, the study took into consideration a new categorization of HIV infected patients in terms of the potential care needed: (a) those with full-blown AIDS, (b) patients with a T-cell count under 200; and (c) and those over 200, indicating that those with AIDS should include not only people with the full-blown syndrome, but also those with a T-cell count under 200. It is further indicated that there are about twice as many people with the HIV infection without AIDS as those with AIDS, and the former category is roughly equally divided between those under and those above the 200 T-cell count level [18a].

Four calculation methods were used (two statistical extrapolation models and two back calculation models - those labeled as "traditional" in the study discussed above) in projecting the *number* of AIDS patients based on the number of cases reported to the CDC. The four methods used by the author yield remarkably close results for the years 1992, 1993, 1994 and 1995: 66,296-66,667 (1992); 76,187-78,370 (1993); 86,790-86,532 (1994), and 91,363-97,805 (1995). The CDC's 1990 projection ranges for 1992 and 1993 were 58,000-85,000 and 61,000-98,000, respectively. The number of fully-blown AIDS patients alive and likely requiring inpatient hospital care, or equivalent, was projected as 176,811 (1992), 203,191 (1993), 231469 (1994), and 260,846 (1995).

The cost of HIV infected treatment is projected in three categories: (a) the cost of treating AIDS patients, (b) that for HIV infected patients with a T-cell count under 200, and (c) those over 200. The total healthcare cost of *patients with AIDS* is the sum of inpatient hospital cost (IC) and that of outpatient hospital costs (OC); IC=ALOSxAHCxH, where ALOS is the average length of stay during each hospitalization, AHC is the average hospital charge per day, and H is the number of hospitalization instances. OC=OP+LT+HC+D, where OP is the frequency of outpatient visits, added to long-term care (LT), to home care (HC), and drug utilization (D). Thus, the annual cost of AIDS patient care is IC+OC. Among the components, in New York, the cost distribution was found to be as follows: IC (82%), outpatient hospital (8.7%), long-term care (.7%), home care (2.6%), and AZT and other drugs (5.6%). The average medical cost of treating AIDS patients, alive during any part of a given year, is $38,300. If during that given year, the average number of months lived by an AIDS patient is 7.5, the average monthly cost comes to $5,100, and the average survived lifetime cost over an estimated 20 month period is $102,000[19].

In addition to AIDS patients, the other two categories of patients include those infected with the HIV, but do not have full-blown AIDS symptoms yet, may be divided into those with a T-cell count under 200 (already seriously ill), and those with a T-cell count equal to or over 200. The average annual cost, in 1991 dollars, of treating a person with *AIDS* is estimated at $28,700 (inpatient hospital), plus $$9,600 (outpatient - made up of $$3,660 for office visits, $420 for long-term care, $1,460 for home health care, and $4,060 for drugs), for a total of $38,300. The same cost factors, also in 1991 dollars, for other HIV infected patients with *T-cell counts of less than 200*, were $7,603 (inpatient), and $5,922 (outpatient). For HIV patients with *T-cell count equal to or greater than 200*, these estimates are $2,323 (inpatient), and $4,121 (outpatient). The demarcation of these disease stage-based categories appears to be justified by the ratios of the costs involved. AIDS patients are three times as expensive per annum to treat as HIV patients with less than 200 T-cell count, and some six times as expensive as those with T-cell count equal to or over 200. Much of this difference is attributable to the cost of *inpatient hospital* care ($28,700, $7,603, and $2,323 for the three categories respectively). In the outpatient categories, the numbers are relatively comparable for office visits, long-terms care is estimated only for AIDS patients, home healthcare utilization costs do, however, dramatically increase as the disease progresses ($1,460, $423, and $81, for the three categories respectively). Since drug therapy is used from the discovery of the disease, and although it intensifies as the disease progresses, the differences among the three stage categories of the disease, in terms drug costs, are relatively small ($4,060 for AIDS, and $2,498, $1,405 for the other two respectively)[20].

One way or another, society bears the explicit and opportunity costs of treating people with the three identified stages of the HIV infection. The costs are high, they are increasing, and they contain a multitude of components, some of which are more measurable and identifiable than others. The annual cumulative cost burden on society depends on the number of patients surviving and the cost of treating those patients during any given year, or a part thereof. Based on published data, the cumulative projected annual cost (in $ billions) of treating patients with *AIDS* during 1992-1995 is estimated at $6.8(92), $7.8(93), $8.9(94), and $10 (95). For those with an HIV positive diagnosis and a T-cell count *under 200*, these estimates are $2.4(92), $2.7(93), $3.1(94), $3.5(95). For those with equal to or *greater than 200* T-cell counts, the corresponding estimates are $1.1, $1.3, $1.4, and $1.6. Thus, the total projected costs of treating all HIV infected patients, regardless of the stage, although diagnosed as HIV positive, for these four years, are $10.3, $11.8, $13.5, and $15.1. These projected costs will have increased annually between 12.7% and 15%[21].

As we indicated earlier, in addition to increases in inpatient costs because of hospital daily charge and LOS increases for HIV patients, some outpatient cost components have also increased. However, we also noted that increases in the cost of the various drug therapies were also important. In the following section, I will take a closer look at how and to what extent drugs are contributing to the cost of HIV infection treatment, and in particular, how these drugs have been developed so far.

HIV/AIDS Drug Development and Their Cost

Governments have been blamed for many social and economic ills of the past. Indeed, government participation in endeavors otherwise deemed commercially feasible has been viewed by many economists as the second best solution, and it may very well be. Political campaigns, election platforms, and similar missions have been predicated upon removing "big government" from the everyday lives of people, advocating the efficiencies and self-interest motivations of the private sector to produce and distribute in most areas of endeavors. This anti-government posture, however, may, at least partially, need to be reexamined when one discovers the role of government in the development of HIV/AIDS related drugs. In fact, government displayed extensive involvement in the development of drugs presently used for mitigating the actual and potential ravages of the HIV infection. Government scientists, under a National Cancer Institute Grant seeking remedies against tumor developments, discovered AZT in 1964, much before AIDS or HIV has ever been heard of. And it was government scientists who first risked human tests to establish AZT's affect on the HIV virus[22].

We will note shortly that in addition to AZT, two other drugs are also prominent in society's attempts to deal with HIV/AIDS: ddI, and ddC. These drugs also grew out of government research, although, with considerable implications for drug costs, and in contrast to AZT, the government applied for patents on ddI and ddC presumably to secure some return on initial outlays by way of licensing and royalty opportunities, and to retain at least an opportunity to control market pricing for these drugs. Thus, ddI's licensing to Bristol-Meyer is supposed to protect the patient by providing for reasonable pricing[23].

In addition to thus far having discovered all three major drugs administered to HIV/AIDS patients, the government to a large degree also covers their retail cost by being a major third-party payer, through it Medicare and Medicaid programs. Furthermore, the Social Security Administration in 1990 alone expended some $200 in disability benefits to HIV/AIDS patients[24]. Let us take a closer look behind the development and current pricing, and cost structures, of HIV/AIDS drugs.

In April 1984, the human immunodeficiency virus (HIV - or T-cell lymphotrobic virus type III, HTLV-III) was discovered. By mid-1984, the National Institutes of Health, along with the National Cancer Institute, implemented a drug screening system, requesting pharmaceutical companies to offer drugs from their inventory so that they may be tested on the HIV virus. Borroghs-Wellcome (BW) sent a drug that was first created in 1964 funded by the National Cancer Institute in order to control tumors - azidothymidine (AZT)[25]. After experiments with AZT, during 1985 the National Cancer Institute found it to inhibit the multiplication of the HIV and made an agreement with BW to continue to supply the drug while NCI would supply BW with an important component of the drug, thymidine, until BW found its own supplier. Further controlled experiments indicated that with AZT the survival period of AIDS patients, in particular the time period between the presumed infection with the HIV and the onset of full-blow AIDS has been considerably extended. Thus, after less than three years after the NCI search for the drug, AZT was approved in 1987 for widespread human applications.

Along with AZT, two other drugs were developed by government scientists, and by 1991 were administered to AIDS patients: dideoxyinosine (ddI) was licensed to Bristol-Myers Squibb which manufactures it under the trade name VIDEX; and dideoxycytidine (ddC), licensed to Hoffman-LaRoche. The latter could be administered if patients have already found AZT and ddI ineffective[26]. Although other drugs, including genetically engineered ones, are also under development, these three drugs remain the mainstay of anti-AIDS/HIV threrapy. Furthermore, because of developed resistance to these drugs, and their side-effects, they are often administered in combination with each other[27]. Although the three mentioned drugs make up the mainstay of the anti-HIV/AIDS drug therapy, close to a hundred other drugs are under trials and experiments addressing mainly the problems such as carcinomas and infections that set in after the immune system has deteriorated to the its relatively final stages. Thus, by late 1991, close to a hundred drugs and vaccines were in clinical testing against HIV and AIDS related diseases[28].

The government's active support for AIDS/HIV related drugs by way of research, development, financing, and accelerated approval was augmented by the government's legislative support through the *Orphan Drug Act* (ODA)[29]. An "orphan drug" (OD) is one that is development for a disease or a condition affecting less than 200,000 patients, hence the development of which, and the expenditure of its development costs, would simply not be warranted by its potential profitability. ODA provides two major financial umbrellas for the developer of the drug: (a) once the drug is approved for sale, the developer/manufacturer has a 7 year marketing exclusivity; (b) the cost of clinical research can be recovered by tax credit[29]. By early 1991, the FDA granted OD designations to some 400 drugs, which, in the same time, generated significant windfall profits for manufacturers, and may have substantially, and possibly unjustifiably, contributed to pharmaceutical price inflation, particularly since a condition which affects 200,000 people at the beginning, may ultimately afflict millions. Over half of the drugs approved or under trials for HIV/AIDS and related illnesses enjoy OD status, thus preventing the emergence of competition, and possibly allowing for conditions of price gouging[30]. While the number of people afflicted with an AIDS-related condition may be under 200,000 at the time of developing the drug, and even during its clinical trials, by the time the drug reaches the market, the actual and potential number of customers may reach many times the designated 200,000 ceiling. This situation is made even more difficult to control since an OD designation to a drug is assigned based on the number of users estimated at the time the designation is petitioned. Furthermore, if cost or market conditions have changed so that the development costs have been recovered, reasonable profits have been made, and the size of the market has notably increased beyond the initially estimated 200,000, there appear to be no provisions for a timely withdrawal of the OD status from a drug, so that effective competition could enter into the market, and costs could come under market control. Given consistent increases in sales of HIV/AIDS related drugs because of the spreading of the epidemic, drug related profits could be controlled, drug prices lowered, if they were released from the protection of the ODA. Taxpayer assistance accorded to drug manufacturers by way of the government scientists' initial contribution, by way of accelerated approval processes, and by way of legislative protection through the ODA, needs to be reciprocated by commensurably lower drug prices to the consumer.

When lawmakers queried from BW why AZT, at least initially, cost some $10,000 per annum, per patient, various items such as the cost of anti viral research, care for clinical trial participants, potential competition, and input costs, were mentioned without any specific dollar amounts[31]. Since the government conducted most of the developmental research, initial tests and clinical trials, and continues its active role in the process, AZT's developmental costs, including large supplies of its raw materials, up to the marketing stage was largely born by the taxpayer. AZT was approved in 1987, and the first patent protection to 2005 was granted in 1988. The patent was preceded several years by ODA protection granted to BW. In 1987, AIDS activitist prevailed on BW to reduce the price of AZT by 20%, and in 1989 by another 20%. Yet, the value of AZT shipments grew from $158 million in 1988 to some $600 million by the end of 1991[32]. The cost of one year's supply of AZT for the average patient is now at about $6000, and the market has grown from an initially estimated 60,000 to over one million in the United States alone, added to that some 6-8 million world-wide, and the recent approval of the drug for pediatric AIDS treatment[33].

References

1   Fee, E. and Fox, D.M. "The Contemporary Historiography of AIDS" Journal of Social History, Vol. 23, 1989, pp.303-14. See also Fox. D.M. "AIDS and American Health Polity:The History and Prospects of a Crisis of Authority", in AIDS:The Burdens of History, Fee. e. Fox. D.M. (eds), University of California Press, Berkeley CA. 1988.

2   Center For Disease Control, "Quarterly Report to the Domestic Policy Council on the Prevalence and Rate of Spread of HIV and AIDS - US" Mortality and Morbidity Report, Vol. 37, 1988, p.551. For comments suggesting that these projections were high, see Hay, L. "Projecting the Medical Costs of AIDS and ARC in the US" Journal of Acquired Immune Defficiency Sysndrome", Vol. 1, 1988, p.466

3   Sisk, K. "The Cost of AIDS: A Review of the Estimates" Health Affairs, Vol. 6, 1987, p.16; Bloom, D. and Carliner, G. "The Economic Impact of AIDS in the United States" Science, Vol. 239 1988, p.604; See also Scitovski, A.A. and Rice "Estimates of the Direct and Indirect Costs of AIDS in the US, 1985, 1986, and 1991" Public Health Reporter Vol. 102, 1987, p.5; and, Hellinger, F.J. "Forecasting the Personal Medical Care Costs of AIDS from 1988 through 1991" Public Health Reporter, Vol. 103, 1989, p.309.

4   CDC "HIV Virus Infection in the US: A Review of Curent Knowledge" Mortality and Morbidity Weekly Reports. - Supplement, S-6, 1987. However, see also Osmond and Moss "The Prevalence of HIV Infection in the US: Reappraisal of the Public Health Service Estimates" AIDS Clinical Review, Vol. 1, 1989.

5   Hardy, A.M., Rauch, K. Echenberg, D. Morgan, W.M. and urran, J.W. "The Economic Impact of the First 10000 Cases of AIDS in the US" JAMA, Vol. 255, 1986 pp. 209-11

6   Scitovsky, A.A. Cline, M. and Lee, P.R. "Medical Care Costs of Patients With AIDS in San Francisco" JAMA Vol. 256, 1986, pp.3103-6

7   Seage, G.R. Lander, S. Barry, . Groopman,J. Lamb, G.A. Epstein A.M. "Medical Care Costs of AIDS in Massachussetts" JAMA, Vol. 256, 1986, pp. 3107-9

8   Johnson A.M. Adler, M.W. Crown, J.M. "The AIDS and Epidemic of Infection with HIV: Costs of Care and Prevention in Inner London District" British Medical Journal Vol. 293,1986, pp. 489-92

9   Institute of Medicine, National Academy of Sciences "Cost of Healthcare for HIV Related Conditions" published in Confronting AIDS:Directions for Public Healthcare and Research, National Academic Press, Washington DC 1986, pp.155-73

10   Wachter, R.M. Luce, J.M. Turner, J. Volberding, P. and Hopewell, P.C. "Intensive Care of Patients with AIDS. Outcome and Changing Patters of Utilization" *American Review of Respiratory Diseases*, Vol. 134, 986, pp.891-6. See also Arno, P.S. "The Nonprofit Sector's Response to the IADS Epidemic: Community Based Services in San Francisco" *American Jounral of Public Health*, Vol. 76, 1986, pp.1325-30

11   See Arno

12   Jaffe, H.W., Darrow, W.M. Echenberg, D.F. O'Malley, P.M. Getchell, I.P. Kalyanamaran, V.S. Byers, R.H. Drennan, D.P. Braff, E.H. Curran, J.W. and Francis, D.P. "The AIDS in a Cohort Homosexual Men" *Annals of Internal Medicine* Vol. 104 1985, pp.210-4

13   See Hardy et al

14   Wells, N. The AIDS Virus: Forecasting Its Impact, *Office of Health Economics*, London 1986.

15   Bloom, D.E. Glied, S. "Projecting the Number of New AIDS Cases in the US" *NBER Working Paper* # 4189, October 1992.

16   See Bloom & Glide, Table 6.

17   See Bloom & Glide, p. 12

18   Hellinger, F.J. "Forecasts of the Costs of Medical Care for Persons with HIV: 1992-95" *Inquiry* Vol. 29, Fall 1992, pp.356-65

18a HIV can destroy the human immune system which to a large extent is made up different classes of blood cells. These blood cells identify so called antigens (foreign microorganisms) in the blood stream, and respond by producing antibodies. The latter bind to antigens and aid in their removal. The helper T-cells (T-helper lymphocytes), a type of white blood cells, produce certain chemical signals to alert and activate specific disease-fighting cells and the antibodies (it "calls to arms"). The HIV invades these "early warning systems", the T-cells, and destroys them. It invades the T-cells by camouflaging itself as a substance similar to the outer-coating the T-cell. The "early warning system", the signals to produce antibodies, the immune system, ceases to function. Parasitic infections and other maladies, including various forms of cancer, set in, most of which could normally be dealt with by a healthy immune system, with fatal results. A person testing positive to HIV, means only that, that he/she is likely to have the virus, the person is "seropositive", infectious, and can transmit. It does not mean that the person has AIDS. These people are likely to appear totally healthy, and asymptomatic for many years. In fact, it appears at this time that not all those infected with the HIV will develop full-blown AIDS in the near future, although AIDS related complex (ARC), a non-fatal but nevertheless clearly symptomatic condition may develop as a result of HIV infections, involving recurrent fever, fatigue, progressive weight loss, swollen lymph glands, profuse night sweats, and diarrhea. See, *Mayo Clinic Medical Handbook*, 1992. p.987. Jaret, P. "War Within" *National Geographic*, Vol. 169, 1986, p.702. Laurence, J. "The Immune System in AIDS", *ScientificAmerican*, December 1984,pp.84-90; CDC, USDPTHHS,

Voluntary HIV Counselling and Testing: Facts, Issues and Answers, 1990; Surgeon General's Report, *Acquired Immune Defficiency Syndrome*, 1986.

19   See Hellinger, p.360

20   See Hellinger p.361.

21   See Hellinger p.362

22   Mitsuya, J. "Credit Government Scientists With Developing Anti-AIDS Drug" *New York Times* September 1989, A26.

23   Chase, K. "Borrows-Wellcome Reaps Prifts, Outrage from its AIDS Drug, *Wall Street Journal,* September 15, 1989. Marx, L. "New AIDS Drugs Passes First Clinical Tests" *Science*, Vol.245, 1989, p.353

24   Office of the Secretary of Health,AIDS - Total FederalGovernment Spending (2/23/1990); HCFA, Estimated Federal Medicaid and Medicare Costs of AIDS.

25   Yarchoan, J. and Broder, A. "Development of Antiretroviral Therapy of the Acquired Immuno deficiency Syndrome and Related Disorders: A Progress Report" *New England Journal of Medicine*, Vol. 316 1987, p.557. See also AIDS, Drugs , Need and Greed, *New York Times*, September 29, 1989, A34.

26   Pharmaceutical Manufacturers Association, *AIDS Medicines in Development*, 1991.

27   Stroud, K. "Will New Drugs Help Tame the AIDS Virus?" *Investors Daily*, June 9, 1990.

28   See PMA, p.1

29   Public Law 97-414, 96 Stat.2049 (1983)

30   Food and Drug Administration (FDA), Office of Orphan Products Development, *Orphan Designation Through August 31, 1991.*

31   AIDS Issues Part I: *Cost and Availability of AZT.* Hearings Before the House Subcommittee on Health and Environment, Committee on Energy and Commerce. 100th Congress, 1st Session 31 (1987).

32   BW, Annual Reports, 1987-1991.

33   Lavella, K. "AIDS Drug Brings Providers Challenge of Distribution" *Modern Health Care*, September 29, 1989, pp.38-39. See also Cimons, L. "AZT Cleared for Children's Use. First Such AIDS Drug" *Los Angeles Times* May 4, 1990, p.A4; Oram and Walsh "Wellcome AIDS Drug Wins US Approval" *Financial Times*, March 3, 190.p I4. Okie, S. "Complacency Seen Hurting AIDS Fight" *Washington Post*, Nov.2 1989; Gladwell, M. "AIDS Forecast Focuses on Third World" *Washington Post* June 18, 1991.

Chapter 26
POLITICS, POLICY, REGULATION AND COST CONTAINMENT

A society's responsibilities may be presumed to include a concern for the health of its legitimate members (lately, much was said in the news media about the cost of providing healthcare for illegal immigrants), what healthcare services to provide, how much to provide, how to provide, and, for whom to provide healthcare in certain particularly underprivileged segments of society - in fact, the same set of questions may apply to healthcare distribution that are often reiterated in principles of economic courses for the economy as a whole. However, because a person's life and welfare directly depends on his or her health, and care for that health, healthcare has been deemed by many as a special commodity to which all members of society should have access, to some degree, at some time, and at some or no cost. If you are human, and if you are sick, you should be cared for. Yet, if you are the same human but lack money, food, clothing, or shelter, then to a large extent and often completely you are on your own. If you cannot provide for yourself by eating properly, by clothing yourself properly, or by having protection over your head from the elements, i.e. if you are homeless, then you are likely to get sick. Thus, healthcare problems emerge through the front door, and through the backdoor. And, to the extent that we create and allow the existence of conditions to proliferate which cause illnesses, we ourselves compound our problems associated with the production and distribution of healthcare. So, as a society, we want to create a healthcare system with hopefully equal *access* for all, the *cost* of which is *fairly distributed* among members of society, to secure a fair income level for providers who will supply high *quality* services with minimum administrative costs, with the overall cost of the system to society under control at a desirable level.

In order to achieve socially acceptable healthcare production and distribution patters and costs levels, a number of options may be available. Given the pending reforms offered by the Clinton administration, it may be healthful to review some of the options. (a) One way to produce and distribute healthcare is by completely relying on *unimpeded market forces*. The government stays out of the picture, no publicly funded plans for anyone, and no tax-system supported subsidies for health care at any socio-economic level of society. There are many providers coordinated or possibly competing to some extent with each other. (b) *Impeded market* forces by limited government participation for the benefit of those who would otherwise have no access to healthcare. Government participation takes the form of publicly funded insurance programs, and selectively applied tax-breaks. There are many providers coordinated or possibly competing to some extent with each other. Not unlike the system that prevailed in the US for the past few decades, particularly prior to the early 1980s. (c) Legislatively mandated *employment-based* or employer financed healthcare plans or insurance, with the government filling the gap for those not falling in the private sector category. Once again with many competing providers present[1]. (d) Rationed healthcare by way of government vouchers for everyone, optionally supplemented by using private funds to enhance choice, used to procure care through private insurers or directly from providers, without any other tax-based subsidies, but with the government supplying care for some selected needy segments of the population[2]. (e) A single-payer system, possibly by way of a national health insurance system, and tax-based funding system is supplemented by mandatory employer contributions. Additional care may purchased by using private funds[3]. (f) same as (e), except with the proscription of additional care procurement with private funds so as not to strain supply capacity. (g) A *single-payer* system funded by taxation, where outpatient or ambulatory services are offered by many private individual providers, and hospital care is supplied by institutional providers directly supported by the government, with additional privately funded purchases permitted in the outpatient private sector, but not in the institutional hospital sector[4]. (h) A *British-style* national health service which directly employs private providers, and administers institutional providers and hospitals, making healthcare accessible and affordable to everyone, although supplementary care may be procured privately from individual providers with private funds.

The present system in the US may benefit from selected elements of most of these alternatives. Medicaid does provide care of some quality for many of the poor. However, other poor and "near-poor" people are left out, and need to rely on overcrowded and often poorly (both in terms of quality and quantity) staffed emergency rooms where their care, in turn, is "financed" by other patients and payers of the hospital by way of various modes of "cost-shifting", the scope of which is likely to be progressively limited as managed care proliferates, and privately (insurance or out-of-pocket) funded care becomes the exception rather than the rule. With Medicare not covering long-term care, the elderly in nursing homes "spend-down" themselves of their life-earned savings and life-time of hard-work generated wealth, until they become eligible for Medicaid, ironically after which they absorb a substantial portion of Medicaid funds initially designated for a totally different (poor) segment of the population. Rationing of healthcare, to be discussed extensively later in this chapter, has often been considered as a remedy, and, in fact, is already being utilized, even within the US (in addition to Canada and elsewhere)[5]. In addition, part-time workers of most companies, large or small, are typically uninsured. Other families not having insurance for many years until illness set in, suddenly find themselves in a difficult predicament by either not being able to get coverage because of existing conditions, or not being able to get care for lack of coverage. An argument to the effect that such predicament is simply the price a person or family has to pay for lacking foresight and prudence by securing coverage while they were well runs into social, moral, and ethical barriers in our society with an inevitable return to references to the unique nature of healthcare as a commodity as distinct from other commodities, to the rights of all members of society to have access to that commodity, and the moral obligation of society to provide that commodity to its legitimate members. So, we are back to where we started, indicating at least some of the complexities of the healthcare predicament. The following sections of this chapter will examine some of the regulatory, policy, legal and marketing implications of this predicament.

Healthcare Regulation in Society's Interest

In terms of its ultimate management, the healthcare scene has been under the influence of largely two schools of thought: one advocates the importance of competition as a managing agent in some viable healthcare market place, while the other, relying on administrative or discretionary measures, regulates to mandate certain range of operational or financial conduct. These two intellectual approaches to solving perennial cost related issues in the practice of American medicine have existed along with each other for some two decades now. Ironically, at the present time, and in spite of, and probably even after the introduction of, the pending reforms from the Clinton Administration, the healthcare system has elements of both, competition to an ever increasing extent, along with regulation which, due to the heavy participation of third-party, particularly government, payers for healthcare also increasingly imprints its constraints. Yet, the cost-spiral dilemma continues, as does the continued weighing of the competitive approach against regulations of various forms.

Although in terms of standard economic principles, and the economic tradition of the United States, competition is often seen as a more desirable medicine to administer against continuously escalating healthcare costs, regulation has long been a governing mainstay on the healthcare scene. This is so, in spite of two decades of a relatively conservative Republican administration, and in spite of the fact that during these past two decades many other sectors have become deregulated, such as banking, the airlines, other transportation industries, telecommunication with the cable industry being the most recent example. Yet regulation has not arrested cost increases, and competition, to the extent it exists, has not done so either. Clearly, enunciated reasons would rest with the camp consulted: regulators would argue for more administrative measures, while competition advocates would push for larger doses of that remedy.

It should, however, be noted that the regulation of US medicine, in contracts to similar regulatory measures abroad, tended to control not the global budget aspects of healthcare but rather the conduct of providers. Thus, US healthcare regulation was largely conduct, instead of global budget, oriented. Rather than concentrating on the fees of physicians, particularly at least until the recent implementation of RVBVS reimbursement system in Medicare, and upon budgetary constraint for hospitals, medical regions, various provider segments and elements, as often done outside the United States, regulatory measures in this country focused on individual and institutional provider behavior, case-specific control, peer and utilization reviews. It is difficult to determine the exact reasons for these regulatory trends, however, it may be that the political scene in this country may still be more conducive for conduct rather than legislatively implemented global budgetary regulation. The reasons may also rest with specific interest groups that tend to dominate purchasers of healthcare on the one hand, and providers, on the other. Providers may have been adversely preoccupied with the growing sentiment for regulation, and chose the lesser of two evils, accepting conduct regulation over the implementation of specific budgetary constraints amounting to caps on their income. Consumers, on the other hand, may be seen as being divided between those in the government sector who politically disavow regulation but are fiscally forced to implement it, and an even more conservative private group stubbornly adhering to market-based principles[6].

Regulatory efforts of recent decades on the healthcare field, in terms of their gravity of implementation, may be divided into two major categories: decentralized and centralized, each of which, in turn, may be directed at financial, and not directly financial targets. Since these measures have already been discussed in the volume, we may simply list the items involved. *Decentralized* but not directly financial measures include professional standards review organizations (PSROs), health system agencies (HSAs), and certificate of need (CON) controls. The directly financial measures in this category were implemented largely by rate setting. *Centralized*, but not directly financial efforts, on the other hand, include peer review organizations (PROS), practice guidelines, and outcomes research, while the directly financial ones were prospective payment systems (PPS), and the recently implemented medicare payment systems to physicians by way of the resource based relative value scale (RBRVS)[7].

Concern for the quality of healthcare was a basis for the 1989 creation of the *Agency for Health Care Policy and Research* (AHCPR)[8]. Its mandate focused on scrutinizing the outcome and effectiveness of medical care and research, intensifying an already elaborate conduct regulation system in place. With the blessing of such medical groups as the AMA, the American College of Physicians, and the American Society of Internal Medicine, the Agency is charged with the development and dissemination of medical practice and standards guidelines. It can carry out research, develop guidelines, implement activities and systems of information, regarding health services, specifically regarding their effectiveness, efficiency, quality and results. It can do the same regarding clinical practice and ambulatory care, utilized technology, facilities and equipment. It can review costs, productivity and the market environment. It can examine preventive measures, health promotion, disseminate statistics, and report on medical liability. Much of the information dissemination would be by way of subject specific computer databases, and particular reports. At least initially, its operation was to be guided by a seventeen member advisory board, National Advisory Council for Health Care Policy, Research and Evaluation, made up of physicians, economists, lawyers and healthcare related business specialists[9].

The creation of the agency was in large part motivated by concern for the poor scientific basis for many areas in medical practice and much of medical care, inadequate congressional support for medical research, and the cost of running Medicare. The first concern, was based on studies which appeared to have revealed a lack of scientific basis for much of medical practice[10]. It was noted that services received by patients contained a substantial number of random factors, including the physicians "practice style", making the establishment of third-party payment criteria difficult[11]. The remedies for these problems were seen to rest with adequate research on medical practice outcomes. Lack of congressional support was seen as related to the first problem, and a major program supporting outcomes research was likely to ease up congressional finances. Finally, the third problem, the financial crises facing the Medicare program, may have precipitated preoccupation with the first two, particularly with medical practice outcomes research.

Healthcare Policy by Managing Competition and Not Just Care

At the writing of this chapter, the Clinton administration released a major healthcare reform proposal package. Once passed by Congress and signed into law by the President - pursuant to major transformations brought about by various political ineterst groups, it is unlikely to yield significant fundamental structural changes in the system. A sector that employs some nine million people now, and more as it continues to grow as it indeed will, traditionally based on market though not always competing principles in the United States, is not likely to be transformed into a single-payer nationalized healthcare system, such as the likes of Canada and Japan[12]. There is no question about the existence of problems associated with rapidly rising healthcare costs, and regarding the presence of some 37 million people without any or adequate health insurance. However, and without meaning at this point to invoke the various elaborate social, moral, ethical and political arguments regarding the rights of all to healthcare, some 85% of the US population *is* insured, with their health insurance being financed largely or completely by their employer by way of tax-free financial benefits. Their vested interest in fundamental structural healthcare reforms could be in doubt. Indeed, even those who lack coverage can receive care if they seek it, although under less desirable circumstances with the costs shifted onto those who can afford it, or absorbed by the provider. Incidentally, cost shifting is not new or unique to the healthcare profession. The airlines have been, and to some extent still are, doing it between various short and long-distance markets, and they have particularly been doing so prior to deregulation. During initial stages of the campaign, candidate Clinton frequently advocated a "play-or-pay" approach - employers either covering employees directly, or indirectly way of paying a tax. Political pressures, however, have caused him shift emphases to the notion of "managed competition", and the same with a budgetary cap from above as an alternative.

The political, ideological and real tasks facing the healthcare system include controlling cost inflation, making the system accessible to all, and maintaining or improving the quality of care. Managed competition, and managed care - discussed at length earlier in the volume, confused at times but differ from each other. We may recall that *managed care* is supplied by HMOs and PPOs by limiting the patient's choice of among providers within an organized care system, and by conventional commercial insurers offering indemnification insurance plans with a relative freedom of provider choice, but nevertheless "managing" care by monitoring, screening and frequently denying claims. In general, managed care plans control costs by managing provider conduct in various ways. Thus, group and staff model HMOs provide generally defined care by way of multispecialty group practices with full-time salaried doctors functioning at HMO owned facilities. IPAs, a network of independent but nevertheless HMO affiliated providers devoting at least part of their time to HMO/IPA subscribers under an IPA established system of care and payments to providers. Virtually all forms of HMO combine the delivery and insurance aspects of care and assume the financial risks for a contracted pre-payment of fixed premiums, attempting to control costs by prevailing, through various often unpopular means, upon physicians to practice with cost containment in mind. No such close control and practice monitoring or modifying efforts were normally imposed on physicians by the managed care plans of indemnity insurance companies, beyond paying the doctors' bills, although PPOs in general often choose a group of participating physicians based on the latter's practice patterns from cost and efficiency points of view. A predominant portion of those insured through employer sponsored plans (over 150 million people) are delegated to managed care plans of one type or another, although less than 10% of some 60 million people covered by Medicaid or Medicare belong receive their benefits through managed care organizations. At any rate, it is now apparent that managed care delivery alone, no matter how widely proliferated, has not and is not likely to control costs, and may interfere with efficiency and quality due to most managed care plans' designed interference with the practice of medicine itself.

Under the traditional fee-for-service healthcare distribution system, the patient, not using his or her own money, chose the physician, and normally a third-party (typically some health insurance organization) paid the doctor for services rendered, with the former having had no bargaining power over the latter. The physician chose any option he or she wanted for prescribing medicine, once again without any control over contents and costs from the payer. Having no bargaining power, nor the incentive to lower price due to the presence of third-party coverage, the patient rarely engaged the doctor in any negotiations regarding fees and had little knowledge or understanding of the nature and certainly the quality of services to be rendered.

The concept of *managed competition* in healthcare has been in the making and continuous refinement for almost two decades. Back in 1978, Professor Enthoven of Stanford suggested that the benefits of managed care may be combined with those of market competition, yielding what became to be known as "managed competition". The essence of the idea may first be briefly summarized as follows: managed care organizations were seen to compete in terms of price and quality for contract with so called "sponsors" (employers, other third-party payers including the government, and health insurance coalitions) under the watchful eyes of public regulatory agencies who would approve managed care plans, enforce open enrollment, monitor quality, and define the portfolio of standard benefits. The cost of the lowest priced plan would be tax deductible, and the cost differential between the lowest level and anything above, if chosen by employers or individuals, would need to be covered by taxable income. Plans would be subject to quality control and periodic outcome studies. The "sponsors" would make a predetermined contribution that would apply to the cost of coverage for the patients for whom they coordinate the available plan options.

Managed competition attempts to overcome the consumer's traditional impotence in healthcare markets by way of systematic purchasing arrangements designed to control costs and maintain quality. An entity, the "managed competition coordinator" (MCC), which may be public, private, or a healthcare purchasing cooperative, consolidates the purchasing power of a large group, or groups, of consumers (subscribers) by selecting healthcare plans, and otherwise ensuring eminence of price/quality competition among providers and insurers. Thus, the MCC is basically a higher level umbrella healthcare intermediary which contracts with health plans regarding prices, coverage, and other terms of the contract. However, being the MCC entails more than just an administrative purchasing agent for healthcare consumer groups, for it needs to negotiate by using judgment, market finesse in a very imperfect market environment[13]. Thus, it needs to possess the necessary data and expert advice in order implement competition at lower levels of healthcare intermediation. Managed competition in implemented *not* at the particular provider level but at the levels of healthcare intermediation by way of third-party financing and healthcare delivery plans. The competitive impact of managed competition upon providers is to divide the latter into competing groups, within and among communities, thus prompting them to behave in a manner more consistent with the neoclassical principles of microeconomic competition, primarily in terms of price, quality and efficiency[14].

Price competition is implemented in terms of annual premiums charged to subscribers for health plan participation, and not at the provider level. This creates the environment where the provider prescribes the services and medication needed by the patient, yet the cost of these services to the patient (the price) is embodied in the annual premium they pay for the health plan, a price they can readily understand, interpret and compare among health plans. Copayments and deductibles, set by service and easily understood by patients, also prompt patients to once again to make informed price-based decisions[15].

In contrast to frequent traditional health insurance practices of choosing subscribers based on experience, namely healthy people accommodated and at a much lower cost than those with serious pre-existing conditions ("experience rating"), prompting the latter to often go without insurance, MCCs, simultaneously dealing with a number of health plans bidding for business, can ascertain that the coverage is uniform in cost and availability within each plan, although there may be cost and coverage differences among health plans in comparison to a basic plan, in which case the subscriber simply pay the difference. The MCCs would be in the position to implement community rating and a continuous coverage within each plan, once again with cost differences among plans allowed for and paid by the subscriber. In order to implement this system, the MCC would be the sole gateway for subscribers to any health plan in the region (as we now find with large employer sponsored insurance plans) Thus, if any legitimate screening (for whatever reasons) is called for, and there may be few or none, it would be done by the MCC, rather than the health plans motivated by their profit potentials. The health plans may nevertheless benefit financially and directly by at least foregoing the administrative cost of marketing to individuals and small groups which has been estimated at some 40% of filed claims[16]

An important function attributed to the MCC is to transform the healthcare market from its traditional price-insensitive state to one with significant price sensitivity, i.e. from a one where the revenues moved in the same direction as price because of low price elasticity of demand to one where revenue moves in the opposite direction to price. Under these circumstances, there would be an incentive to lower price as the consequent increase in quantity demanded is proportionately greater than the percentage drop in price, causing a net increase in revenue and, subject to relatively constant cost conditions, and increase in profits. There would be an incentive to compete, and there should be enough flexibility in price, with permissible cost levels and profit margins, for health plans to compete among each other for MCC contracts. The health plans within each region work with any given MCC would be standardized, facilitating mostly price and some quality comparisons, and reduce economic waste by product differentiation, and prevent market segmentation which gives emphases to coverage instead of price. Under these circumstances, patients can periodically, for administrative cost reasons no more often than once a year, migrate from one plan to another motivated largely by price instead of major differences among the plans, and without being concerned that a cheaper plan offers inferior coverage. Finally, the MCC would periodically publish medical practice outcome reports for providers in each of their respective health plans, as product information made available to their subscribers[17].

In view of the largely dispersed composition of the employed labor force, employers would be often incapable of acting as MCC for their employees. Some 40% of the employed labor force is with employers with a total number of employees 100 or less. Spreading the risk of coverage by a health plan over such a small group is not possible, yielding in the past, due mostly to their dominant experience rating, large variations among premiums paid by these various smaller groups. Furthermore, covering small groups preclude significant administrative economies of scale, yielding administrative expenses as high as 40% of claims for groups of 1-4 people, contrasted with 5.5% for groups covering 10,000 or more subscribers[18]. By way of a remedy, small employers' and individuals' purchasing power could be pooled and made substantially more market potent by a network of MCCs, so called *Health Insurance Purchasing Cooperatives (HIPCs)*. As nonprofit corporations, HIPCs would contract with small employers in their respective region, could not decline coverage for health related reasons to any group or individual, and its board of directors would be elected by participating employers. Thus, and HIPC would function as an MCC on behalf, and in the collective interest, of its subscribers. As other MCCs, HIPCs would amalgamate various risk levels combining those low and high cost experience groups, an unlikely combination otherwise, and would generate participants the same economic benefits as other MCCs do, such as individual plan choice, competition among plans for subscriber patronage, stable premiums, and administrative scale economies[19].

A universal system of coverage is thought to be workable financially by mandated full-time employee/employer participation, payroll taxes on part-time employees, taxes on other solvent non working persons. Every household would be held to a "play-or-pay" principle, by either mandated to join an HIPC, or pay a cost equivalent tax, thereby cross subsidizing the premiums of low or no-income households. In other words, the financial foundation of the system could be based on some type of payroll or other form of taxation[20]. From the providers' point of view, particularly for hospitals that often had to resort to cost-shifting whenever that was possible, the system would likely generate satisfactory income levels, because payment for all of their services would be assured, although at a level more controlled by competition managed and implemented by MCCs or HIPCs at health-plan levels[21].

Managed competition, as proposed and thus far discussed, may not provide an effective solution to the healthcare cost crisis. First, in its original and most often discussed form, it does not provide for a global cap on the healthcare budgets involved. No limit on total healthcare expenditures was envisioned in the model. Insurers can stay competitive at relatively high price levels instead of a socially more desirable low levels, allowing for consistent increases in their prices without any one of them getting out of line - a conduct not unusual, in fact typical, in oligopolistic markets with few competitors. Furthermore, while conscious parallelism behavior on the part of a few oligopolists has been frowned upon by antitrust enforcement agencies, price-leadership situations were repeatedly accepted in antitrust history as a way life. Secondly, even if prices were successfully contained, the providers' profit motive would, in the face of relatively fixed prices, likely turn to service curtailment, either in quantity or quality, although the contrary could be true in terms of quantity if they were to offset fixed prices by larger volume, which, in turn, could further curtail quality.

Before moving on to another perhaps more radical form of healthcare cost control, i.e. healthcare rationing, we should note that managed competition has been advanced in a variety of forms, in addition to the standard one, if we may call it that, first advanced over the years by Professor Enthoven. As we discussed, the essence of the Enthoven theory of cost containment by way of managed competition is to have market power-based large MCCs ("sponsors") force insurance companies and HMOs to lower their premiums, with the latter, in turn, constraining and keeping in line provider (individual and institutional) conduct and cost with the threat of excluding non performers from contracts. With much of the patient market ultimately assumed to be included or covered by managed care plans, the threat of contract denial to a provider by an HMO or insurance carrier would be tantamount to the latter's professional and business, at least within the context of clinical practice. In addition, Professor Enthoven originally envisioned employees paying for 20% of the least expensive plan's premium, plus to cover (co-pay) 20% of the cost of covered services, further mandating employers to offer this basic plan to all employee, otherwise pay a tax to a public fund. The financial impact of this plan on employers was seen by Enthoven as mitigated by an 8% reduction in the legal minimum wage. The marginal cost to the employer of a plan, if offered, better than the least expensive one would constitute taxable employee income - a built-in incentive for employees to join the least expensive plan, and to prevent the "moral hazard" related consequences of being protected from premium costs. Government would assume the responsibility for the coverage of self-employed and unemployed individuals, and a negative tax of a sort would finance a basic coverage for the poor. Although at this writing the Clinton plan has not been formally introduced, it appears that some sort of state-based healthcare expenditure targets are seen desirable by the President, although it is unclear how those targets will be implemented, and, particularly, enforced under a complex multi-payer (in contrast to a single-payer, normally by way of government, system). In addition, President Clinton does not appear to plan lowering the legal minimum wage.

A liberal version of the Enthoven plan was advanced by Senator Bob Kerrey, having employers pay into a public fund which would function as a universal MCC and contract with individual plans for the most cost-effective coverage. The marginal cost of plans above the minimum contracted by the government would be covered by the private sector, and those benefits provided or financed by the employer above the minimum would constitute taxable income. The conservative version of managed competition, advanced by President Bush's administration, would exempt employers from contributing to the public fund, replacing it by tax incentives to private persons or employers who would secure their own coverage from large healthcare coverage purchasing organizations, such as MCCs.

Cost Containment by Healthcare Rationing

Healthcare is an economic good. As such, it is the product of relatively scarce resources - limited amount of resources relative to an unlimited volume of human wants, so teach the first few pages of most textbooks of economic principles. In order to allocate scarce resources and their commodity or service products, we rely on the *market*. Uninhibited markets are capable of answering the basic questions of any economy (what, how much, how, and for whom) by transmitting the consumers' "dollar vote" to the producers, who make production decisions with a profit incentive in mind. Thus, some goods or services are "worth" producing, and some are not. Products and services will be produced, not produced, substituted, foregone, temporarily in excess supply, or temporarily in shortage - depending on the efficiency of markets. The market price suggests who will get what ("can afford"), and in what quantity. The market engages in perpetual rationing. Something we want it to do, something that we rely on it to do. Rationing in standard markets has been an accepted, even desirable, notion. It has commanded the faith of more people, governments and countries, than any other forms of resource allocation - and most others have, in fact, failed, or are under transformation toward market rationing of scarce resources and their products. So, why is the rationing of healthcare services, just another economic good (or, is it?) attracting so much emotion, contention, and, in general, public and private attention? In fact healthcare rationing is seen some time as something new, revolutionary, and a solution for yet unsolved problems. On the other hand, when we look at the healthcare scene, we cannot help noting that healthcare *is* already rationed. We have already noted some 67 million Americans who are either uninsured or have inadequate insurance. They are, to varying degrees, rationed out of the system - unless one assumes the unlikely that they have voluntarily withdrew from the system, with the latter being probably inconsistent with most definitions of rationing. For all intents and purposes, healthcare is already being rationed by price, geography, and in other terms. Yet, because healthcare is not viewed by most as a "standard" product or service, and the right and access to healthcare is often viewed as a social rather than private concern, rationing healthcare has become a major policy issue that is, at this stage of the volume, worth a brief look.

Health demands can easily be infinite. The marginal utility of healthcare, that is, the return on an additional unit of needed treatment, assuming a perceived or actually competent and honest provider, is always positive. Since society cannot devote all of its resources to the supply of healthcare, for if it did those resources would surely be absorbed, rationing must inherently be involved. Healthcare expenditures in the US have long been suspect, and having grown at a rate 250% higher than the general rate of inflation[22], they are viewed as unsustainable. We have invented more medicine, diagnostic and therapeutic tools and methods, than we can afford. Furthermore, this problem should be assessed not only in terms of perspectives, but also in terms of the prospective age composition of the population, slowed if not stalled economic growth, and the enormous national and international debts on the books. American medicine now sees virtually no limit to what it can do to treat or sustain an aging, or a young but severely injured, person. We, as a society, have a problem, and a relatively new one at that: we must balance often enunciated convictions in traditional personal choice and values regarding healthcare against scarce social resources and consequent inevitable priorities. Thus, rationing healthcare may be viewed as the price we must pay for our achieved successes in that field. The target is clearly to procure the maximum of amount healthcare for most of the people, under perennial resource availability constraints. The problem is compounded, indeed dramatized, by the distinction between the health of a nation, and that of an individual. Thus, once again, rationing enters the picture. As we will note in the next chapter, the US spends about 50% more on healthcare than some of the other major industrialized countries such as Japan, Canada, and the UK. Yet, we do not appear to have data to support any contention to the effect that Americans enjoy better health than people in those countries.

Thus, at what level should rationing healthcare be administered: "basic", "necessary", or "appropriate" level. How do we measure and identify these terms? Thus, do we stop with what is "necessary" - for survival, or do we deem necessary that is needed for general well being, and call that "basic", but not necessary? If by some criteria we include those that are "basic" into "what is necessary", we are bound to spend perhaps an extra $100 billion, which otherwise, restricting rationing to necessary for survival, could be saved. To further complicate matters, even if we were to be able to define these yardsticks, who is to implement them, and how? At what level with the criteria be defined, implemented and enforced? Who will bear the consequences, and how, of having implemented the inappropriate level of care under some circumstances? This list of queries could continue, and are certainly relevant to rationing. However, generating answers for them is, fortunately for the author, beyond the scope of this even this chapter, let alone the volume[23].

We can deal with some institutional issues, however. Rationing healthcare could be *implemented* at several levels. Physicians can do some of the rationing, or at least could substantially contribute to a rationing process by their application of technical know-how, wherever present, and by assessing the consequences of various treatment levels for the patient's potential welfare. Another contributor to the process could be the patients themselves, and perhaps they already do that by, for instance, staying away from treatment centers, creating living wills that specify the extent of healthcare they expect to receive with the probable consequences, and how long they wish to be kept alive, and in what condition, in emergency or traumatic situations. In addition, consumers can determine the entire policy of rationing by simply voting in majority through their law-makers. And when the doctor finds himself by the bed-side of a patient who cannot communicate his or her decision regarding rationing, it will be up to the physician to balance his duty to the patient and his possibly statutory obligation to society to preserve scarce resources as much as possible and, probably, prudently. Mechanisms will need to be placed in motion to ascertain that when a patient dies, it was not the result of malpractice but rather of a conscious and professionally prudent decision on the part of a physician not to apply, in his or her judgment futile, treatment in favor of preserving society's resources.

Some countries such as Canada and the United Kingdom implement rationing by central administrative decision-makers - "totalitarian healthcare", if you are so inclined. Decision makers decide on budgetary caps for financial institutions, and supervise service rationing. A somewhat similar perhaps related process involves rationing implemented by politicians through the legislative process. Given the large and increasing proportion of healthcare and related research funded and regulated by either federal or local, or both, governments, medicine may now be viewed as a social (if not public) good.

Once the source of implementation is decided, the *methods of rationing* needs to be explored. In this country we typically ration most commodities and services, including healthcare, by price, except in some parts of the country where availability, or physical access, may play a role. Other countries, such as the Untied Kingdom, outright limit quantity at some levels of care. Finally, existing insurance coverage and plans may themselves constitute a form of rationing which may fall somewhere between those based on price and access. This type of rationing may be divided into two categories: *low stratum rationing* implemented mostly at the primary care or ambulatory levels, and *upper stratum rationing*, implemented mostly at the tertiary care level. In the US, rationing in this context takes place mostly in low stratum categories by way of limiting access through having the patient pay in full (no coverage) for some primary services, or through high coinsurance and deductibles applied to primary care services, while typically covering more elaborate and expensive tertiary care services. Medicare does not, at least as of this writing, cover prescription drugs, and Medicaid rations healthcare among the poor by low physician reimbursement rates. Where upper stratum rationing is applied, such as in the UK and Canada, a national system of coverage for everyone rations tertiary care by limiting quantity or delaying treatment, allowing generally ready access at the primary care level[24]. Finally, whatever method of rationing is implemented, it may be applied formally or informally. The Oregon method of rationing (to be examined briefly below) is a direct form of organized distribution, governed by regulation and statutory rules. Informal rationing is typically contingent on provider and administrative discretion and may be based on professional or personal judgments, delays, and geographic discrimination.

The State of *Oregon* passed its Basic Health Services Act in 1989, providing access to uniform levels of healthcare for all uninsured state residents, and ranking medical procedures. The Oregon Plan is based on the premise that society has an obligation to provide a "basic level" of medical care benefits to its legitimate members at no cost financed by the state for those with incomes under the Federal Poverty Level, and through employment based plans for those above it, hence presumably employed. Much of the concern has existed over what constitutes a "basic level" of care, in addition to, and separately from, issues relating to the source of its financing. The passage of the Basic Health Services Act recognized that residents have the right to basic healthcare, that the funds covering the cost of such healthcare is limited, and some necessary care may be omitted from the "basic" package. The Oregon Health Services Commission was charged with setting a priority list for efficient and cost-effective medical care. The variables considered by the Commission in ranking services include measurable yardsticks of well-being (health), quality adjusted life years, actuarial costs, possible outcomes with and without treatment, and social standards. The Commission initially developed a subsequently ill-fated formula contrasting various disease categories with and without treatment, their respective expected outcomes, and cost estimates of specific treatments.

This formula proved to be unfunctional due largely to lack of data, the omission of screening, preventive, and morbidity related variables, problems with measuring quality adjusted life-years, and other related problems. Presently, alternative methods of ranking are being tested[25].

The problems that preceded the Oregon experiments, problems with pervasive presence throughout the United States, were aptly summed up in the Oregon Legislature by a local physician, also a member of the state legislature, as follows:

> When money is spent on one set of services, it is, by definition, not available to spend on other services. Health care services must compete with all other legitimate services state government must provide. An explicit decision to allocate money for one set of services means that an implicit decision has been made not to spend money on other services. That, in essence, constitutes the rationing of health care. State legislatures do it with every budget cycle. We are spending vast amounts of money on some people and virtually none on other people. We spend about three billion dollars a year on neo-natal intensive care while we deny pre-natal care to hundreds of thousands of women. We spend fifty billion dollars a year on people in the last six months of their lives while we are closing pediatric clinics because we claim that we do not have the resources to keep them open. We are rationing by default[26].

References

1   See for instance Enthoven, A. and Kronick, R. "A Consumer-Choice Health Plan for the 1990s: Universal Health Insurance In a System Designed to Promote Quality and Economy, Parts I and II" *New England Journal of Medicine*, Vol. 320, 1989, pp. 29-37 and pp.94-101.

2   See, Enthoven, A. "Consumer Choice Health Plans, Parts I and II" *New England Journal of Medicine*, Vol. 298, 1978, pp.650-8, and pp.709-720

3   See, Beauchamp, D.E. and Rouse, R.L. "University New York Health Care: A Single Payer Strategy Linking Cost and Universal Access" *New England Journal of Medicine*, Vol. 323, 1990, pp.640-44

4   Not unlike the Canadian system. Because of frequent comparisons between the US and Canadian healthcare delivery systems, citing the latter as a posible example to follow in the US, I will review the Canadian system in the next chapter.

5   The Oregon Medicaid rationing experience specifically will also be discussed later in the chapter.

6   Brown, L.D. "Political Evolution of Federal Health Care Regulation" *Health Affairs*, Vol. 11, No. 4, Winter 1992, pp 17-37

7   Brown discusses these at some length at pp.22-30

8   AHCPR was in fact created by the Omnibus Budget Reconciliation Act (OBRA) of 1989, Title IX of the Public Health Service Act, Section 6103 of OBRA, also amending Title XVIII of the Social Security Act - Medicare. It effectively replaced the National Center for Health Services Research and Health Care Technology Assessment (NCHSR). Its organizational level corresponds to those of the CDC, NIH, FDA, and the Health Resources and Services Adminsitration

9   Gray, B.H. "The Legislative Battle Over Health Services Research" *Health Affairs*, Vol. 11, No. 4, Winter 1992, pp.38-65

10   Wennberg, J.E. "Dealing With Medical Practice Variations: A Proposal For Action", *Health Affairs*, Summer 1984, pp.6-32 - cited in Gray. See also *Variations in Medical Practice*, Senate Appropriations Commitee Hearings, 1985. Roper, W.L. et al. "Effectiveness in Health Care: An Initiative to Evaluate and Improve Medical Practice" *The New England Journal of Medicine*, November 3, 1988, pp. 1197-1202. Bowen, O. Burke, T."New Directions in Effective Quality of Care: Patient Outcome Research" *Federation of American Health Systems Review* September/October 1988, pp.50-53. All cited in Gray.

11   Gray, at p.41

12   The following chapter will take a quick look at the Canadian, some of the European, and Japanese systems.

13   Enthoven A.C. "The History and Principles of Managed Competition" *Health Affairs*, Supplement 1993, pp. 24-48

14   Enthoven, at p.29. Enthoven uses the term "sponsors" instead of "coordinator".

15   Enthoven, at p.30

16   Enthoven, at p.30

17   Enthoven at pp.31-32

18   "Private Health Insurance: Options for Reform" House Ways and Means Committee on Health, 101st Congress, 2nd Session, Committee Print 101-35. US Government Printing Office, Washington D. C. 1990. Cited by Enthoven p.48.

19   Enthoven at pp.35-37. HIPCs would perform similar functions in relatively remote geographical areas with few or no population concentrations.

20   Enthoven at pp.42

21   For more detailed and varied discussions and hypotheses regarding HIPCs and other dimensions and issues of managed competition, the reader is referred to the entire issue of *Health Affairs*, Supplement 1993.

22   US Department of Commerce, *Statistical Abstracts of the United States*, 1990, Tables 141, 467, 756

23   For some of the issues, see Relman, A. S. " Is Rationing Inevitable" *New England Journal of Medicine* Vol. 322, 1990. p1809-10

24   For some discussion of these categories of rationing, see Merril C.J. and Cohen, A.B. "The Emperor's New Clothes: Unraveling the Myths About Rationing" *Inquiry* Vol. 24 1987 pp.105-7

25   For further particulars regarding the history and present status of the Oregaon Plan, see two articles by Crawshaw, R. :"Society Must Decide - Oregon Health Decisions: Bioevaluations Beyond Bio-Ethics" *The Western Journal of Medicine* 1986, pp.246-48, "Organ Transplans - A Search for Health Policy at the State Level", *The Western Journal of Medicine* 1989, pp.361-63; and, Crawshaw, R., Carland, M. Hines, B. and Anderson, B. "Developing Principles for Prudent Health Care Allocation: The Continuing Oregon Experiemnt" *The Western Journal of Medicine* 1990, pp. 441-46, and Crawshaw, R., Garland, M., Hines, B. and Lobitz, C. "Oregon Health Decisions" *JAMA*, 1985, pp. 3213-16. Oregon Health Services Commission, Prioratization of Health Services: A Report to the Governor and the Legislature, Salem OR 1991. Menzel, P. *Strong Medicine: The Ethics of Rationing Health Care* Oxford University Press, New York, NY. 1990. Rawles, J. "Castigating QALYs" *Journal of Medical Ethics*, Vol. 15, 1989 pp.143-47. Welch, H. and Larson, E. "Dealing With Limited Resources: The Oregon Decision to Curtail Funding for Organ Transplantation" *The New England Journal of Medicine*, Vol. 319, 1988, pp.171-3. Carr-Hill, R. "Background Material for the Workshop on QALYs: Assumptions of the QALY Procedure" *Social Science and Medicine*, Vol. 29, 1989, pp.469-77; Oregon Health Services Commission, *Preliminary Report: March 1, 1990.* Salem OR, 1990.

26   Statement by Senator John Kitzhaber, Hearing on S.27 Before the Senate Health Insurance and Bio-Ethics Commission, 65th Legislation, Regular Session, 1989 Oregon p.16-7.

Chapter 27
HEALTHCARE COST
COMPARISONS ABROAD

For the past two decades, the rate of growth in US healthcare spending far exceeded growth in other sectors of the economy. In spite of spiraling healthcare costs, questions have been raised regarding access to care by tens of millions of people, the prevailing state of health and well-being in this country, along with the increasing proportion of GNP devoted to healthcare. Between 1970 and 1990, national income devoted to healthcare increased by over 50% (from 7.3% of GNP in 1970 to 12.3% in 1990), and, if nothing is done, may easily reach 16% by the year 2000, in the same time as the number of people without health insurance increased from about 30 million in 1979 to over 37 million in 1987. This predicament often prompts a comparison between the United States healthcare scene and that in other major industrialized countries such as Canada, France, Germany, and Japan. These countries spend a smaller share of their national income on healthcare than the US does, yet they appear to have secured universal access to basic healthcare services, and registered no inferiority in any basic measure of health status (e.g. infant mortality and life expectancy).

The French, German, and Japanese healthcare systems have several major characteristics that are similar to those of the US. In all three countries, healthcare is provided by private physicians, and by a conglomeration of public and private hospitals. Patients have a free choice of doctors. Much of health insurance coverage is employment-based. Health insurance plans are procured from multiple third-party intermediaries. However, there are major differences as well. Insurers are predominantly nonprofit. They are required to provide minimum coverage but for a wide range of services. Everyone must enroll in a health plan in general with minimum or no choice among plans. Employer-based coverage is paid for by contributions from employees and the employer, and the premiums are based not on individual group ratings, but on the expected cost of a broader population segment. Mandated health insurance is accompanied in all three countries by centrally controlled and standardized reimbursement rates to private and institutional providers. These rates are generally determined pursuant to negotiations among private and institutional providers, third-party payers, and the government. In addition, all three countries apply healthcare macro budget controls, with various degrees of enforcement rigor, designed to cap expenditures for physician and hospital services. Thus, healthcare financing in all three of these countries, as in the US, is based on a *multipayer* system, in contrast to the Canadian healthcare financial scene, to be discussed later, founded on a *single payer* system. Let us now take a closer look at the three countries with multipayer systems.

Multiple Payer Systems[1]

As I already indicated, the three industrialized countries being contrasted here, France, Germany, and Japan, have healthcare institutional characteristics similar to those of the United States: healthcare delivery is essentially a private industry, where patients can choose their own physician, and receive ambulatory (outpatient) care from private individual providers. While institutional care is provided mostly in public entities, private institutions also provide a significant proportion of inpatient beds, some one-third in France, about a half in Germany, and some two-thirds in Japan[2]. Health insurance is typically employment-based.

Private office-based physicians are remunerated by fee-for-service, as is still often the case in the U.S., although we now have frequent alternatives to fee-for-service, such as HMO capitated payments instead of payment for each service provided, relatively rare in the three countries being examined. On the other hand, physicians in a hospital setting normally function as salaried employees of the hospital, and enjoy considerable clinical freedom. Utilization reviews in these countries tend normally to concentrate more on the propriety of billing than on assessing the propriety of treatment.

As does the US, all of these three countries have multiple payer-based financing systems anchored largely at the place of *employment*, although the implementation of the systems is different from that in the US. Thus, at the base of employment, it is the employer, instead of the employee as is mostly the case in the US, who procures (brokers) the coverage from the carrier/third-party payer based often on the employee's occupational status at the company or in the labor force. And, while in the US employee procurement of coverage through the employer is at least at the present time optional, and the employee can, and often does, procure coverage directly from an intermediary, the system in these three countries in general does not permit direct procurement of coverage by employees in place of the availed employment-based plans.

The insurance industry is relatively unconcentrated in Germany and Japan, with a large number of insurers, as in the US. In fact, Germany and Japan each have about 1000 independent healthcare intermediaries providing coverage via specific companies or employer categories (e.g. small businesses), geographic areas, and trades or occupation categories. France, on the other, has a more highly concentrated healthcare intermediary market-based in a highly concentrated insurance market in general, with only a few types of payers with one being entrusted with covering some 80% of the population[3].

In the US, we have for-profit and *not-for-profit* healthcare intermediaries. In general, the latter category of third-party payers have a somewhat smaller percentage of the coverage markets that for-profit payers. Thus, the predominant not-for-profit programs in the US, the Blue-Cross/Blue-Shield Plans, has about 40% of the covered market[4], while in Germany nonprofit payers cover about 90% of the population, and in France and Japan virtually everyone is covered by operators of nonprofit plans. Looking at the employment-based coverage category specifically, nonprofit plans are the virtually the only source of coverage for employees in these three industrialized countries (in France and Germany they are called "sickness funds") procured through the employer as well for retirees, self-employed, or unemployed people, who cannot get employer-based coverage. In contrast to the US, for-profit plans have only a very small share of the coverage market in these three countries, normally concentrating in specialized areas such as supplementing mandated employment based coverage, or, as in Germany - where people with high incomes are not mandated to obtain employment- based coverage, providing personally designed private coverage, or, as in Japan, providing coverage for specific ailments, and other specialized benefits.

While the nonprofit plans in the US may be viewed as generically private, the extent of government regulation applied to nonprofit plans in France, Germany and Japan call the degree of their "privacy" in question. This is true to the greatest extent in France, where nonprofit funds are actually part of the social security system. In general, the plans have private legal status and administrative autonomy, but they are heavily subsidized and regulated by the central government. US health insurance regulations are selectively implemented at the state level, mandating specific benefits rather than blanket coverage, allowing considerable competition among plans in terms of their other provisions, such as terms of reimbursement, covered benefits, and pricing. Outright government public programs in the US, such as Medicare, Medicaid, and the Medical Program of the Uniformed Services, cover about 23% of the US population, in contrast to about one percent in France (covering indigents not members of the sickness fund), and virtually zero percent in Germany[5]. The reason clearly rests in the mandated functions of nonprofit plans in these countries which include the coverage of the indigent and the elderly.

The virtually *universal coverage* that exists in these three industrialized countries are enforced by laws mandating employment-based insurance coverage for employees and their dependents, having public or nonprofit plans insuring the rest of the population. In addition to mandating access to health insurance through employment, the employer is required to co-finance an insurance plan containing a minimum portfolio of benefits that normally include a wide range of services, and employees are required to enroll in the employer subscribed plan, that also includes coverage for their dependents. This leaves little choice for the employee as to the insurer, nor does this allow insurers to discriminate among employees in any terms, including their risk levels. The mandated level of minimum coverage in these countries includes a broad range of services and supplies, such as physicians services, hospital care, laboratory tests, prescription drugs, and limited amounts of dental and optical care. There are no deductibles, although copayments for physician and hospital services can range from zero (Germany) to 30% (France and Japan), with Japan limiting copayments of regulated fees for catastrophic medical expenses to about $400 per month[6].

The financing of mandated employer-based health insurance in these countries is mainly payroll-based. In contrast to the US, where financing of most coverage is implemented through a system of premiums reflecting actuarial estimates of expected future illnesses and healthcare related expenses of the covered group, these three countries utilize mandatory payroll contributions from both the employer and the employee. In addition, France and Japan also use general tax revenues to supplement payroll-based financing. The proportion of payroll-based contribution falling on the employees and employers varies by country. Thus, in France, the mandatory payroll contribution, as determined by the central government, indicates a 12.6% share of the total wage bill for the employer, and 6.8% for the employees. Similar mandatory payroll contributions, but determined by individual sickness funds, in Germany sets the shares of both the employees and the employers equally at an average level of about 13% (ranging from 8% to 16%) of the total wage bill. In Japan, the mandatory payroll contribution is determined by the individual insurance carrier, which constitutes an average of about 8% (range: 3.5% - 13.3%) of a standard monthly salary, with the employer co-contributing at least 50% of that amount[7].

In order to cap healthcare spending and set reimbursement rates for providers, a government agency in each country sets broad healthcare budgetary targets either as guidelines or by way of biding rulings. In addition, a collaborative process among healthcare intermediaries, the government, and private as well as institutional providers set reimbursement rates for providers. In general, reimbursement rates are the same within each service category. The procedures for implementing healthcare budgetary caps vary somewhat among countries. In France and Japan, the central government sets the goals, but while in the former the goals also constitute budgetary targets for public hospitals, the latter ties the rate of healthcare budgetary increases to the growth in the GDP, without aiming at any specific healthcare sector. In Germany, general and rather specific (hospitals, physicians, prescription drugs) healthcare spending targets are set semi-annually by a quasi-public organization, called the Concerted Action, made up of representatives from major participant groups in the healthcare system, such as private and institutional providers, pharmacies, private insurers, sickness funds, drug manufacturers, business and labor, state as well as local governments. Although there are various measures in place for healthcare budgetary controls in these countries, these arrangements are by no means static, and are likely to change. Political interest groups representing providers and employers perennially exert pressures upon governments to alter the regulatory framework in their own economic interests[8].

The *Germans* imposed two types of budgetary control on physician care costs. Between the late 1970s and 1985 there were spending targets, while spending caps were implemented since 1986. Spending targets on ambulatory physician services were not binding. They simply set spending goals based on previous year's expenditures, expected demand for services, and the projected income of enrolled patients. These targets coexisted with price controls, discussed below, but there was no coordination between them. In fact, over the years the targets were normally exceeded, necessitating the imposition in 1986 of binding expenditure ceilings on physician services. These ceilings are adjusted upward in accordance with changes in subscriber income. On the other hand, the "flexible fee" provision in the enforcement process allows downward adjustment in per-unit fee for a service if the increase in volume threatens consistency with the predetermined ceiling. In 1986, German hospitals were also required to formulate annual spending budgets, although adherence to these budgets were not enforced in the manner similar to France. The government, through an advisory body on national health policy, recommends annual spending targets for hospitals, as individual hospitals negotiate their budgets with the sickness fund in their particular region. There does not appear to be a formal enforcement mechanism in place.

The global budget constraints imposed on public hospitals in *France* since 1984 replaced a prior per-diem price control. The public hospital arrives at its annual budget, covering operating costs and the cost of debt incurred by way of construction and capital equipment, by negotiating with the sickness fund and national government experts, where in particular the latter oversee that the negotiated budgets remain within government set national hospital spending targets. As I indicated earlier, *Japan* has no budgetary policies or significant constraints addressing specific healthcare sectors, although it has a central government imposed national healthcare expenditure policy [9].

Provider *price controls* are almost always politically volatile subjects. Physicians in particular, and providers in general, are reluctant to subscribe to, and perennially oppose, regulations which would limit, possibly even reduce, their income. Price controls have typically been applied either by way of fee schedules setting geographically uniform rates, or by way of per-diem rates by which third-parties reimburse hospitals. In *France*, physicians are subjected to specific service-based rates set uniformly across that country in private physician or private hospital settings, although physicians can privately bill patients above these rates, but not without some financial disincentives such as being restricted from joining sickness funds for salaried people forcing them to join more limited sickness funds for the self-employed, and losing their own fringe-benefits. Somewhat like the recently implemented RVBS under Medicare reimbursement of physicians in the US, the French fee structure utilizes relative value scale ranking procedures and tests relative to each other, and a factor, annually set in government supervised negotiations between physicians and sickness funds, that converts the relative values into monetary units. French private hospitals are subjected to a fixed per-diem rates (also applied to public hospitals until the global budget system was brought in) not related to the specific contents of the service. While these per-diem rates can vary among private hospitals, they get reimbursed by all sickness funds at a uniform rate - there can be no cost shifting.

The *German physician* is subjected to the same type of price controls, negotiated with sickness funds in the a similar manner, as the French for outpatient services with some major exceptions, such as no billing in excess of the set fees is permitted, instead of a single national fee schedule service rates are set on a regional basis, and the government plays no formal functional role in the negotiations between the physicians and the sickness funds. Regional fee schedules, based on relative value scales and negotiated between the sickness funds and the physicians assign points to specific medical procedures, with the monetary conversion factors also negotiated between the sickness funds and their physicians, through their respective associations.

Since hospitals and physicians there can both provide inpatient and outpatient care, the *Japanese* do not typically differentiate between inpatient and outpatient services for fee setting purposes. Thus, a single nationally set fee schedule, established and administered by the Ministry of Health and Welfare, applies to both, with balance billing not allowed. The fees are set by the Ministry in collaboration with the Central Social Insurance Medical Council made up of providers, payer representatives, and public interest advocates such as lawyers and economists[10].

How did budgetary and price controls fare in limiting costs? It appears that in two healthcare sectors, French hospital services and German physicians, mandated and compliance enforced budgetary spending ceilings were more effective than price controls. Where only spending controls were used without formal compliance enforcement, such as the German hospital sector, healthcare costs did not rise slower than if price controls were utilized. The income effect of price controls on providers, hence cost controls, can largely be neutralized by increasing the volume of service output. A control on total spending, with compliance enforced, can thus be more effective as there is no incentive to increase service volume by providers, and with a given minimum amount of service volume, prices can increase only by an amount subject to the imposed total spending increase. Thus, in Germany, targeted and capped ambulatory physician care expenditures (adjusted for inflation) were 17% lower between 1977 and 1987 than what they would have been in their absence, with a corresponding reduction in the annual rate of nominal spending from 9% to 6%. Similar reductions were experienced in France, where the inflation-adjusted cost of inpatient hospital care in 1987 was some 9% lower than it would have been without the impact of global budgets and sector-wide spending targets. The average annual rate of growth in nominal spending pursuant to budgetary controls were 5%, in contrast to the 9% expected to occur under price controls[11].

While compliance enforced budgetary controls appear to slow the rate of healthcare cost inflation, they do so mostly by artificial administrative channels, instead of through perhaps socially more beneficial efficiency gains. Providers functioning under enforced budgetary ceilings have no incentives to contain waste and inefficiency, so long as they stay within budgetary guidelines, nor are they rewarded for functioning more efficiently by providing a higher volume of at least constant quality service under the budgetary guidelines. In this manner, set budgetary allotments can even keep inefficient hospitals in business which, in a market environment, might simply have to close. In addition to efficiency questions, enforced budget controls may also an adverse quality impact, largely through a lack of time care availability. This is particularly true with limits on hospital reimbursements and capital expansion permits that inhibit patient access to major tertiary treatment procedures requiring sophisticated equipment. In addition, in a severely constrained financial environment, hospital may not be able to maintain their therapeutic equipment in good working order, and may be prevented from developing innovative treatment techniques. Apparently, this was particularly the case during recent years in France where stringent hospital budgetary controls have been applied. Similar constraints on physicians may selectively or in general inhibit the supply of services in that category. Other countries, where a longer experience may be reviewed in terms of budgetary constraints on healthcare providers, such as Canada, Sweden, and the UK, stringent financial constraints on providers, particularly on hospitals, appear to have contributed to a serious deterioration in the quality of care. These quality problems appeared mostly by way of long waiting periods for major tertiary care items, and the consequent rationing of many services by tertiary care hospitals[12].

The Canadian Experience

While often cited as a possible model for the United States, the Canadian healthcare system is by no means an ideal solution, and may not even be a desirable one for this country. This section will briefly examine the evolution and various attributes of the Canadian system with a view to sifting through its pros and cons for our consideration. A health policy analyst recently stated that health insurance systems often reflect on the "cultural beliefs, political priorities and medical imperatives of the countries in which they evolve"[13]. The Canadians apparently feel that the financial responsibility for maintaining the healthcare of the individual, of all individuals, belongs to society.

The historical roots of the current Canadian system may perhaps be traced back to the Great Depression when in1931 a small town in the Province of Alberta established the first group purchase health insurance plan. Members of the plan voluntarily paid $25 to the two physicians in the town for one year's medical care[14]. Although Theodore Roosevelt's initial presidential campaign platform included elements of a national medical care program, and Prime Minister McKenzie King in Canada also campaigned (from around 1919 through the 1930s) for a national health insurance program, much of health insurance in both countries remained in the private sector until the end of the Second World War. During subsequent years, the nature of the Canadian political scene, in particular the predominance of social democratism, contributed substantially to the disparities in the evolution of healthcare delivery systems between the United Staes and Canada. The Canadian political scene has for many years ranged from the left-wing New Democratic Party through the Liberals, and to the supposedly Conservatives, with even the latter possessing an ultra-liberal branch called the "Red Tories". Thus, while in the US socialist programs are often advocated in Congress by liberal millionaires, the Canadians have it vested in their fundamental political structure.

The first socialized medical plan in Canada was enacted in 1946 by the governing Cooperative Commonwealth Federation Party of Saskatchewan, which was a government hospital insurance plan. Plans of a similar type and nature followed shortly in British Columbia, Newfoundland, and Alberta. The subsequent 1957 National Hospital Insurance and Diagnostic Services Act covered the 40% population segment that was largely uninsured up to that time. In July 1962, while the author was still an undergraduate student in Ottawa, North America's first Medicare Program, the Physicians Services Insurance Plan was installed by the CCF Party. While in principle the Plan was to be a cooperative effort between the public sector and the providers, it was essentially imposed by the government upon the medical profession. The program was passed subsequent to minimum consultation with providers, and the governing Health Insurance Commission Board had no provider representation. The Saskatchewan plan was based on the principles of prepayment, universal coverage, controlled care quality, government sponsorship, and provider concurrence. The 1965 Royal Commission Report, under the chairmanship of Chief Justice Emmet Hall of Saskatchewan, expounded on similar principles that included portability. The Hall Commission's Report essentially gave birth in 1966 to the Medicare Act, the Canadian national health insurance program, completely replacing private health insurance in that country. Thus, instead of caring for only the indigent segment of the patient population, as it has for some years, leaving the rest to the private health insurance sector, the government took over responsibility for covering the entire population[15].

The Plan allowed physicians the option not to participate. They could bill patients separately according to a fee schedule (set by agreement between the government and provincial medical associations), with the latter recovering the preset amount from the government. Nevertheless, because of the much lower transaction cost of billing one payer (the government), instead of many small ones (the individual patients themselves), most physicians joined the plan. However, problems soon began to develop. The government gradually reduced its percentage of the reimbursement, effectively reducing providers fees, at the same time as discouraging extra billing by physicians. In fact, while the federal government originally agreed to cover 50% of provincial health care costs, it subsequently passed the Canada Health Care Act, effectively barring contributions to provinces that allowed excess billing. The subsequent doctors' strike of 1988 could not help matters, and, by about the end of that year, all doctors were forced to join the plan. The Canadian medical scene has thus become a government controlled bureaucracy. The negative consequences may offset the social benefits.

Recent developments saw the imposition of ceilings on the income of the highest earning physicians. Efforts have been made to limit the number of medical graduates, and residents in specialty programs. Hospitals are being closed. A shortage of convalescent and chronic care facilities force many such patients into acute care hospital beds, further reducing already scarce inpatient capacity. There are long waiting lists for elective procedures, and even for office visits, with some procedures and facilities heavily rationed. Most states in the US individually possess more MRIs than the entire Canada. Similar important diagnostic tools, such as lithotriptors and cardiac catherization units, are also in relative and absolute short supply. Patients frequently take out private insurance to procure diagnostic and therapeutic care in the United States. Budgetary caps on Canadian hospitals, and they are all public, force them to cut corners, potentially compromising quality, reducing capacity or staff, or both. Perennial budgetary constraints are accompanied by increasing demand for hospital emergency room care, further taxing the system. Fines are imposed on first offender excess-billing physicians, with a threat of prison sentence for subsequent offenders[16].

We could contribute to a balanced analysis of the issues by looking at some of the positive aspects of the Canadian system. As to the shortage of some major items of therapeutic equipment in Canada, one could argue that the US, on the other hand, has too much of them, likely contributing to spiraling costs here. However, while this comparison makes sense by identifying a possible source of excessive healthcare costs in this country, it does not resolve or justify the predicament that the other extreme generated in Canada. Yet, there are some more noteworthy points of comparison. In contrast to America's 37 million uninsured, and its 60 million insured under government programs (Medicare and Medicaid) often perceived as inferior plans, Canada has universal coverage. Thus, one may, in a somewhat simplistic manner, reconcile the two systems, by reducing excess technological capacity in the US but not to the point of scarcity, covering uninsured people and those under less desirable plans to protect personal dignity and reasonable levels of wealth, all the while keeping healthcare costs under relative control - relative, that is, to those countries where alternative systems have been experimented with during the past several years and decades, and relative to the past cost history of the United States. It appears that the Canadian system in its entirety could not and would not work in this country. The system is getting weaker in Canada itself, increasingly begging for the infusion of private resources to sustain itself at civilized levels[17]. So, what does the US-Canadian healthcare balance sheet look like? In the shadow of what already was said, let us briefly and systematically review the Canadian healthcare scene.

The Canadian healthcare system is publicly funded. It actually consists of 10 separate provincial (and 2 territorial) plans with some common features. Coverage is universal for all hospital and physician services. Coverage is also virtually completely portable, and is largely unaffected when a persons moves from one job to another. In each province, a public agency administers the plan, and is responsible for health planning, as well as for the reimbursement of providers. Thus, the provincial governments are the single payers of providers, and largely the sole formulators as well as implementors of healthcare policy in each of the provinces. The provincial governments bear the political and financial responsibility for the status and functioning of healthcare delivery systems in their respective provinces. Provincial governments set hospital budgets, physician fees, and control major capital and service procurements. In contrast, US providers are reimbursed by a multitude of direct or third-party payers - private, for-profit, nonprofit, federal and local governments, and, in some limited number of cases, the individual patient himself or herself. Procedures and coverage vary by the payer, and there is no single organization that uniquely coordinates the healthcare delivery system. Some plans include sizable deductibles and copayments with the coverage, others limit them. The Canadians have no deductibles and copayments for covered services, nor is there alternative coverage for those services covered by the public single payer. Services not covered by the provincial plan, such as routine dental care, cosmetic surgery, and extra amenities in hospital rooms, can be insured from private sources with the premium covered by the patient.

It may be that the installation of a single payer system in the US would save enough in administrative and various types of transaction costs to cover the presently uninsured 37 million people, and may even permit a substantial reduction of copayments or deductibles. Such a single payer system could likely control healthcare costs, as those costs have risen substantially slower in Canada than in the US, probably the outcome of stringent controls on hospital budgets, physician fees, and on capital equipment procurement, present in Canada but largely absent in the US.

In Canada, there appears to be a relatively easy access to primary care services. Canada has more physicians per person than does the US, and the average Canadian uses more primary care physician services than does an average American. Yet, the per capita cost of physician services in Canada is typically about 33% lower than that in the US. Thanks to the stringent controls. Although emergency cases are treated out of turn, there appear to be serious problems with access to specialty and tertiary care services. There are waiting lists for specialty care items such as cardiac by-pass surgery, lens implants, MRI diagnosis utilizations, and the like[17]. Because of fundamental differences between provider and financer institutions in the two countries, a reformed US system is not likely to take on an unmodified Canadian form. However, some features of the Canadian system, such as single and uniform payer system, universal access, and capital expenditure controls may have potential applicability[18].

While in terms of the presence of universal coverage, the functioning of a single payer, and lack of cost sharing by way of deductibles and copayments, the Canadian systems does substantially differ from that of the US, however, there also are substantial similarities. In fact, the Canadian healthcare system may be closer to that of the US than the system of any other major industrial country. Thus, as the US, Canada does not have a socialized system of health care delivery. Virtually all healthcare resources in Canada are in the private sector. A government based single payer disburses to private providers. Most private providers are independent and get paid on a fee-for-service basis. Almost all physicians in Canada work for themselves and not for the government. In addition, some 90% of the hospitals are also private not-for-profit corporations, although the veterans hospitals and provincial psychiatric hospitals are federally owned and operated.

The Canada Health Act covers all residents in all provinces for necessary care in a physician's office or in a hospital. Private health insurance duplicating provincial plans are prohibited. In the US, coverage is typically employer-based, or is provided by public plans to the elderly or the indigent. Since policies are often not portable, and some employers do not, or cannot afford to, provide coverage, there are millions of people in this country without coverage, and perhaps many more are discouraged from improving their working conditions or from otherwise bettering themselves by changing jobs for fear of losing their and their family's health insurance coverage. Not a typical predicament in Canada. Furthermore, the Canadian concentration of administrative responsibilities for provider reimbursement in the hands of a single provincial agency, in contrast to a large number of private companies and public bodies - as in the United States, generates substantial administrative savings by way of greater administrative efficiencies, and focused control over disbursements. Thus, in 1989, Canadians spent some US$670 less on healthcare per person than did Americans, largely as a result of the controls built into their system[19]. In addition, financial barriers to access in Canada is eliminated by prohibiting direct patient payment to providers, copayments or deductibles, all of which occur frequently in the US.

As for controlling healthcare expenditures, Canada has been more successful than the US, although at a price and trade-off, as we noted above. In 1971, when the Canadian system reached full implementation, the *proportion of GNP* devoted to healthcare was roughly the same in both countries. By 1989, Canada was only spending 8.9% of its GNP on healthcare, compared with 11.6% in the US. Furthermore, the Canadian single public payer system eliminates the need to market competing plans, and avoids corresponding marketing, billing, collection, and risk evaluation costs. Consequently, as of 1987, the Canadians spent no more than about 20% of per capita expenditures in the US on *insurance administration*. Per capita *expenditures on physician* services have also been lower in Canada than in the US, by some 34%. In fact, between 1971 and 1985 inflation adjusted Canadian physician fees have declined by 18%, in contrast to a corresponding increase of 22% in the US, once again reflecting on the provinces' control on reimbursement rates. Although increases in physician fees is annually negotiated between physician associations and the provinces, the latter has virtually complete statutory power to control cost increases. While the gross income of Canadian physicians is lower, their net income does not reflect the same difference due their lower office and administrative overhead associated with reduced paperwork and simplified reimbursement collection. No office staff is needed for direct billing of patients, insurance record keeping, and collecting bad debts. The proportion of physician gross income spent on administrative expenses in Canada during 1989 was 36%, compared to 48% in the US, although part of this saving by the physician may not end up as his or her profit, instead, may be negotiated away by the single payers and thus be transferred back to the tax-payer[20].

Canadian hospitals also function cheaper than comparable US institutions. In 1987, per capita hospital services in Canada cost 18% less than comparable services in the United States. This difference is largely due to lower administrative costs, the single payer system of reimbursements, to global hospital budgeting, and to limits on technological acquisitions. Most of the billing functions and related expenses plaguing US hospitals are not present in Canada. The provincial ministry of health typically negotiates with each hospital its annual operating budget, and rations among hospitals the right to acquire high-technology equipment and, therefore, the ability to provide high cost specialized services.

While access to primary care is relatively easy and directly free to the patient, tightly controlled hospital operating budgets and technological procurements limit access to more specialized levels of care. Immediate or life-threatening needs are usually met promptly, or without much delay, however, there are several month long waiting lists for elective and diagnostic procedures. Thus, in October 1990 there were about 1000 patients in Ontario on the waiting list for cardiac surgery. Emergency patients were treated immediately, so called "urgent" cases waited up to a month[21].

A 1991 study by the General Accounting Office indicates that if the US were to shift to a Canadian-style single-payer universal coverage system, savings in administrative costs alone would cover the additional cost of universal coverage. In the short run, $35 billion would be *saved* in insurance overhead alone; $33 billion would be *saved* in hospital and physician overhead costs, minus the cost of data recording for future analyses for which the Canadian system may not provide very well; *new* insurance policies would *cost* some $18 billion; and, if copayments and deductibles are eliminated, additional services will likely be demanded costing about $46 billion, according to a GAO 1991 estimate[22]. It is further suggested that the US may want to retain some elements of cost sharing in order to control utilization. The GAO suggests that long-run controls on payments to providers by way of compliance enforced limit budgeting, negotiated but constrained physician fees, and rationing of high tech equipment could substantially reduce the growth in healthcare expenditures.

The question whether the Canadian system, as is, should be adopted in the US calls for a comparison of the current US healthcare scene with that in Canada at the time it was implemented there during the early 1970s. The US already has a well developed and large health insurance industry, not to be found in Canada during the early 1970s. Additionally, the possession of medical technology of the highest caliber and potency is pervasive in most states of the US, medical centers, and university affiliated hospitals as well as teaching centers; again, not a situation that could apply to the early 1970s Canadian scene. In other words, the moneys have largely been spent, although similar expenditures in the future can be closely controlled. Questions like whether we should deprive those who want to benefit from this type of technology in the future if they are willing and able to pay for them, is one of several of the same type that will be dealt with in chapter 28, the final chapter, of this volume. Another major difference between today's American healthcare scene, and that of Canada's in the early 1970s is the presence in the US of a well developed system of alternative healthcare delivery mechanisms (HMOs, PPOs, and the like) which have already contributed somewhat to healthcare cost control. Thus, what we may want to look at closely in the Canadian system, and possibly adopt some versions of in an appropriately adjusted manner, are (a) *universal access*, a principle the importance of which no one denies, (b) some sort of uniform payment system, possibly from a single or institutionally organized and coordinated payer, and (c) direct and possibly enforceable controls on healthcare expenditures. These improvements need to be implemented within the context of the already existing strengths and positive attributes of the US healthcare system. These include world class research facilities and talent, continued technological innovations, and inherent structural flexibilities in the system to accommodate the changing medical needs of society and implement new and innovative delivery systems in the future.

A final note on the German system and its implication for the US healthcare reforms. In spite of an excellent record in healthcare cost control and universal accessibility, in 1993 Germany decided to impose emergency budget ceilings, and commenced a review of the structure of its healthcare delivery system. Germany has long had universal coverage and an effective administrative structure to scrutinize provider fees, and service utilization. Nevertheless, cost pressures from the increasing aging component of the population, expanding demand for high-tech medicine, and a perennial demand for ever improving medical care from the population are mounting. And, although Germany's success with healthcare cost controls and universal access may be a model for the US during the current healthcare reforming efforts, Germany's current efforts to change and further improve the system and to deal with emerging problems indicates that there may not be such a thing as a "terminal healthcare reform" which, once implemented will yield medical care bliss for all members of society for decades to come. The healthcare scene is a dynamic one. Its composition and society's needs constantly change. Thus, healthcare reforms now or in the future cannot be viewed as terminal processes. Instead, they are likely to be a perennial process of adjustments and readjustments between *what* it has to offer, *how* it should offer it, and society's *needs*.

References

1   Much of this Section is based on United States General Accounting Office, Report to Congressional Requesters, *Health Care Spending Control: The Experience of France, Germany and Japan* [GAO/HRD-92-9], November 1991.

2   GAO, November 1991, at p. 23

3   GAO at pp. 24-25

4   Health Insurance Association of America, *Source Book of Health Insurance*, Washington DC 1990; cited in GAO, at p. 25.

5   GAO at p. 27

6   GAO at pp. 29-30

7   GAO at pp. 32-33

8   GAO at pp.42-48

9   GAO at pp.42-45

10 GAO at pp. 41-43. See also Rodwin, V. et al. "Updating the Fee Schedule for Physician Reimbursement: A Comparative Analysis of France, Germany, Canada, and the United States" *Quality Insurance and Utilization Review* Vol. 5 (February, 1990), p.17, cited in GAO.

11 GAO at pp.45-48

12 GAO at p.52. The Canadian experience is discussed in the next section of this chapter. See also Saltman, R.B. "Competition and Reform in the Swedish Health System" *The Milbank Quarterly*, Vol.64 (1990), pp.597 618. See also, Gilbert, B. *The Evolution of National Insurance in Great Brittain: The Origins of the Welfare State*, Michael Joseph, London 1966

13 Iglehart, J.K. "Canada's Health Care System Faces its Problems" *New England Journal of Medicine*, Vol. 322, No.8, 1990, pp.262-68.

14 Editorial. "Medicare's Humble and Earthy Beginnings", *Canadian Doctor*, June 1990.

15 Health and Welfare Canada, *National Health Expenditures in Canada, 1960-73*, Government of Canada, Ottawa, April 1975. See also, Panitch, L. {ed.) "The Role and Nature of the Canadian State" in *The Canadian State: Political Economy and Political Power*, University of Toronto Press, Toronto, 1977.

16 Rublee, D.A. "Medical Technology in Canada, Germany and United States" *Health Affairs* (Millwood), Vol. 8, No.3 1989, pp. 178-81. See also Munro, I.R. "How Not To Improve Health Care" *Reader's Digest*, September 1992.

17 This section relies substantially on United States General Accounting Office (GAO), Report to the Chairman, Committee on Government Operations, House of Representatives, *Canadian Health Insurance: Lesson for the United States*, June 1991, GA)/HRD-91-90. pp. 2-3

18 It would also be incorrect to assume that the US already possesses, or historically possessed, no attributes of the Canadian system. Thus, many states have long had, although ironically several have lately abandoned or relaxed, certificate of need programs (CONs), requiring state health department approvals for major capital projects.

19 GAO, June 1991, at p.4

20 GAO, at p.5

21 GAO at p.6

22 GAO at p.7

Chapter 28
HEALTHCARE COSTS AND THE LAST REFORM OF THE 20TH CENTURY

During 1992 the US state and federal election campaigns, healthcare costs, access to healthcare, as well as a myriad of related issues have become a cornerstone of many political campaigns, and often the basis of voter decision[1]. This chapter will later note a number of the proposals that have come out of various political, quasi-political, professional (including the AMA), and trade groups all having their own ideas of, and interests for, reforming the US healthcare system. At this writing, the next year, or even well into 1994/95, will witness which of the various proposals will have survived, and which of the many suggestions will have been transformed or vanished, at least for the time being. At least for the time being, because campaigning for, and suggesting variations on, healthcare reforms are by no means new phenomena. Healthcare reform proposals have been advanced for many decades, but rarely succeeded politically in this country, largely due to the political might of the AMA. By the second decade of this century, most western European countries had some type of national health insurance. Yet, when President Coolidge wanted to increase federal spending on healthcare (from only 3% of then GNP), the AMA labeled the action as an attempt at socialism. The AMA also prevailed upon Franklin Roosevelt not to include major aspects of healthcare in the New Deal, and spent some $1.3 million (over $7 million in today's dollars) to defeat Harry Truman's plans for a national health insurance. Even Medicare, which later turned out to be rather helpful not only to those who are covered by it but also to many providers, was initially labeled by the AMA as "socialized medicine". Indeed, enactment of

Medicare and Medicaid were the last two major health policy actions that resulted in substantial improvements in access to healthcare for large population groups. It appears that while historically there were a number of attempts to increase federal spending on the healthcare scene, most of these were oriented more towards issues of access and availability than toward cost containment.

We have noted a number of times that healthcare expenditures and healthcare costs are not only a direct function of demand, but also appeared to be a direct function of supply: unlike in markets for nonmedical goods or services, both demand and supply had an increasing impact on healthcare expenditures. During the 1960s and early 1970s, third party payers showed little concern for either the price or quantity aspects of total healthcare expenditures, which are, of course, the product of the two. Even when expenditures were controlled, voluntarily or otherwise, such as that which occurred for the indigent segment of the population, the savings, or non-spending, was made up for by shifting the costs onto another healthcare segment. Some of the efforts of the 1970s were directed at the suppliers of healthcare services, such as state-based CON regulations. Others were directed at price, such as the Medicare prospective payment system imposed on hospitals, and the more recent relative value-based reimbursement of physicians by Medicare. While the DRG-based hospital rate setting efforts did result in some cost cutting, the federal-state regulatory machinery aimed at controlling healthcare costs has essentially failed to achieve it designated functions. Thus, the 1980s Reagan campaign to deregulate the economy at least partly also embraced the healthcare industry itself: health systems agencies that ran health planning and regulation at local levels, and CON controls have largely petered out. The failure of efforts to control costs were accompanied by politically even more volatile difficulties on the coverage and access fronts. For the past fifty years, employment-based health insurance became the main channel of access and source of coverage, and also the source of many problems as well as social concerns.

The Employment-Based Coverage Predicament

Employment-based health coverage systems gained prominence after World War II due to prevailing political and economic conditions. They were not covered by the wage control policies of the times, hence became important in labor management bargaining processes. This coverage system remained popular even after the removal of wage controls, since the benefits were tax exempt. Although the system subsequently became a way of life for most people, it was never really designed to, nor could it, achieve universal coverage. Yet, much of private healthcare coverage is still employment based, and many of the pending or historically considered reforms, such as mandatory coverage, or "play-or-pay", and many others, were and are based on that system. Today, some 90% of private coverage is employment-based, either through third-party payer or by self-insurance, with most or often all of the premiums paid by the employer[2]. However, the trend for complete employer coverage of premiums has lately been declining, and the frequency of cost sharing by employees by way of copayments and deductibles has been on the rise.

A fundamental problem with the system has long been that it is based on the principles of voluntary participation, both on the part of the employer and the employee, but particularly that of the employer, with the voluntary nature of the latter's participation even including the composition of the plan, that is, the services that would be covered. Thus, there have been wide differences among the plans offered by various employers. In general, the breadth and generosity of the coverage plan, as well as the extent to which it was employer financed, varied directly if not proportionately with employer size. Recent research indicated that only some 40% of employers with fewer than 10 employees even offered health insurance coverage, forcing their employees to seek coverage elsewhere, and leaving about 30% of employees in this category completely without health insurance coverage[3]. Over 66% of those without any coverage are people with full-time jobs and their families[4]. Although coverage was available, it was often not comprehensive, and excluded essential services such as those meeting dental and optometric needs, prescription drugs, preventive services and the like. Even when some of these items were included, selective limits as to covered services were often applied[5].

All of these issues thus far addressed those people, and possibly their families, who are employed. What about those who, for whatever reasons, are not? In many cases, the spouses and children even of those who are employed were not covered. Only recently was there an expansion of Medicaid to cover pregnant women, regardless of their marital status[6]. Some retired persons have had their pre-retirement benefits extended, but many have not been accorded this opportunity.

Medicare was enacted to cope with the plight of the uninsured elderly of 65 and over. Some retired people under 65 not qualifying for Medicare may be left out as if they were never employed. It has been estimated that no more than about half of those currently employed are potentially covered after retirement[7]. Although, since 1986 they could purchase their preretirement coverage for a limited time period[8]. Those who do not work, and under Medicare or retirement age, in general must meet certain poverty requirements, or must reach that wealth level after a spending-down process, unless they are single parents with young children, disabled, or blind. The rest of the unemployed under retirement age need to rely on whatever healthcare they could get on public agencies and institutions, such as community health centers, public health departments, and indigent care programs. Finally, as we indicated earlier, there is always the possibility of receiving primary care in hospital emergency rooms, and tertiary care by way of provider service donations.

Another problem with employment-based health insurance coverage is the fact that it protects those who likely need protection the least, that is, those who are healthy enough to work. On the other hand, when they get sick, hence cannot work, they often get squeezed out of coverage when they need it most. If they attempt to procure coverage after having become unemployed, they may or may not succeed at a price comparable to that which employed people pay, depending on prevailing insurance "rating systems". Under "community rating", the premiums are based on community-wide averaged risk which may be comparable to group rates accorded to employees of large corporations. In affect, a social group's healthier members subsidize those who are less well, with the basic degree of subsidization by those who are directly related to their well-being, and vice-versa. On the other hand, health insurers tend to maximize revenue wherever possible by way of "experience rating", that is, setting premiums for smaller restricted groups according to their specific risk levels. Thus, those employed, younger, or having better and healthier working conditions, and enjoying better health, would get a lower rate, while those out of work, for some reason or another in less healthy environment, hence carrying a higher risk, are charged higher premiums. Medical underwriting, as the process of risk/rate determination is called, thus antisocially, but in a private business sense perhaps soundly, discriminates between those with lower risks and those with higher risks and often entirely excludes those with the highest risk and those who are already ill and need healthcare the most.

In essence, the employment-based system, at best, covered those healthy enough to produce for the employers, and left the rest for the entire society, i.e. the public sector, to cover. Theoretically, it may be that if the public sector was well enough organized to pick up the slack, the system might work: employers providing coverage for those working for them, and society as a whole caring for the rest. A major imperfection that exists in this scenario is the currently still voluntary nature of employer coverage, discussed above. Some employers, the smaller ones, simply do not provide coverage, hence seek to rely on society to cover health insurance for their employers and, in fact, subsidize their private business enterprise: society finances the wellness of their employees, hence generates a transfer payment contributing to business profits, and to the wealth of absent (in case of public traded companies) or, more likely, resident owners (in the case smaller private firms). This may be viewed as an "adverse distribution" of healthcare costs. These practices may prevail subject to labor market conditions, particularly during recession and higher levels of unemployment when most workers prefer being employed without health benefits to not being employed at all. This predicament was targeted by the "play-or-pay" proposal during the initial stages of the 1991 Clinton presidential campaign which would have either had all businesses provide a certain degree of coverage for their employees, or pay into the public treasury to help finance public coverage. As the healthcare reform proposals of the new President evolved, the "play-or-pay" option has largely receded into the background, with modified and modernized versions managed competition gaining more attention.

Clearly, something has to be done. The employment-based system, supplemented to an extent and rather imperfectly by social programs, does not work. The number of people without any insurance has in recent years been expanding at rate of one million per year, leaving at least one out every six persons in the US without insurance. Furthermore, some 60% of these uninsured are either the fully employed or their dependents[9]. The financial concerns of business with healthcare expenditures are also noteworthy. Employer healthcare spending has increased just over 2% of wages in 1965 to over 7% in 1987. Looking from another dimension, further highlighting the employers' predicament, corporate employee health spending as a percentage of profits increased from 9% (pretax) and 14% (after-tax) to 49% and 94% respectively between 1965 and 1987[10]. Consequently, businesses have turned to self-insurance and service utilization intensive managed care. By the end of the last decade, less than 20% of those covered by employer-based plans were under unmanaged fee-for service care, almost half were in fee-for-service programs but with preadmission certification, and just over 30% in HMO and PPO environments. Furthermore, utilization was discouraged by intensified employee cost-sharing through sizable deductibles and copayments, with the latter often reaching 20%. And, when even managed care does not reduce costs as expected, benefits are reduced or elements eliminated, and dependent coverage terminated[11].

Small businesses cannot afford insurance. Even if they had coverage at a reasonable cost before, if their risk rating increases because an employee get seriously ill, their premium cost will increase to the point where they have to terminate coverage. Yet, people get sick. So do the uninsured. And most, if not all, get care from many individual providers, and particularly from institutional providers, such as large urban medical centers. The latter, in turn, attempt to shift the cost of unreimbursed care to those plans that can or will pay. But the cirle of cost aversion continues, as employers and third-party payers attempt to fend off cost-shifting by intensive price oriented negotiations and contracting with providers. However, the bubble can only take so much air, after which it will burst. The ever decreasing numbers and scope of private insurance, and the imperfectly designed and administered public insurance system, can no longer cope; chaos will, if it has not already, set in. Some reforms to assure universal or near-universal coverage are clearly called for. So are healthcare cost-containment efforts. Employment-based health insurance plans yielded little by way of universal coverage, and less by way of cost-containment. I will review current reform proposals, and the Clinton administration's model before Congress at the time of this writing, after a quick but systematic look at the major target variables for cost-containment.

Models of Cost Containment

The rest of this chapter, after this section, will examine the reform proposals of the present administration along with some alternative proposals, and will attempt to draw some tentative conclusions as to what the long term solution is going to be. The previous section above dealt with some of the problems inherent in efforts to make healthcare universally accessible under the current system. While at various stages in the volume, many these issues were discussed, at this point, just before discussing the pending reforms, the reader will be well served by reviewing various cost containment alternatives and related policy targets in a systematic and consolidated manner. In general, cost control targets may be divided into three broad categories: (a) the providers, (b) consumers, and (c) both, the providers and the patients.

Some *provider* targeted cost control measures directly involve hospitals and physicians, while others constrain both indirectly by controlling overall expenditures. One of the earliest *hospital* targeted cost control measures in this country involved certificate of need regulations CONs. These were implemented by local health systems agencies and required hospitals to seek pre-approval for capital expenditure projects, including investments to expand the number of beds and to procure new equipment, above a certain size, the threshold often being $100,000. As part of a regional health planning effort, CONs were approved if they were shown to substantially improve healthcare quality and quantity for the region. An underlying justification for CON regulations was vested in the view that a control on the number of hospital beds was in essence a control over healthcare expenditures. Nevertheless, CON-based cost control efforts have by-and-large failed. A reason for its ineffectiveness was the conduct of the hospitals prior to the imposition of the CON controls: when they learned of, and expected, the controls to take effect, they simply loaded up on capital equipment, thus avoiding much of the CON control's intended impact. In addition, CON approval bodies, boards, and state health departments, often looked at the expansion of hospitals in their areas as highly desirable, and, more importantly, had themselves individually or as institutions no financial interest or incentive to actually control healthcare expenditures, they were at no risk or bore no financial burden if the controls failed.

If the regulator's performance is directly assessed in terms of the policy's success, that is, if they assume certain risks, particularly financial ones, for the failure of their policy, then the outcome may be better. Thus, we saw in the previous chapter that in Canada, while the provinces implement their own healthcare cost controls, the federal government's contribution to each province is fixed, hence the financial consequences of province-based excessive healthcare expenditures fall on provincial shoulders. Thus, healthcare technological expansion in Canada is the direct financial responsibility of the provincial governments by not only granting regulatory green lights for capital expansion, but also funding such expansion, and, even if a hospital obtains private financing, e.g. by way of major private donations, the hospital's reimbursement for using such technology must come from the province, giving the latter virtually single-handed control over medical technology related healthcare costs.

Reduced availability of medical technology simply yields reduced utilization, hence reduced, or at least controlled, costs. We have noted in the previous chapter that this method of technological cost control does extract its price: rationing by way of long waiting lists for many medical procedures would be intolerable for most Americans, instead of rationing by price, presently found in the US. It is also questionable whether it would be wise to essentially leave the decision as to what medical services will be provided and for whom up to the government, instead of the profession and to better informed patients themselves.

Some states have experimented during the past two decades with hospital rate- setting policies aimed at indirectly controlling hospital expenditures[12]. The controls were by no means uniform. In some states, the controls were mandatory and applied to all third-party payers, while in others they were voluntary and applied to only a selected group of intermediaries such as Medicaid or Blue Cross. Of the 25 states with such a program, only eight implemented them on a mandatory basis, and even of these only three applied them to all intermediaries. Furthermore, studies conducted of these hospital rate-setting programs indicated that to be effective, they had to be mandatory and in effect for at least three years[13]. Even then, selectively enforced hospital rate setting policies have little chance for succeeding, for if they apply to some payers and not to others, hospitals can simply shift costs by raising prices to uncontrolled payers, or by increasing the quantity of services rendered to both groups. Rate setting programs applied to all payers, such as those in effect during the 1980s in New Jersey, Maryland, Massachusetts, and New York, did show some impact on hospital costs.

Another healthcare cost containment method targeted at hospitals, the 1983 Medicare Prospective Payment System (DRGs), has also been discussed extensively earlier in the volume. We recall that under this system the hospital is paid a fixed sum per admission, and the payment itself is based on patient diagnosis categories (diagnostic related groups, or DRGs). The payment to the hospital is thus unrelated to the patient's length of stay. The program has shown some success in controlling costs, but also resulted in some major changes in institutional healthcare provider structures. Although one would have expected that if the amount of per-patient revenue is limited to hospitals that they would have simply increased the volume by increasing admissions. No such increase in admissions occurred, in fact, studies suggested the opposite, an 11% decline in admissions during the six year period immediately following the implementation of the DRG system[14]. This reduction may have in part resulted from a marked shift where possible of some dispensable inpatient care to an outpatient environment. Thus, between 1984 and 1987 Medicare expenditures on hospital inpatient services rose only by an annual rate of 4%, while outpatient expenditures by hospitals increased by 20% per annum. In addition, it appears that DRGs may have also caused a shift to post-hospital nursing home care, and an increase in expenditures in that healthcare sector[15]. Thus, any decreases in hospital care expenditures pursuant to the implementation of DRGs should be viewed in terms of these possibly compensating increases in healthcare expenditures in other sectors. Furthermore, assuming at least equal quality and lower input costs, a redistribution of resources from in-patient hospital care to outpatient care and nursing homes may very well have resulted in a more efficient allocation of healthcare resources. As would be expected, average length of hospital stays have dropped significantly shortly after DRG implementation but appear to have stabilized in recent years. I might add here that the consequences of DRGs for healthcare quality have also been reviewed with mixed results. While a study of some 16,000 Medicare patients between 1981 and 1986 found a decline in mortality rates, it also found that patients were discharged in less stable, or in outright unstable, condition[16].

Finally, hospital targeted cost controls are also implemented by way of global hospital budgets, as is the case in Canada, discussed in the previous chapter. Hospitals negotiate their annual and binding operating budgets with the provincial government each year. This practice has not, as of the date of this writing, been implemented in the United States.

Another group of provider targeted healthcare cost controls is aimed at *physicians*. These could be implemented through controlling physicians' fees, physician supply, and globally controlling expenditures on physicians' services. The US does offer some history of attempts at controlling physician fees. Such controls were implemented during the 1971-74 wage and price controls, Medicare fees were frozen for a while during the 1980s, and, in Colorado, some Medicare physician fees were reduced while others increased at one time. The response to physician fee controls in general appeared to have been an increase in the volume of services, largely offsetting a fee reduction's possible income effect. On the other hand, if the elasticity of demand for physician services is very low, significantly under one, then even an attempt to compensate for lower fees by increased volume will not increase physician revenue, hence expenditures on physician services[17].

There is some question as to whether or not physician supply control limits healthcare cost savings. If one looks at the issues from a market competitive point of view, the logical conclusion would be that competition would vary directly with the number of physicians, decreasing physician monopoly power, and negatively impacting on healthcare costs. If we assume away competition in physician markets, as the case often tends to be, and attribute "induced demand" to physicians, a notion extensively discussed earlier in the volume, then an increase in the supply of physicians is likely to be accompanied by an increase in costs. In other words, given society's insatiable appetite for healthcare, more physicians will simply provide, and bill for, more healthcare. In addition, the composition of physician labor force is also significant. Specialists bill higher than family or general practitioners. And, although the recently implemented Medicare physician reimbursement system may in the long-run reduce the growth in the supply of specialists and make general practice financially more attractive in the US, at present only 15% of physicians in this country is in general practice, compared to 50% in Canada[18].

Consumer oriented healthcare cost controls can be implemented in a number of ways. Copayments, normally by way of an initial deductible plus a proportion of incurred medical expenses up to a certain limit, imposed on patients are basically designed to discourage utilization. Medicare's copayment involves over $600 deductible on hospital stays, between $150 and about $300 copayment for hospital stays after 60 days, and about a $100 per annum deductibles on physician fees, along with a 20% coinsurance on reasonable charges. Medicare does not limit out-of-pocket expenses. Furthermore, the use of copayments as cost-containment tools are becoming more frequent. The percent of people with employment-based coverage and without deductible fell from 15% to 5% during a ten year time period between 1977 and 1987, as did the proportion of those with under 20% deductibles[19]. The Rand Corporation Health Insurance Experiment, often referred to and discussed extensively earlier in this volume, found that copayment clauses in health insurance policies tended to discourage utilization. Whether or not increasing copayments, based on the Rand study, is likely to arrest healthcare cost increases is questionable, partly because due to the limited scope and size of the Rand experiment only small a proportion, if that, of most physicians' patient pool and income would have been affected, and partly because if in fact there would be an impact by way of reduced number of patients, it could be compensated for by rendering more service. Finally, it may be that if the value of healthcare benefits were taxed to the employee, they would be voluntarily reduced, yielding reduced utilization.

Both *providers and patients* are affected by the management of alternative healthcare delivery systems (ADS), HMOs, PPOs, and a number of others discussed earlier in the volume. They use a combination of price controls, service rationing, utilization management, financial incentives, (or disincentives), aimed at physicians to control costs. Since ADSs use a variety of techniques, and receive their income on a per capita basis with the incentive of reducing costs in the face of fixed income, one would think that they should constitute a large part of the answer to healthcare cost control questions. Furthermore, since HMOs, for instance, have been around for a long time, if effective, their impact on healthcare costs should have been at the least noticeable, if not gratifying. Yet, that is not the case. There may be several reasons for this anomaly. First of all, the studies that attributed significant savings to HMOs, concentrated on prepaid group practices, instead of IPAs, and savings associated with the latter form of HMOs is unclear, although the predominant form HMO enrollment is in IPAs[20]. Secondly, HMOs tend to benefit from favorable selection in their marketing efforts, thus might demonstrate lower costs than would be the case if their membership would represent a cross-section of the population. Thus, it was shown that HMO enrollees were lower service utilizers prior to enrollment than were those in a fee-for service system[21]. Thirdly, it may be that HMOs may be more economical than fee-for-service arrangements with zero cost sharing, but not so when compared to the latter with copayment provisions. Furthermore, while HMOs may reduce hospital rates and hospital utilization, there is no evidence that they have substantially contributed to slowing healthcare cost inflations. Finally, even if they were to save substantially, the HMOs's impact on overall healthcare spending is largely a function of their market share. But HMOs are by far not the prime choice for healthcare coverage, and fall far short of fee-for-service arrangements which normally allow freedom of provider choice. This sentiment surfaces when most (75%) people support some form of national health insurance coverage, but the support drops to 30% when the provision for free choice of provider is removed[22].

Preferred Provider Organizations are no panacea either. While they do incorporate, as we have seen before, what appears to be the best of both worlds which HMOs do not, namely freedom of provider choice and limited practice interference (utilization review), and they ostensibly generate cost savings, questions have been raised about the true financial impact, and even the authenticity, of the negotiated discounts which constitute the basis for contractual arrangements with PPOs. They do receive discounts from affiliated hospitals and physicians, in return for generating patient volume to these providers. They can practice some utilization review to control quantity and quality, and they can choose to deal with providers whom they deem to be the most efficient and the most likely to be cost-effective. But questions could be raised regarding the authenticity of the discount given, that is, do they reduce a standard market price, or are they simply applied to an artificially elevated fee structure? Furthermore, while one payer may get true discounts, those could be compensated for by charging a higher rate to another payer ("profit-shifting"), thus netting no savings in healthcare costs to society as a whole. Finally, PPO utilization management is normally not as intensive as could be found with HMOs, in fact, most PPOs have been found not to even discipline over utilizing providers, as HMOs often do[23]. Under these circumstances, the true savings that PPOs generate on the healthcare scene may be questioned. In fact, if reduced copayments which PPOs often offer generate increased demand for healthcare services, PPOs could constitute a source of increased rather than decreased healthcare costs.

Earlier in the volume, in connection with healthcare regulation, we discussed the recent establishment of the Agency for Health Care Policy and Research (AHCPR), an aim of which is to minimize differences in "practice styles" among physicians within and among geographical regions. These measures are expected to be implemented by way of formulating *medical practice guidelines*. In terms of future healthcare costs reductions, these guidelines might mean that services not included in them will simply not be reimbursed, or statutorily reimbursable, by third-party payers. But that is so only if the new practice guidelines will contain less by way of the number of services for any given illness than was practiced before. This may not be the case. In fact, instead of suggesting a lower number of services, the new guidelines might increase the portfolio of services considered the norm in dealing with various diseases. And, if so, when it comes to malpractice litigation, the courts, instead of considering today's norm, that is "the standard of medical practice" in the community, will simply have the physician account for whether or not he or she applied all practice options included in those guidelines, which will need to be done if the finding of liability is to be avoided. That the new practice guidelines will likely include more than less by way of required services for an average medical predicament is suggested by a recent government study which found present treatment patterns in connection with some cancers less than adequate, and not up to standards set by the National Cancer Institute[24].

Finally, before looking at the pending healthcare reforms themselves, let us quickly glance at the impact of *medical malpractice litigation* on current and future healthcare costs. In this category two alleged culprits were often identified; the cost of malpractice insurance, and the additional expenditures associated with so called "defensive medical practice" allegedly needed to avoid malpractice law suits, or if they do nevertheless occur to mount a more potent defense. Studies conducted thus far, however, by no means present a consensus in support of a hypothesis that medical malpractice litigation contributes, or contributes substantially, to healthcare cost inflation. The AMA study of the cost of medical malpractice for the year 1984 estimated its total cost as $14 billion, $3 billion in physician premiums, and $11 billion by way of defensive medicine. Other studies found these estimates far too high, and considered some of the practice items (such as follow-up visits, more time spent with patients, and more tests) included by the AMA into defensive medicine as simply manifestations of prudent medical practice benefiting the patient and improving healthcare service quality. Furthermore, the future importance of this issue is augmented by the fact that apparently only a small proportion (no more than about 10%, according to a New York State study) of actually committed medical malpractice instances sparked lawsuits[25]. Thus, there are reasons to expect an increase, instead of a reduction, in the frequency of medical malpractice litigation, unless they get legislated away. On the other hand, there are some mitigating indications, such as the reduction in medical malpractice premiums by 5% to 35%, although it is noteworthy that these reductions were brought about by legislative limits imposed by some states on malpractice suits[26]. Thus, much will depend not only on the politicians, lawyers, and the litigious tendency of the population, but also on the extent to which the medical profession itself is willing and able to objectively police its members' own conduct and competence.

The Healthcare Reforms: Pending, and Those That May or May Not Come

Ever since World War II, good health and healthcare has come to be known as a right, instead of a privilege. The view that people should get healthcare, good healthcare I suppose, has become pervasive to the extent that some people might have the notion that healthcare, in contrast to other goods and services, may be, or should be, a free good. The argument often follows along the moral rights of the patients and similar moral obligations on the part of a society to provide care for its members. Acknowledging the fact that these arguments are by no means unique to the US, and most industrialized nations, as we particularly noted in the previous chapter, provide heavily subsidized or even what appears to be "free" healthcare for their citizens, and without necessary convictions in this regard on the part of author, one can view these arguments as manifestations of a "healthcare paradox". After all, where does one draw the line for delineating "healthcare"? Should it be necessarily drawn at the stage where the healthcare providers' services are actually utilized, or needed, that is, when someone gets sick and needs care? As we will note later on in the chapter, elements of "preventive care" are likely be incorporated into reforms that may ultimately end up on President Clinton's desk for his signature, even if he may not recognize much of the rest in the light of his recently announced reform propsals. But if so, how do we delineate "preventive care"? Does it need to originate in the offices of a healthcare or allied healthcare provider, such as a family physician, a nurse practitioner, a mid-wife, or a nutritionist? How about those who are too poor and become ill because they have no roof over their head, or cannot eat a "balanced" meal regularly, or cannot afford to cloth and protect themselves from the elements, or are addicted to illicit, or even licit (such as alcohol and nicotine) substances? Would preventive measures have to extend to these situations? Once again, where does "healthcare" begin? In or about the providers' environment, or in the offices and within the responsibility of those who design and implement social policies? On what grounds does society find itself morally or otherwise justified to be more preoccupied with only those who are already sick than with those who are top candidates to become sick because of their living conditions? This contradiction can easily spill over to related cost consideration. It may be that substantial "healthcare" (in a traditional sense) overall cost savings could be realized if the definition of "healthcare" is expanded so as to incorporate what could be called "social care". More will be said regarding this issue later in the chapter.

As healthcare concerns and conventional wisdom stands today, the debate continues, and will likely continue for a long time, regardless what shape the Clinton Proposals will ultimately take for the President's own signature. The general concerns typically include: (a) universal insurance coverage (so that moneys that we do not in the first instance spend on the welfare of the poor will ultimately be spent for their insurance and care); (b) freedom of provider choice - presumably including not only freedom on the patient's part to select the providers, but also some type of freedom on the part of the provider to select what she or he considers the most appropriate service; (c) and, we need to do all this along with controlling the cost of what we are doing - not necessarily by reducing cost, but arresting the annual rate increase. These goals are largely inconsistent with each other. The first goal, universal access, when viewed along with the third one, under the present institutional and employment-based circumstances, is a victim of a "vicious coverage circle" which may make it impossible to secure universal access and control costs in the same process. We have already noted that in our employment dominated coverage system, businesses are the major purchasers of healthcare coverage. They have to pay insurers for those, or for much of those, policies from their earnings. The latter, in turn, is a function of their earning power in a usually competitive market place. To remain competitive in the market, businesses must control their cost of doing business, a substantial and increasing part of which is healthcare costs, that is, the cost of insuring employees indicated above. Thus far, businesses had a difficult time controlling their healthcare costs because of a proliferation of services augmented by ever increasing and improving costly medical technology, and due also to the government's politically motivated preoccupation with its own financial problems prompting it to shift more of the healthcare financial burden to the private sector by limiting reimbursements. So, the ball is back in the court of the business sector. Business' response has been to reduce or, in some cases, completely eliminate coverage, adding to a Marxian-like "reserve army" of the uninsured, or inadequately insured, a problem which has long been social, and has now become acutely political.

A long history of healthcare reform efforts in the United States has now culminated a in set of proposals to Congress by a newly elected President. As these proposal are introduced and discussed, a number of other proposals are also on the table. In order to illustrate the diversity of some of the views on Capitol Hill alone , let us first review some of the alternative proposals of this time, and then discuss in detail the President's Health Security Plan, as it was formally introduced. We will close the chapter with some prognoses for the future.

The general dimensions of concern by the various proposal alternatives to the President's in general are (a) access on a voluntary or involuntary basis, (b) the portfolio of benefits covered, (c) the incidence of financing, (d) broader financing provisions, (e) sources of cost containment, (f) medical malpractice considerations, (g) and the administrative agency. Representative *McDermott's* Canadian style single payer proposals would avail a standard medical benefits package to all legal residents. The government would cover provider costs, and it would be administered by the states. The benefits would include completely covered physician and hospital bills, prescription drugs, mental health substance abuse, and other medically necessary treatments. The coverage would be free to individuals, but employers would pay payroll taxes into the healthcare treasury, with the latter replacing the current insurance premium payment system. The plan would further establish annual national healthcare budgets, and the portfolio of benefits as well as their pricing standards would be set by a national health board.

Two other members of the House of Representatives, *Cooper and Michel*, have also put forth some widely noted proposals. Representative Cooper suggested setting up purchasing cooperatives in order to reduce insurance costs, while the US Government would pay for the care of people below the poverty level, and subsidize people with incomes between the poverty level and the level twice above that. The benefits package would be determined by a national health board. Representative Michel would have employers offer their employees at least one insurance plan and a tax-free medical savings account. Smaller employers could obtain these options from insurance companies. Community and migrant healthcare centers would increase access to care. The health benefits would be set by the National Association of Insurance Commissioners. Both law makers would exempt employers from payment requirements, and would impose no controls on premiums, copayments or deductibles, and they both would proscribe higher insurance rates or policy cancellation for pre-existing conditions. They also expect market competition to generate some savings. As to medical malpractice litigation, both lawmakers would introduce mediation and alternative dispute resolution, have losers pay the winner's court and legal costs, and limit pain and suffering, as well as attorney fees to around 20%.

Senator *Chafee* from Rhode Island, in charge of the Republican formulation of healthcare reforms, proposed that employers should be required to offer insurance for a standard health benefit package, and employees should be required to get it. Employees, and non employees, could also procure coverage through purchasing alliances. Healthcare services for the poor would be distributed by using vouchers to become available and financed pursuant to system generated savings. There would be two alternative benefit plans, one for catastrophic care, and the other would include physician, hospital, prescription and some mental health coverage. No employer payments would be required, and there would be no control on premiums. Co-payments and deductibles would be set by a benefits commission subject to Congressional approval. The premium of those with pre-existing conditions would be capped. Major savings are envisioned by cutting some $200 billion from Medicare and Medicaid growth by the year 2000, and from increased market competition. The solution to the medical malpractice dilemma is seen as essentially the same as those proposed by Representatives Cooper and Michel. The benefits would be set by a national health board. States would set up health insurance purchasing cooperatives for small businesses and individuals. Multistate employer plans would be regulated by the US Department of Health and Human Services. Finally, Texas Republican Senator *Gramm* would have employers offer employees at least three options which would include their present policy, a membership in an HMO or in another plan, and a tax-exempt savings account to cover medical expenses over $3,000. He did not specify included benefits, and would not require employers to pay, nor would he control premiums, copayments, or deductibles. He would either limit or subsidize premiums for pre-existing conditions, except for those caused by smoking or excessive alcohol consumption. Senator Gramm would reduce the growth of Medicaid by $113 billion, and of Medicare by $62 billion between 1994 and 1998. Self-employed health insurance expenses would be tax-deductible up to the average cost of all full-time employees in the business. Further savings are expected by increased competition in the market place. Senator Gramm's medical malpractice proposals are essentially the same as those of his colleagues in Congress.

There are some other noted proposals or models for reform. A model that could be considered for national adoption has long been used right in Washington DC. for over 30 years, and provides medical coverage for some 9 million federal employees, retirees and their families: *Federal Employees Health Benefits (FEHB) Program*. The Program's two underlying premises are consumer choice and market competition. In contrast to the circumstances of private sector employees where the employer chooses the plan without an incentive for the employee to seek economical alternatives, federal employees may choose their own health plan nationally from among 400 healthcare intermediaries, including the major commercial plans, the Blues, and from over 300 managed care plans. Since most federal employees are likely choose from a collection of plans right in their area, they prompt a competitive bidding among the insurers in terms of coverage and pricing variables. Annual premiums range from $350 to $2,000 for single employees, and twice that when family coverage is included, with the government paying over half of the premiums. The availability of choice and competition seem to have kept costs under control, with recent annual increases falling below corresponding increases in the private sector. We will note that health alliances under the President's proposals also attempt to consolidate purchasing power in the hand of organized consumer groups, a principle not unlike the FEHB. For federal employees, there is an "open season" every year during which, armed with information and data obtained from provider advertising soliciting their business and from various advisory services, they can go coverage "shopping", and make the same choice decisions by themselves, and apparently more economically, as do employers make for their own employees.

The *Hawaiian* model may also be seen as a possible general pattern to follow. Even before the notion of managed competition, aimed preserving private health insurance with some government control over healthcare costs, gained momentum on the mainland, Hawaii already had a simpler but similar mechanism in place. Hawaii mandates a minimum benefit package to be provided by employers. Competitive bidding for the employers' health insurance business substantially reduced the number of insurers to the point where today there is a virtual oligopsony in the Hawaiian health insurance market with the Hawaii Medical Service Association (a Blue Cross/Blue Shield Plan) insuring about 60% of the population, and the Kaiser Permanente Staff HMO covering some 20%. In this market environment, healthcare costs appear to have been kept under relative control, particularly since the two dominant insurers virtually set the rates at which providers are reimbursed[28]. Medicaid and the State Health Insurance Program (SHIP) takes up the gap.

The *Clinton Plan* differs from the above in a number of dimensions[29]. A major element of the President's proposals is to utilize financial incentives that would prompt consumers to join low cost HMOs, and to prompt providers and insurers to form functional networks. The underlying purpose is to generate healthcare financial responsibility on the part of the consumer, and competition prompted cost and service quality sensitivities on the part of health plans. The growth in healthcare spending would be constrained either by competition or by capping insurance premiums. Thus, the President's proposals essentially rely on the US healthcare system's existing institutional service delivery structure, and attempts to control costs by introducing or intensifying fiscal responsibility on the part of providers, insurers, and on the part of consumers. Let us a take a look at some of the details.

The employer would pay at least 80% of the average cost of the regional premium, and would support coverage for dependents. The employees would contribute an average of 20% to cover the cost their own insurance premiums, plus deductibles and copayments. Persons self-employed, or not working, would be required to procure their own coverage paying full cost, unless they qualify for government subsidies. The cost of health insurance policies would be 100% tax-deductible, in contrast to the 25% deductibility at the present time. The government would subsidize coverage for small and low-wage businesses, and for persons not in employment with income under 150% of the poverty line. The elderly and the disabled would continue to be covered by Medicare, and Medicaid would utilize the health alliances to pay for the coverage of the poor plan.

The Clinton Plan focuses on the functions of so called *health alliances*. These are envisioned as regional purchasing groups run by the states under federal government supervision. They would collect and distribute premiums from the insured, negotiate fees with providers for services outside HMO's, constrain premium growth rates to federally set guidelines, collect and disseminate data on the performance of the various health plans in their regions, and would certify health plans prior to offering them to consumers. In essence, the alliances would avail access to all legal residents and citizens. They would set the target range for average premiums charged by plans in their particular regions. Any plan than met state requirements could contract with the alliance in its region. Plans available through alliances would generally fall into three categories: HMOs, fee-for-service, and a combination of these two. A plan cannot turn patients away, unless it has been oversubscribed. The information and plan-specific performance data published by the alliances would help potential subscribers to engage in comparison shopping. The number of alliances and their size in each state would vary, depending upon the state's population distribution and density, with each large city likely to have one alliance. States would have an autonomy in determining the structure of alliances, that is, whether they would be state agencies or non-profit corporations with one constant: consumers and employers would have equal representation in the management of an alliance.

Large corporations would have an option to by-pass alliances and negotiate directly with insurers for their employees' coverage, although they would still have to pay at least 80% of their employees' premium. Thus, although large employers could form their own alliances, they would still have to offer the minimum guaranteed benefit package and a choice of plans. In such cases, however, employees are likely to have a choice of fewer providers.

Although most alliances would offer a large selection of plans, they must include at least one fee-for-service option offering free choice of providers. While the cost of a plan would likely vary by region and by type, the average cost would be about $1,800 per individual and $4,200 par family. Costlier plans would require subscribers to pay a higher share of the premiums. Furthermore, plans could offer coverage beyond the standard minimum for items like extra dental or mental health benefits the cost of which could optionally be covered by employers, or by employees with tax-deductible dollars.

Plans contracted by alliances would fall into three cost categories. The least expensive ones would be the HMOs, requiring a $10 fee per visit only to affiliated physicians. However, visits to physicians outside the HMO would require a 40% copayment from patients. The middle expense category includes plans that would combine HMOs and fee-for-service coverage, and would allow patients to consult other, not included, physicians with a 20% copayment. The highest cost category plans would include fee-for-service coverage exclusively, where much of the premium and cost contribution would cover the widest freedom of provider choice. Thus, a $200 and $400 deductibles would be included for individuals and families respectively, along with a copayment of 20% for office visits and hospitalization, capping the personal responsibility for costs at $1,500 for individuals and $3,000 per family.

A guaranteed *benefit package* would be available upon presentation of a health security card. These basic benefits would include preventive dental care for children, with similar benefits for adults phased in by the year 2000. Prescription drugs, and routine vision and hearing examination, although eye glasses only for children. Professional services in private offices, emergency care and other outpatient hospital services, laboratory tests, and ambulance. Speech, occupational, and physical therapies in an outpatient setting to restore skills lost due to illness and injury, but would need to be re-assessed every 60 days. Hospital stays in semi-private rooms, as well as private rooms if medically warranted. As an alternative to hospital inpatient stay, nursing homes and rehabilitation centers for a maximum of 100 days per year. Also as an alternative to hospital inpatient stays, home care to be reassessed every 60 days. For terminally ill patients, hospice care. Medical equipment by way of braces, artificial limbs or prosthetic devices in order to improve functional abilities or to prevent deterioration. Preventive services by way of immunizations, mammograms, Pap smear, prenatal care and cholesterol screening. Limited amount of outpatient and inpatient services for substantive abuse. Explicitly excluded are medically unnecessary and inappropriate services such as cosmetic orthodontia, hearing aids, contact lenses, sex-change procedures, citing just a few.

The President would appoint a seven member *National Health Board* and charge it with monitoring state compliance and the functioning of health alliances, interpret the standard benefit package, and monitor changes in technology and emerging medical needs. This body would also be entrusted with setting regional healthcare spending limits. It would further be entrusted with developing yardsticks and methods for measuring health plan performance in terms of the various quality dimensions of care, and to disseminate this information to consumers so as to enhance informed choice among competing plans. A separate committee would be established to monitoring drug prices.People in different employment situations would be affected differently by the implementation of the Clinton Plan, as proposed. Employees already in HMOs would note little change, except that they would have a choice of plans. Employees presently without insurance would be required to purchase coverage and pay 20% of the cost of an average plan, and less if they choose a cheaper plan, and would be subsidized on a sliding scale if their family income is under 150% of the poverty line - which in 1992 was at $14,340 for a family of four. Those not working with little income would receive full coverage at a minimum cost, while those with unearned family income would contribute on a sliding scale reaching full cost contribution when income exceeds 250% of the poverty line. Part-time workers employed from 10-30 hours per week would be employer subsidized on a prorated basis in comparison with those fully employed. Cheaper group rates would in general replace the high premiums paid by extra-group individuals at the present time. A complex formula treats self-employed persons like a small business.As employers, they would contribute between 3.5% to a maximum of 7.9% of their business income, depending on the income level, but would also pay their employees 20% share. When both spouses in a family hold full-time jobs, they each benefit separately from their respective employers'

80% contribution to their individual plans, but can joint together to cover one 20% family share of employee contribution in an average priced plan. Retirees under 65 not yet eligible for Medicare, and not included in a former employer-based healthcare or pension plan, would be subsidized by the government and would get coverage through their alliance for paying 20% of the cost of an average premium, as if they were employed; subsidies would be adjusted if the retiree worked part-time, or if the spouse had income.

Current elderly Medicare receptionist would get the same or better benefits, since now prescription drugs and home-care would also be included. A state can bring Medicare beneficiaries into a health alliance with equal or better benefits, provided a fee-for-service alternative plan is also offered. Present Medicaid beneficiaries could sign up for a plan, with premium at or below the regional average, through an alliance, with the federal and state governments making fixed subsidy contributions to the chosen healthcare plan - instead of paying the providers based on a per service fee schedule. Students would be expected to sign up for coverage through an alliance in the region of their attendance, financed by a portion of family and its employer premium payments transferred from the home alliance to the alliance of the student's choice. Finally, illegal aliens would be excluded from health alliances, although could continue receiving emergency care as they do under the current system, financed mostly by social welfare and community organizations, or simply donated by providers.

Progress and Prognoses

Although at the time of writing the Clinton health plan has not been submitted to Congress, several major companies experienced major reductions in the annual growth of their healthcare costs. Major cost savings were achieved by making greater use of managed care plans such as HMOs and PPOs. Companies such as Chevron, DuPont, Ford, and Merck reduced the annual rate of increase in their healthcare costs by an average of some 3%-4%. Wal-Mart, spending about $450 million per year for the health benefits of 212,000 employees, estimates a per-capita increase of only 3.2% in 1993. McDonnell Douglas Corp. was able to extract discounts of about 40% from of its contracted providers[30]. Because of the number of employees, hence potential healthcare customer groups, these and other large companies represent, they can in fact confront providers with purchasing market power similar to those envisioned for alliances in the President's pending proposals.

It appears that even the anticipation of the implementation of at least some of the reforms prompted an increasingly cost-conscious atmosphere, and a more aggressive posture by large employers towards providers and insurers. Thus, the CEOs of three American auto makers, GM, Chrysler and Ford, for the first time ever wrote a joint letter during May 1993 to about a dozen healthcare intermediaries demanding a 10% cut in premiums. HMOs are going through transformation as well to control costs. For instance, the Henry Ford Health System has sufficient number of subscribers, a large enough market, to train and support its own group of general practitioners, leaning toward the staff model HMO. Furthermore, elaborate vertically integrated systems are utilized to reduce costs. Thus, Henry Ford integrates financing and care, six hospitals, 37 ambulatory care centers, and two nursing homes. Henry Ford expects a 4% healthcare cost inflation during 1993. In Minneapolis, 14 large employers formed a healthcare purchasing cooperative to buy in volume and set the standards for care. Federal Express in Tennessee saved millions of dollars by inviting bids from health plans[31].

Thus, even at the beginning of the healthcare debate in Congress, fundamental changes are being implemented in the healthcare industry. Although these changes facilitate cost reduction efforts by large companies with substantial market power, they do not solve the problem of the 37 million or so uninsured, that is, they do not automatically bring about universal access - a principle that turned out to be bipartisan one. Furthermore, notwithstanding the existence of well-worn statistics regarding the level and the historical annual rate of increase in healthcare costs, and the increasing proportion of GNP it represents in the United States, some valid questions may be raised regarding the potential efficacy of the healthcare reform proposals even if implemented in their entirety. First of all, in spite of its alarmingly high level, the average growth of healthcare costs in the US, in real terms, between 1960 and 1990 has, at 1.1%, by no means been the highest in the world; Austria, Netherlands, Australia, Norway, and Switzerland experienced a higher real rate of growth in their healthcare spending than did the US. Furthermore, and importantly, Canada's corresponding rate of healthcare cost growth, in spite of its many years' of experience with a tightly controlled single-payer system, was the same as in the US.[32]. Thus, the culprit for persistent healthcare cost levels and annual increases may need to be sought out somewhere else, at least in addition to the concerns indicated by the reform proposals. It may be that the high cost of healthcare service production to a large extent is inherent in the nature of the production process itself. Because of its high labor intensity, with the utilized labor in general tending to be highly trained and skilled, but nevertheless inhibited by inherently low levels of productivity since physicians cannot produce faster than is prudently necessary to maintain some desirable level of quality, the ultimate fruits of any cost control effort may very well be limited. Improvements in medical technology may improve some on the physician productivity, but many items of medicine's technological marvels are diagnostic, instead of therapeutic, hence add little to improvements in physician productivity. Healthcare productivity will likely increase slowly, hence overall healthcare costs may continue to accelerate, if possibly somewhat lower than experienced in recent years.

References

1   The election of Pennsylvania Democrat Harris Wofford into the US Senate over former Attorney General Richard Thornburgh based on the former's intensive campaign for healthcare reforms is a vivid illustration of the public concern for the country's healthcare system. Indeed, as we all know, President Clinton's platform prominently dealt with, if was not dominated by, promises to reform the healthcare system.

2   Employee Benefits Research Institute *Issue Brief*, No. 104, Washington DC, 1990. See also USGAO, *Health Insurance: An Overview of the Working Uninsured*, GAO/HRD-89-45, Washington DC

3   USGAO, *Health Insurance: Cost Increases Lead to Coverage Limitations and Cost Shifting*, GAO/HRD90-68, Washington DC

4   See, Employee Benefit Research Institute.

5   Starr, P. *Social Transformation of American Medicine*, Basic Books, New York, 1982. And, US Small Business Administration, *The State of Small Businesses: A Report to the President*, Washington DC 1987

6   Omnibus Budget Reconciliation Act of 1989, P.L. 101-239

7   Chollet, D. and Friedland, R. "Employer-Paid Retiree Health Insurance: History and Prospects for Growth" in Employment Benefits Research Institute, *The Changing Healthcare Market*, Washington DC 1987. See also Swartz, K. *A Chartbook: The Medically Uninsured*, The Urban Institute Washington DC 1989.

8   Consolidated Omnibus Budget Reconciliation Act of 1985, P.L. 99-272, Title X, Private Health Insurance [26 U.S.C. 162 (k)],

9   Congressional Research Service, *Health Insurance*, Library of Congress, Washington DC 1990. See also Swartz, 1989.

10 USGAO, *Health Insurance: An Overview of the Working Uninsured*, GAO/HRD 89-45, and, GAO *Employee Benefits: Company Actions to Limit Retiree Health Costs*, GAO/HRD-89-31BR, Washington DC 1989.

11 Gabel J. et al. *Employer Sponsored Health Insurance*, Health Affairs, Vol. 9, 1989, pp. 161-75

12 Thorpe, K.E. "Health Care Cost Containment: Reflections and Future Directions". In Kovner, R.A. (ed.) *Health Care Delivery in the United States*, Springer Publishing Co., New York, 1990.

13 Sloan, F.A. "Rate Regulation as a Strategy Control: Evidence from the Last Decade" *Milbank Memorial Fund Quarterly*, Vil 61, No.2, 1983, pp.195-221. See also Steinwald, B. and Stone, F.A. "Regulatory Approaches to Hospital Cost Containment: A Synthesis of the Empirical Evidence", in Olson, M. (ed) *New Approach to the Economics of Health Care*, American Enterprise Institute for Public Policy Research, Washington DC 1981. Ashby, J.l. "The Impact of Hospital Regulatory Programs On Per Capita Cost, Utilization and Capital Investment" *Inquiry*, Vol 21, Spring 1984, pp.45-59.

14   Wilensky, G.R. "Medicare at 25: Better Value better Care" *JAMA* Vol. 264, No.15, 1990,pp.1996-7.

15   Morrisey, M.A. Sloan, F.A. and Valvona, J. "Medicare Prospective Payment and Posthospital Transfer to Subacute Care" *Medical Care*, Vol. 26, No.7, 1988, pp.685-98. See also, US Congress. House, Committee on Ways and Means. *Background Material and Data on Programs Within the Jurisdiction of the Committee on Ways and Means*, 1989 Edition. Government Printing Office, Washington DC. March 15, 1989.

16   Kahn, K.L. Keeler, E.B. Sherwood, M.J. Rodgers, W.H. Draper, D. Benton, E.J. et al. "Comparing Outcomes of Care Before and After the Implementation of the DRG-based Prospective Payment System" *JAMA* Vol. 264, No.15, 1990, pp.1984-88. See also, Kosecoff, J., Kahn, K.L. Rodgers, W.H. et al "Prospective Payment System and Impairment at Discharge, *JAMA* Vol. 264, No.15, 1990, pp.1980-83.

17   Health Care Financing Administration, "Relative Value Scales for Physicians Services", in *Medicare Physician Payment*, Washington DC, October 1989. This study found that each one percent decrease in physician fees is accompanied only by a 0.5% increase in the volume and intensity of services. See also, Gable,J. and Rice T. "Reducing Public Expenditures for Physician Services: The Price of Paying Less" *Journal of Health Politics, Policy and Law*, Vol. 9, No.4, Winter 1985, pp.595-609; and, Holahan J. and Scanlon, W. "Physician Pricing in California: Price Controls, Physician Fees, and Physician Incomes from Medicare and Medicaid" *Health Care Financing Grants and Contracts Report*. HCFA, Baltimore MD 1979; Mitchell, J.B., Wetig, J. and Cromwell, J. "The Medicare Physician Fee Freeze" *Health Affairs*, Vol. 8, No. 1, Spring 1989, pp.21-33.

18   Iglehart, J.K. "Canada's Health Care System Faces Its Problems" *New England Journal of Medicine*, Vol. 322, No. 8, 1990, pp.562-68. See also Public Health Service, *Health US 1987*. DHHS Publication No.PHS-88-1232, Department of Health and Human Services. Hyattsville MD March 1988.

19   DiCarlo, S. and Gabel, J. "Conventional Health Plans: A Decade Later" *Research Bulletin*, November 1988, pp.1-29

20   Welch, W.P. "The New Structure of Individual Practice Associations, *Journal of Health Politics, Policy and Law* Vol 12, No. 4, 1987, pp,.723-39. See also Luft, H. *Health Maintenance Organizations: Dimensions of Performance*, John Wiley and Sons, New York, NY 1981; Manning, W.G. Leibowitz, A., Goldberg, G.A. Rogers, W.H. and Newhouse, J.P. "A Controlled Trial of the Effects of a Prepaid Group Practice on Use of Services" *New England Journal of Medicine*, Vol. 310, No.23 June 1987, pp.1505-10

21   Hellinger, F.J. "Selection Bias in Health Maintenance Organizations: Analysis of Recent Evidence" *Health Care Financing Review*, Vol. 9, No.2, Winter 1987, pp.55-63. See also Langwell, K.M. and Hadley, J.P. "Evaluation of the Medicare Competition Demonstrations" *Health Care Financing Review*, Vol. 11, No.2, Winter 1989, pp.65-80.

22 Blendon, R.J. and Donelan, K. "The Public and the Emerging Debate Over National Health Insurance" *New England Journal of Medicine*, Vol. 323, No.3, July 1990, pp.208-212

23 deLissovoy, G. Rice, T. Gabel, J. and Gelzer, H.G. "Preferred Provider Organizations: One Year Later" *Inquiry*, Vol. 24, Summer 1987, pp.127-35.

24 General Accounting Office, *Cancer Treatment, 1975-85: The Use of Breakthrough Treatments for Seven Types of Cancer*, January 1988, Washington DC.

25 Reynolds, R.A. Rizzo, J.A. and Gonzales, M.L. "The Cost of Medical Professional Liability" *JAMA* Vol.257, No.20, 1987, pp.2776-81; see also Eisenberg, J.M. *Doctors' Decision and the Cost of Medical Care*, Health Administration Press, Ann Arbor MI 1986; Sloan, F.A. and Bovjberg, R.R. "Medical Malpractice: Crises, Response and Effects" *Research Bulletin*, Health Insurance Association of America, Washington DC. May 1989; and, Physician Payment Review Commission, *Annual Report to Congress* Washington DC 1990.

26 Pear, R. "Malpractice Insurance Rates Are Going Down", *The New York Times*, September 23, 1990.

27 These views have been abstracted and consolidated from the news media of this time period, The New York Times, Wall Street Journal, Washington Post, Philadelphia Inquirer during the months of September and October, 1993.

28 In 1991, per capita healthcare expenditure in Hawaii was $1,889, or 8.9% of per capita income. While this is lower than comparable figures in most other states of the US, the percentage of per capita income expended on healthcare in Hawaii was nevertheless higher than in New Jersey (7.4%), Connecticut (8%), Maryland (8.7%), Illinois (8.8%), New Hampshire (8.3%), Virginia (8.6%), Washington (8.7%), Vermont (8.2%), Wyoming (7.6%), and Idaho (8%); and, was the same as in Oregon, which, as we discussed in the previous chapter, has been rationing healthcare. DHHS, Census Estimates - published in the *New York Times*, October 7, 1993, p. A24.

29 President Clinton's proposals are based on The White House Domestic Policy Council, *The President's Health Security Plan: The Clinton Blue Print*, Times Books, Random House, New York, NY 1993. This volume, in turn, contained the complete text of the *Working Group Draft*, dated September 7, 1993, by the White House Domestic Policy Council. When the financial version of the American Health Security Act finally came on the market through bookstores of the GPO, the major changes from the original plan were as follows: (a) expected date of universal coverage delayed by a year to January 1, 1998; (b) the coverage for mammograms and pediatric dental care expanded; (c) services for children under Medicaid expanded; (d) FTC given new powers to regulate insurers and assure fair competition among them; (e) HMOs and other plans must offer all patients

te option of free providers choice, although at an additional cost; (f) alliances may reject a healthcare plan only if it does not meet state standards of quality and care, or if their budgets exceed the average of others in the region by 20% or more; the number of fee-for-service plans cannot be limited; (g) the administrative obstacles to a state attempting to create a single-payer system have been reduced; (h) a limit of 3.9% of income has been set for low income workers' premium; (i) companies subsidized for the premium cost of early retirees may need to rebate some of their savings. In addition, a tentative calendar for reform implementation has been advanced: 1993-1994 - Congress will act on the administration's plan; late 1994-mid-1996 - transitional period for states to establish healthcare programs for their residents; mid-1996-end of 1997 - January 1, 1998 is the present deadline by which all states have their plans approved and the guarantee for coverage would commence.

30 "Big Companies See Health Costs Slowing: Employers Push Managed Care, Seek Discounts", *Wall Street Journal*, October 22, 1993, p.A2

31 "Why Wait for Hillary?, Thanks to Competition, Business Has Started the Healthcare Revolution Without Washington", *Newsweek*, June 28, 1993, pp.38-39

32 O.E.C.D. *Health Date File*. Cited in Baumol, W. "Health Reform Can't Cure High Costs", *The New York Times*, August 8, 1993, p. 13

Index

About the Author

Dr. Seplaki is an associate professor and chairman of the department of economics at Rutgers University - Camden Campus, where he has taught undergraduate and graduate courses for the past 21 years. After obtaining his PhD from University of California (Riverside), he spent one year at the University of Chicago as a post-doctoral fellow in economics and industrial organization. Subsequently, he received a Fellowship from the Harvard Corporation, and was a Fellow in Law and Economics at the Harvard Law School, concentrating, in addition to some basic legal education, on antitrust courses and graduate seminars in that specific field. Recently, Dr. Seplaki was a Visiting Scholar in the Economics Department and at the School of Public Health at Columbia University, where much of the research for the instant volume was conducted, and also did some Fulbright financed visiting in Japan and gave seminars at the Schools of Public Health at Kyoto and Tokyo Universities, and at the Japanese Ministry of Health and Welfare.

Dr. Seplaki published some 40 articles in the field of economics, antitrust and related field, and a book on antitrust.

In addition to his academic and scholarly endeavors, Dr. Seplaki has also functioned as a consultant in a number of antitrust cases over the years, including several rather large ones in the healthcare field.